Heart Diseases in Children

Ra-id Abdulla
Editor

Heart Diseases in Children

A Pediatrician's Guide

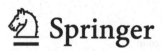
Springer

Editor
Ra-id Abdulla
Center for Congenital and Structural Heart Diseases
Rush University Medical Center
Chicago, IL, USA
ra-id_abdulla@rush.edu

ISBN 978-1-4419-7993-3   e-ISBN 978-1-4419-7994-0
DOI 10.1007/978-1-4419-7994-0
Springer New York Dordrecht Heidelberg London

Library of Congress Control Number: 2011921345

Printed on acid-free paper

Springer is part of Springer Science+Business Media (www.springer.com)

Foreword

Heart Diseases in Children: A Pediatrician's Guide fills an important need in pediatrics and occupies a valued spot on the bookshelves of practicing cardiologists and pediatricians. This outstanding new reference work is in part the byproduct of my colleague Dr. Ra-id Abdulla's decade of editorship of the journal *Pediatric Cardiology*, his creation of one of the most visited internet Web sites in his field, and his leadership of outstanding fellowship training programs at the University of Chicago and Rush University. Dr. Abdulla is a consummate educator in the field of pediatric cardiology. His mastery is evident in the abundance of understandable illustrations, images of actual cases, and personal observations of real life practice that fill this book.

The management of children with heart disease – whether asymptomatic or symptomatic, diagnosed or undiagnosed, congenital or structural, corrected or palliated, acute or chronic – requires collaborative teamwork between the pediatric cardiologist and the primary care pediatrician. With this in mind, each of the chapters in this book has the dual authorship of an academic cardiologist and a practicing general pediatrician, a format which is unique among textbooks in the pediatric subspecialties. Many of the pediatric coauthors are recent graduates of our categorical Pediatrics and Internal Medicine/Pediatrics residencies at Rush. Their contributions provide a fresh and practical viewpoint that reflects their experiences in the hospital and in practice. The result is a text whose content is both authoritative and relevant.

This book proves useful as an accessible resource for teaching the fundamentals of pediatric cardiology, a handy resource for both cardiologists and pediatricians, and a rich trove of illustrative materials. As a pediatric chairman who knows most of the authors personally in their roles as faculty and trainees at Rush Children's Hospital, this book fills me with a sense of scholarly (and fatherly) pride. Its authors have tried to create a useful contribution to the care of children with heart disease and their families. I think they have succeeded admirably.

Chicago, IL

Kenneth M. Boyer, MD

Foreword

Going back to my days when I was a medical student at Jordan University and later as a house officer in pediatrics at Yale New Haven Hospital, it was hard for me to find the proper book for learning everything I needed in pediatric cardiology. Over the last decade or so, the field of pediatric cardiology has evolved causing many pediatric residents to develop great interest in pursuing this specialty. A major part of the reason for this interest is the great advancement in imaging (echocardiography, MRI, CT), interventional cardiology, and electrophysiology. Such advancements contributed to the improved survival of children with congenital cardiac defects.

This book provides a comprehensive review in pediatric cardiology, starting with an approach to heart disease in children and the interpretation of cardiac symptoms. Further, this book provides detailed discussion on how to interpret chest radiographs and the role of echocardiography and catheterization in diagnosing congenital heart disease. The beauty and elegance of this book is the case scenarios discussed in detail in every chapter. Such scenarios teach the reader (be it a student or resident) the flow of the case and how to reach a proper diagnosis.

All forms of congenital cardiac defects are discussed in detail in a systematic fashion, starting with incidence, pathology, pathophysiology, clinical manifestations, laboratory findings, and management. Each defect discussed is followed by case scenario. This format should teach the reader how to think and go about the case.

For the students and practitioners today, the information in this book provides a wealth of practical material, which is invaluable for the current management of congenital heart disease and also provides a systematic approach to each cardiac defect. This book should be a reference for all those who are interested in taking care of patients with congenital heart disease.

Chicago, IL   Ziyad M. Hijazi, MD, MPH, FAAP

Preface

The role of pediatricians in caring for children has become daunting. The ever expanding knowledge in disease processes and the wide and complex therapeutic options available makes keeping up with all nuances of the management of childhood diseases exceedingly difficult. As the subspecialty fields expand, the role of pediatricians change as they work with subspecialists in caring for children with ailments, such as heart diseases. Pediatricians are the primary care providers for children and are entrusted with the discovery of early signs of heart diseases, particularly in the newborn period when presentation is frequently obscure and occasionally with devastating consequences if not discovered and managed promptly.

The issue of how much a pediatrician should know about diseases typically managed by subspecialists is frequently raised. Educators in charge of training pediatric residents as well as regulating bodies providing certification of educational competency to pediatricians continue to emphasis the need for pediatricians to acquire and be considerably proficient in issues relating to heart diseases in children. This is primarily because pediatricians are the frontline practitioners who could identify early signs of heart diseases and are the primary care providers who follow children with ongoing cardiac diseases undergoing medical and surgical management.

Pediatricians are not expected to come up with precise diagnoses of cardiac anomalies in a child; instead, their role is one of identifying the possibility of cardiac anomalies and their potential urgency, or lack of. Furthermore, pediatricians are expected to understand issues relating to ongoing therapy or staged interventional procedures to provide general pediatric care that augments the therapeutic measures underway for the cardiac lesion. Perhaps a good example of the latter includes the knowledge of lesions requiring subacute bacterial endocarditis prophylaxis or the management of a child requiring anticoagulation therapy.

The purpose of this textbook is to provide comprehensive, yet easy to understand details of heart diseases in children. Therefore, the construction of this reference was based upon three principals: Provide comprehensive details of most heart lesions encountered in this field, detail pathophysiological principals of each lesion so as to provide the reader with knowledge that could apply to a wide spectrum of presentations of the same lesion, and finally illustrate each concept and lesion through case scenarios and images.

The art of teaching is a fascinating process. To be able to convey knowledge in a clear and meaningful way is not always easy. Educators should be well versed in the material they intend to teach; but perhaps more importantly is their ability to gauge what the audience already knows and how to build upon their existing knowledge to what is desired. To achieve this, we have followed a unique model in authoring each chapter. Topics were initially written by a pediatric cardiologist knowledgeable in the issues presented; this was then reshaped by a second author, a pediatrician, to suit the needs of the generalist, rather than the specialist. Each chapter traveled back and forth between specialist and generalist until a satisfactory format was reached providing ample information and packaged to what a pediatrician may need.

Significant effort was made in producing the large sum of illustrations in this book. The heart diagrams depicting various congenital heart diseases were based on a normal heart diagram created by Jeremy Brotherton, a talented medical illustrator. Jeremy crafted a normal heart diagram using a computer-based drawing program, thus allowing me to alter it to depict the various congenital heart disease illustrations in this text. The ECG rhythm strips were generated through a computer drawing program which I designed some time ago and found very useful in showing typical electrocardiographic rhythm strips for teaching purposes. The 12 lead ECG images were of actual patients, however, edited to enhance the pathological features without excessive annotations. The chest X-ray images were enhanced to clarify subtleties of abnormalities of cardiac silhouette or pulmonary vasculature though illustrations inserted over the original chest X-ray image providing clarity and details difficult to do with annotations. Variations of many of the images used in this book were previously used in the pediatric cardiology teaching Web site I constructed at Rush University (http://www.pedcard.rush.edu). The echocardiographic images in this book were limited to those which provide a clear understanding of how echocardiography is used in assessing children with congenital heart diseases. The purpose of these illustrations was to demonstrate the different tools available through this imaging modality. The echocardiographic images were made by Stephen Stone, MD who during an elective at Rush University showed an uncanny understanding of the 3-dimension nature of the heart as depicted through 2-dimension images of echocardiography. Furthermore, his ability to illustrate what echocardiographic images produced is a collection of illustrative images which he used in the chapter he coauthored.

Teaching pediatric cardiology to the noncardiologist is an exciting endeavor which I learned to love from my mentor, Dr. William Strong. I witnessed him during my fellowship at the Medical College of Georgia lecturing medical students the principals of pathophysiology in congenital heart diseases, I was awestricken. Dr. Strong captured their attention from the first word he uttered to the conclusion of his talk when he was always warmly applauded by the medical students who were finally able to put all the basic knowledge they have attained in synch with the clinical sciences they are striving to learn. Once I became a faculty member, I too embraced his approach of tracing back cardiac symptoms and signs to their pathophysiological origins, thus demystifying clinical presentations and investigative studies of children with heart diseases. I have experienced many masters of education, but non like Bill Strong, a true scientist, thinker, orator, and above all a remarkable teacher to whom I owe much of what I have learned.

Chicago, IL   Ra-id Abdulla, MD

Contents

Contributors

Ra-id Abdulla, MD
Center for Congenital and Structural Heart Diseases, Rush University
Medical Center, Chicago, IL, USA

Shada Al-Anani, MD
Center for Congenital and Structural Heart Diseases, Rush University
Medical Center, Chicago, IL, USA

Shada J. Alanani, MD
Department of Pediatric Cardiology, Rush University Medical Center,
Chicago, IL, USA

Sawsan Mokhtar M. Awad, MD
Department of Pediatrics, Rush University Medical Center,
Chicago, IL, USA

Sean Barnes, MD, MBA
Department of Pediatrics, John Hopkins Medical Institutes, Baltimore, MD, USA

Steve Barnes, MD
Department of Anesthesiology, Rush University Medical Center,
Chicago, IL, USA

Yolandee R. Bell-Cheddar, MD, FAAP
Department of Pediatric Cardiology, Rush University Medical Center,
Chicago, IL, USA

William J. Bonney, MD
Division of Cardiology, The Children's Hospital of Philadelphia,
Philadelphia, PA, USA

Kenneth M. Boyer, MD
Department of Pediatrics, Rush University Medical Center,
Chicago, IL, USA

Shannon M. Buckvold, MD
Department of Pediatric Cardiology/Cardiac Critical Care,
The Children's Hospital, Aurora, CO, USA

Jacquelyn Busse, MD
Department of Pediatrics, Rush University Medical Center, Chicago, IL, USA

Edmundo P. Cortez, MD
Division of Pediatric Critical Care Medicine, Rush University Medical Center,
Chicago, IL, USA

Russell Robert Cross, MD
Department of Cardiology, Children's National Medical Center,
Washington, DC, USA

Karim A. Diab, MD, FAAP, FACC
Department of Pediatrics, St. Joseph Hospital and Medical Center,
Phoenix, AZ, USA

Daniel E. Felten, MD, MPH
Department of Pediatrics, Rush University Medical Center, Chicago, IL, USA

Rani Ganesan, MD
Department of Pediatrics, Rush University Medical Center, Chicago, IL, USA

Ismael Gonzalez, MD
Department of Pediatric Cardiology, Rush University Medical Center,
Chicago, IL, USA

Umang Gupta, MBBS, DCH
Department of Pediatric Cardiology, Rush University Medical Center,
Chicago, IL, USA

Austin Hanrahan, MD, MS, BS
Department of Pediatrics, Rush University Medical Center, Chicago, IL, USA

Ziyad M. Hijazi, MD, MPH, FAAP
Department of Pediatrics and Internal Medicine, Rush University Medical Center,
Chicago, IL, USA

Joan F. Hoffman, MD
Department of Pediatrics, Rush University Medical Center, Chicago, IL, USA

Kathryn W. Holmes, MD, MPH
Department of Pediatric Cardiology, John Hopkins Medical Institutes,
Baltimore, MD, USA

Omar M. Khalid, MD, FAAP, FACC
Children's Heart Institute, Mary Washington Hospital,
Fredericksburg, VA, USA

Rami Kharouf, MD, MBBS
Department of Pediatric Cardiology, Mary Washington Hospital,
Fredericksburg, VA, USA

Douglas M. Luxenberg, DO
Pediatric Cardiology of Long Island, Roslyn, NY, USA

Megan A. McCarville, MD, MPH
Department of Pediatrics, Children's Memorial Hospital, Chicago, IL, USA

Surabhi Mona Mehrotra, MD
Department of Internal Medicine/Pediatrics, Rush University Medical Center,
Chicago, IL, USA

Zahra J. Naheed, MD
Department of Pediatrics, John H. Stroger, Jr. Hospital of Cook County,
Chicago, IL, USA

Aloka Patel, MD
Department of Neonatology, Rush University Medical Center,
Chicago, IL, USA

Paul N. Severin, MD, FAAP
Department of Pediatrics, John H. Stroger, Jr. Hospital of Cook County,
Chicago, IL, USA

Beth Shields, PharmD
Department of Pharmacy, Rush University Medical Center, Chicago, IL, USA

Stephen Stone, MD
Medical College of Wisconsin Affiliated Hospitals, Milwaukee, WI, USA

Anas Saleh Lutfi Taqatqa, MD
Department of Pediatric Cardiology, Rush University Medical Center,
Chicago, IL, USA

W. Reid Thompson, MD
Department of Pediatric Cardiology, John Hopkins Medical Institutes,
Baltimore, MD, USA

Laura Torchen, MD
Department of Pediatrics, Rush Children's Hospital, Chicago, IL, USA

Thea Yosowitz, MD
Department of Pediatrics, Northshore University Health, Evanston, IL, USA

Part I
Approach to Heart Diseases in Children

Chapter 1
Cardiac History and Physical Examination

W. Reid Thompson and Surabhi Mona Mehrotra

Key Facts

- In most instances, history and physical examination provide crucial information when determining if a child has heart disease
- Heart disease should be suspected if history reveals:

  - Shortness of breath without wheezing
  - History of central cyanosis
  - Easy fatigability
  - Failure to thrive
  - Family history of heart disease or sudden cardiac death

- Heart disease should be suspected if physical examination reveals:

  - Central cyanosis, clubbing of digits
  - Poor capillary refill and pulses
  - Delayed and weak femoral pulse when compared to brachial pulse
  - Hyperactive precordium, thrill
  - Murmurs louder than 2/6, diastolic murmurs
  - Single S2, fixed splitting of S2, additional heart sounds

Introduction

The wide application of fetal echocardiography in the United States has changed the most common presenting symptom of the neonate in many centers from cyanosis or tachypnea to "history of abnormal fetal screen." While this may be

W.R. Thompson (✉)
Department of Pediatric Cardiology, John Hopkins Medical Institutes,
600 North Wolfe Street, Brady 521, Baltimore, MD 21205, USA
e-mail: Thompson@jhmi.edu

Ra-id Abdulla (ed.), *Heart Diseases in Children: A Pediatrician's Guide*,
DOI 10.1007/978-1-4419-7994-0_1, © Springer Science+Business Media, LLC 2011

advantageous to those newborns, the skills needed to detect heart disease presenting without a fetal diagnosis, as a direct result, are increasingly in danger of being lost. Detection of previously undiagnosed heart disease in infants and children usually begins with a careful history and physical examination appropriate for the age of the child and the likely diseases that may present at that time. Knowledge of the classic presenting symptoms and signs of heart disease and skill in distinguishing the abnormal from the normal physical exam is crucial for the general pediatrician, and remains the primary screening tool for children of all ages.

Cardiac History

Consideration of heart disease as a possible diagnosis is usually prompted by one of a small list of symptoms or signs, including otherwise unexplained tachypnea, with or without failure to thrive, cyanosis, abnormal heart sounds or murmur, chest pain, or syncope. Congestive heart failure (CHF) due to excessive pulmonary blood flow is characterized by "quiet tachypnea," meaning the patient is not distressed, but is breathing rapidly (>60 breaths/min in the infant). A careful feeding history should be taken to ascertain how many ounces of formula are taken per feeding and per 24-h period, how long the typical feeding takes, whether the feeding is interrupted by frequent stops for breathing and ends with apparent fatigue, and whether it is accompanied by diaphoresis. CHF usually results in decreased formula intake because of tachypnea despite increased caloric demands, resulting in failure to thrive. Anomalous origin of the left coronary, presenting usually between 2 and 4 months, is typically associated with apparent discomfort during feedings. When asking about cyanosis, a distinction should be drawn between peripheral acrocyanosis, involving only the distal extremities, and central cyanosis, expressed as blueness of the lips and mucous membranes. Cyanosis with crying may be a sign of tetralogy of Fallot. However, visible cyanosis requires at least 3 g of desaturated hemoglobin per deciliter of blood, thus is relatively more difficult to detect in infants with lower hemoglobin values (for a given arterial oxygen saturation). Frequent and more serious respiratory illnesses may indicate predisposing cardiac pathology. Swallowing difficulties and/or stridor may be a sign of a vascular ring.

The older child is more likely to have either an occult congenital defect, such as an atrial septal defect, coronary anomaly, cardiomyopathy, or valve disease that was asymptomatic and difficult to detect on physical exam in infancy, or an acquired disease (e.g., myocarditis). The history should include questions about physical activities including exercise-induced chest pain, dizziness or shortness of breath, decreased exertional tolerance, or syncope. Most chest pain that occurs at rest in children is noncardiac, with the exception of myopericarditis. Heart racing or palpitations that occur at rest, with sudden onset and resolution, in a nonanxious youngster may indicate supraventricular tachycardia.

Family history of congenital heart disease or arrhythmia should be determined. History of premature death, sudden or otherwise, or significant disability from cardiovascular disease in close relatives under 50 years old may put the child or adolescent at increased risk for familial cardiomyopathy or premature atherosclerotic disease. Specific diagnoses should be inquired about, including hypertrophic or dilated cardiomyopathy, arrhythmogenic right ventricular dysplasia, long Q-T syndrome, and Marfan's syndrome.

Cardiac Examination

The comprehensive cardiac examination in the infant or child should begin with a period of observation, prior to interacting with the patient. Note the respiratory rate and pattern, whether or not accessory muscles are being used or flaring is present (usually more consistent with pulmonary disease or airway obstruction), and what degree of distress the patient is in. Note also the general nutritional status, the color of the mucous membranes, the presence of clubbing of digits (Fig. 1.1a, b), and the peripheral perfusion. Also take note of any specific dysmorphic features that might be associated with known syndromes. Next, carefully assess the vital signs and compare with age appropriate normal data, in the context of the potentially anxiety-provoking examination experience. Blood pressures should be obtained in all four extremities with appropriate size cuffs (Fig. 1.2 a, b). Pulse oximetry should be performed in every newborn and, if ductal dependent left-heart obstruction is possible, upper and lower extremity pulse oximetry should be compared. Lungs should be auscultated, listening for wheezing or rales, though these findings are relatively uncommon in infants with CHF. Also take note of any stridor, especially with crying, that may indicate a vascular ring. The abdominal exam should include careful assessment of the liver position and distance of the edge relative to the costal margin. Hepatomegaly is a reliable feature of significant heart failure in infants (Fig. 1.3). A more central liver edge is found in heterotaxy syndrome. Peripheral edema is relatively uncommon in pulmonary over-circulation lesions (e.g., VSD), and in infants in general. Likewise, jugular venous distention is not usually appreciated in infants.

Cardiac auscultation begins with a general assessment of the chest, looking for signs of hyperdynamic precordium. When palpating the chest, check for the apical impulse which represents the left ventricular (LV) impulse. LV impulse is at the apex of the heart, approximately in the fourth or fifth intercostal space at the midclavicular line. In addition, the right ventricular (RV) impulse can be elicited at the right lower sternal border (Fig. 1.4). Decrease or increase in either or both LV and RV impulse may indicate hypoplasia or hypertrophy (respectively) of that ventricle. Palpation of the chest may reveal the presence of a lift or heave of increased right ventricular pressure or thrill associated with a grade 4 or higher murmur. Use the appropriate stethoscope for the patient's size and listen systematically to each part of the cardiac cycle and at each area on the chest. Start by listening to the first and second heart sounds. S1 is best heard at the apex and marks the beginning of systole, whereas S2 is best heard at the mid to upper sternal border

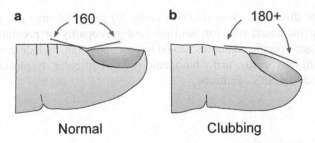

Normal   **Clubbing**

Fig. 1.1 Clubbing. (**a**) The angle at the junction of skin with the nail at the dorsal surface of digits is normally around 160°. (**b**) In children with cyanotic congenital heart diseases this angle becomes wider and may exceed 180°. This is the result of hypoxia in peripheral tissue, which causes the opening of normally collapsed capillaries to better perfuse the hypoxic tissue. Perfusion of these collapsed capillaries will result in expansion of the volume of these peripheral tissues (tips of digits) resulting in clubbing. This phenomenon is seen in other lesions causing hypoxia of peripheral tissue, such as with chronic lung disease and chronic anemia (causing hypoxia through reduction of level of hemoglobin and therefore reduction of oxygen carrying capacity) such as with ulcerative colitis, Crohn's disease, and chronic liver disease

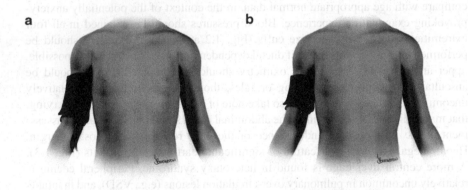

Fig. 1.2 Appropriate size BP cuff. Cuffs used to measure blood pressure should be appropriate in size for the child. (**a**) The breadth of the cuff should extend 2/3rd to 3/4th the distance of the forearm (or leg). (**b**) Smaller blood pressure cuffs will cause falsely elevated blood pressure measurements

and marks the beginning of diastole. By identifying S1 and S2, the systolic versus diastolic intervals can likewise then be distinguished, even though they may be of equal duration (at higher heart rates). In the case of mesocardia or dextrocardia, the apical impulse will be displaced rightward.

S1 is usually single, though in reality is the result of multiple low frequency events, which can often have at least two detectable components ("split S1"). This normal finding is relatively common in older children or adolescents, and is

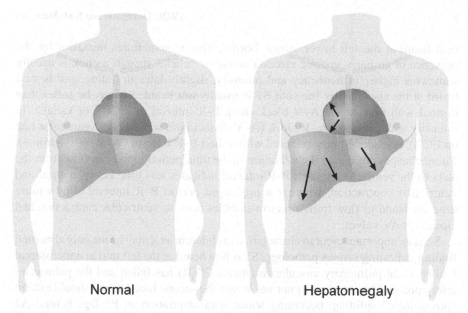

Normal   Hepatomegaly

Fig. 1.3 Hepatomegaly. Increased blood flow in the right heart such as seen in patients with atrial or ventricular septal defects will cause dilation and increase in right atrial pressure. This will eventually lead to congestion of organs draining blood into the right atrium such as the liver, leading to its enlargement

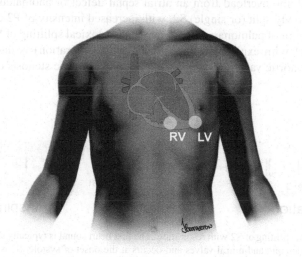

RV LV

Fig. 1.4 RV and LV impulses. The left ventricular (LV) or apical impulse reflects the left ventricular apex, while the right ventricular (RV) impulse reflects the right ventricular apex. LV impulse is normally the left lateral most border of the heart, while the RV impulse is at the left lower sternal border. RV impulse is close in intensity to the LV impulse in the neonatal period. Later in life, the LV impulse is much more prominent

best heard at the left lower sternal border. This is sometimes mistaken for the presence of an early systolic ejection sound or "click," though a click is usually somewhat higher in frequency and intensity, slightly later in timing, and is well heard at the apex, where the split S1 is usually not heard. S1 may be softer than normal with first degree A–V block (long P–R interval on ECG), or variable in intensity with complete A–V block (A–V dissociation with slower ventricular rate on ECG). A louder S1 may be heard with a short P–R interval (W–P–W syndrome). These changes are due to the alteration in the time period blood can flow from the atria to the ventricles. A short P–R interval indicates less time between atrial and ventricular contraction, whereas a prolonged period P–R interval allows more time for blood to flow from atria to ventricles prior to ventricular contraction and closure of AV valves.

S2 is an important event to characterize in children, as it may be the only abnormal finding indicating serious pathology. S2 is best heard at the left mid to upper sternal border. Once pulmonary vascular resistance (PVR) has fallen and the pulmonary artery pressure has reached its normal levels, the second heard sound should exhibit "physiologic" splitting, becoming wider with inspiration as P2 lags behind A2 (Fig. 1.5), then narrower with expiration, and P2 intensity (reflecting pulmonary artery pressure) should be softer than A2 (reflecting systemic arterial pressure). The interval should close with expiration, at least in the sitting position, though may occasionally remain slightly split when supine, sometimes reflecting an incomplete right bundle branch block (normal variant). Wide, fixed splitting of S2 is a sign of right heart volume overload from an atrial septal defect or anomalous pulmonary return. A narrowly split (or single) S2, with increased intensity of P2 component is an important sign of pulmonary hypertension. Paradoxical splitting of S2 (widening of the interval with expiration, and closing with inspiration) is due to delayed closure of the aortic valve (A2) and is often found in aortic stenosis or left bundle branch block.

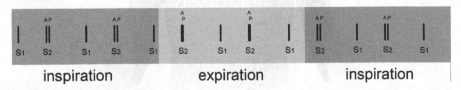

Fig. 1.5 Normal splitting of S2 with respiration. The first heart sound is typically single, reflecting closure of the tricuspid and mitral valves and occurs at the onset of systole. S2 is normally split, consisting of closure of the aortic valve, followed by the pulmonary valve. The aortic valve closes first due to the shorter left bundle branch of the His conduction system. This will allow the left ventricle to contract a few milliseconds before the right ventricle and therefore complete systole a few milliseconds before the right ventricle, hence aortic valve closes before pulmonary valve. This phenomenon is exaggerated during inspiration due to the increase in blood return to the right heart secondary to the sump effect of a negative intrathoracic pressure, thus leading to wider splitting of the second heart sound. The opposite is true in expiration, leading to approximation of the aortic and pulmonary components of the second heart sound, thus sounding as a single heart sound

An intermittent S3 is a common, nonpathologic finding in older children and adolescents, while S4 and/or S3–4 gallop is a sign of left ventricular dysfunction.

Clicks are additional, brief sounds in systole that are usually due to valve abnormalities, but may also be caused by increased flow in a dilated ascending aorta or main pulmonary artery. A constant, early systolic ejection click, occurring immediately after S1 and well heard at the apex, is a sign of bicuspid aortic valve. This click (or "ejection sound") is heard better in the sitting or standing position, but does not vary from beat to beat or shift in timing relative to S1. An early systolic ejection sound that is better heard in expiration than inspiration and best heard at the left upper sternal border is most consistent with an abnormal pulmonary valve. Mitral valve prolapse (MVP) causes a mid systolic click that moves closer to S2 in the squatting position and closer to S1 in the standing position, compared to supine. In diastole, an opening snap is an early diastolic sound made by a stenotic mitral valve.

Murmurs are sounds of longer duration caused by either the passage of blood through the heart and vessels with resulting vibrations of the normal cardiac structures (innocent murmurs) or turbulent flow across abnormal structures such as valves or septal defects (Fig. 1.6a–f). Murmurs should be listened for at all areas of the anterior chest, axilla, and back and described in terms of intensity (grades 1–6), presence in systole, diastole, or continuous, timing within the interval (early, mid, late, pan), contour (ejection or regurgitant), quality (vibratory, harsh, blowing), location on chest best heard and radiated to, and response to maneuvers, such as standing or squatting.

Intensity grade 1 implies a very soft murmur only heard when paying careful attention, grade 2 is easily heard but not loud, grade 3 is loud but without a thrill, grade 4 is loud with a thrill, grade 5 is heard with the stethoscope partly off the chest, and grade 6 is heard with the stethoscope completely off the chest. Whereas, innocent murmurs can be heard in 70–90% of older infants and children on at least one visit (Table 1.1), persistent murmurs that are benign are relatively rare in neonates and young infants. In the older infant or child, innocent murmurs are often more obvious during febrile illnesses or other states of increased cardiac output. Innocent murmurs are usually short, systolic ejection murmurs, intensity grade 1 or 2, not associated with any other abnormal cardiac findings. Innocent murmurs should decrease in intensity or disappear in the standing position due to the reduced volume of blood returning to the heart and thus eliminating a "normal" murmur. The vibratory or musical "Still's" murmur is very common in young children, often heard best at the left lower sternal border to the apex (Table 1.2).

Pulmonary flow murmurs are soft, medium frequency, blowing murmurs heard best at the left mid to upper sternal border. The venous hum is a continuous murmur and the only innocent murmur heard in diastole. The sound is due to blood flowing down the neck veins into the innominate vein and superior vena cava and is louder in diastole and with inspiration. It is usually not heard in the supine position but is easily heard in the sitting position under the right or left clavicle in most 3–5-year-old children, often accentuated by turning the head to one side or the other and extinguished by compressing the ipsilateral neck veins.

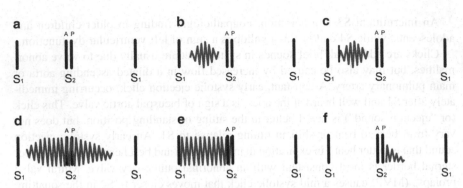

Fig. 1.6 Heart sounds and murmurs. (**a**) Normal heart sounds: once the ventricles start to contract at the onset of systole, the tricuspid and mitral valves close. Closure of the atrioventricular valves contributes to the first heart sound which tends to be single. Aortic and pulmonary valves open soon after S1; however, this is usually inaudible in the normal heart. Flow across the aortic and pulmonary valves follows, which is again usually inaudible in the normal heart. The aortic valve closes first, followed by the pulmonary valve; the delay in closure of the pulmonary valve gives the "splitting" character of the second heart sound. Diastole, similar to systole is quiet; during diastole, blood flows through the tricuspid and mitral valves into the right and left ventricles. (**b**) Systolic flow murmur: increased blood flow across the pulmonary or aortic valve causes turbulence of blood flow which produces a systolic flow murmur heard over the left or right upper sternal border, respectively. In atrial septal defect, increased blood flow across the pulmonary valve causes a systolic ejection murmur along the left upper sternal border. Severe anemia with increase in blood volume to compensate for decreased oxygen carrying capacity causes turbulence of blood flow and consequently a murmur across both aortic and pulmonary valves. These murmurs are distinguished from those caused by stenosis of the pulmonary or aortic valves by lack of a systolic ejection click heard just before the systolic murmurs. (**c**) Pulmonary or aortic valve stenosis: flow across the pulmonary and aortic valves occurs during midsystole; therefore, pulmonary or aortic stenosis produces a systolic ejection murmur preceded by a systolic ejection click. These murmurs are loudest over the right upper sternal borders in aortic stenosis and the left upper sternal border in pulmonary stenosis. The systolic ejection click is caused by the snap sound of opening of abnormal pulmonary or aortic valves. (**d**) Continuous murmur: a murmur heard over systole and most of diastole reflects abnormal shunting across a vascular structure connecting the systemic to pulmonary circulations, such as with patent ductus arteriosus. Murmur caused by PDA may be restricted to systole in children due to the soft and inaudible flow during diastole. (**e**) Early diastolic murmur: during early diastole, blood in the proximal portions of the pulmonary artery and aorta eject to the pulmonary and systemic circulations, respectively. Backward flow of blood into the right or left ventricles due to valve regurgitation will cause an early diastolic murmur. Aortic regurgitation is best heard over the mid or left sternal region. Pulmonary regurgitation is typically inaudible due to low pressures in the right heart and if heard may indicate pulmonary hypertension. (**f**) Mid-diastolic murmur: during mid-diastole blood flows from the atria to the respective ventricles. Excessive blood flow across the tricuspid valve, such as with atrial septal defect, or across the mitral valve such as with patent ductus arteriosus will cause a mid-diastolic murmur heard over the left lower sternal border in patients with atrial septal defect and at the apex in patients with patent ductus arteriosus

Pathologic murmurs can be at any intensity level, though louder murmurs (>grade 2) are more likely to be pathologic. Holo (or pan) systolic murmurs and mid to late systolic regurgitation murmurs are pathologic, and usually indicate either ventricular septal defects or mitral or tricuspid valve regurgitation. Harsh quality (wide frequency

Table 1.1 Distinguishing features of nonpathologic and pathologic murmurs

Features	Innocent murmur	Pathologic murmur
History	Void of any symptoms associated with heart disease	Symptoms such as easy fatigability, shortness of breath, cyanosis may be present
Physical examination	Normal	Abnormal findings such as cyanosis, clubbing of digits, delayed capillary refill, hepatomegaly, thrill over the precordium
Auscultation findings		
– First heart sound	Normal	Typically normal
– Second heart sound	Splits and varies with respiration (single in expiratory phase and split in inspiratory phase)	May be single such as in pulmonary or aortic atresia, truncus arteriosus or transposition of the great vessels. Wide, fixed splitting is present in atrial septal defect
– Systolic murmur	Grade 1 or 2 and rarely 3 of 6, soft (often musical) in nature, short, ejection systolic	3/6 or higher, harsh, may be systolic ejection or regurgitant, often holosystolic
– Diastolic murmur		May be present, such as in atrial septal defect and aortic regurgitation
– Continuous murmur	Soft and heard in the supraclavicular region (venous hum)	Harsh, heard over subclavicular region (PDA) or over the back (aortic–pulmonary collaterals)

distribution) systolic ejection murmurs are almost always pathologic and usually are due to either right or left ventricular outflow obstruction (pulmonary or aortic stenosis). Early diastolic decrescendo murmurs are indicative or aortic or pulmonary insufficiency and are usually best heard at the mid to upper sternal border, especially with the patient sitting and leaning forward. Mitral stenosis usually results in a low frequency mid to late diastolic murmur, often with crescendo at end diastole, best heard at the apex with the patient in the left lateral decubitus position. Systolic murmurs that appear to increase in intensity in the standing position are pathologic, and usually indicate dynamic obstruction (hypertrophic obstructive cardiomyopathy) or MVP with regurgitation. The presence of an abnormal additional finding, such as an abnormal S2 or a click, makes a murmur much more likely to be pathologic than innocent.

Images as well as movie/audio clips of heart sounds and murmurs reviewed in this chapter can be found through the internet at: (http://www.pedcard.rush.edu/murmur).

Heart Disease Presenting in Infancy

Most serious congenital heart defects are present in the neonatal period. Often a syndromic appearance may raise suspicion of specific heart defects (trisomy 21 and A–V canal defect, trisomy 18 and ventricular septal defect, Noonan's syndrome and

Table 1.2 Types of innocent heart murmurs

Pulmonary flow murmur	Features: systolic ejection murmur, soft Location: left upper sternal border Cause: blood flow through normal pulmonary valve, possibly due to thin chest wall and normal rapid heart rate seen in children
Aortic flow murmur (Still's murmur)	Features: systolic ejection murmur, soft Location: right upper sternal border Cause: blood flow through normal aortic valve, possibly due to thin chest wall and normal rapid heart rate seen in children
Peripheral pulmonary stenosis	Features: systolic ejection murmur Location: left upper sternal border with radiation into both axilla Cause: relative small pulmonary arteries in infants less than 8 weeks of age secondary to reduced pulmonary blood flow in utero. Murmur should disappear by 8 weeks of age, otherwise pathologic peripheral pulmonary stenosis should be considered such as with William, Allagile, Noonan syndromes, or secondary to congenital Rubella
Venous hum	Features: continuous, soft murmur Location: over either side of the neck Cause: flow in normal veins
Mammary soufflé	Features: systolic flow murmur Location: over breasts in females, during initial growth of breast (puberty) or during pregnancy Cause: rapid growth of breast tissue with increase in blood flow

pulmonary stenosis, William's syndrome and supravalvar aortic stenosis, DiGeorge syndrome, and interrupted aortic arch or truncus arteriosus).

Left Heart Obstructive Disease

With critical left heart obstructive disease (coarctation of the aorta, critical aortic stenosis, hypoplastic left heart syndrome, and interrupted aortic arch), symptoms and signs of obstruction to systemic flow begin with the onset of ductus arteriosus closure. Tachypnea and poor feeding are the most common symptoms, and result from metabolic acidosis and pulmonary venous hypertension. Prior to ductal closure a difference in pulse oximetry between the upper (higher saturation) and lower (lower saturation) maybe the only clue to the diagnosis of critical coarctation or interrupted aortic arch and may be difficult or impossible to distinguish from persistent pulmonary hypertension of the newborn without echocardiography. After ductal closure, the pulse oximetry differential is replaced by a difference in pulse intensity and blood pressure between the upper (higher systolic pressure) and lower (lower pressure) extremities. A systolic pressure differential greater than 10 mmHg, often with upper extremity hypertension, is a sign of aortic arch obstruction. A systolic ejection murmur may be detected in the axilla or mid left back. Critical aortic stenosis presents with a harsh systolic ejection murmur noted immediately after birth, followed by low systemic output upon ductal closure. Hypoplastic left heart syndrome may be undetected until there is systemic collapse, with a pale, gray appearance indicating both cyanosis and shock. On exam, there is shallow, rapid breathing, hypotension and poor pulses in all extremities, poor peripheral perfusion, and lower than normal oxygen saturations.

Cyanotic Heart Disease

Cyanotic heart disease is due to inadequate effective pulmonary blood flow, resulting from either obstruction of flow to the lungs (tetralogy of Fallot) or from the lungs (obstructed total anomalous pulmonary venous return), or parallel (instead of in-series) circulations (transposition of the great arteries). Infants are usually noted to have cyanotic lips or mucous membranes (depending on the hemoglobin level, as mentioned above), but are not in distress except when severely hypoxemic ($pO_2 < 30$ TORR), or when pulmonary venous return is obstructed (causing classic "ground-glass" appearance of lung fields on CXR). The cardiac exam is specific for the defect. With severe pulmonary stenosis, a harsh systolic ejection murmur is usually heard immediately after birth. If a to fro murmur is heard (systolic ejection murmur with early diastolic decrescendo murmur), the diagnosis is usually tetralogy of Fallot with dysplastic pulmonary valve, especially if the infant appears to be in respiratory distress from airway extrinsic compression (due to enlarged pulmonary arteries). Other rare causes of to–fro murmurs in the neonate include truncus arteriosus and aorta to left ventricular fistula.

Transposition of the great arteries usually has a single second heart sound and no murmur.

Increased Pulmonary Blood Flow

Heart defects resulting in increased pulmonary blood flow (e.g., ventricular septal defects, patent ductus arteriosus, some forms of double outlet right ventricle) typically present when PVR falls, resulting in left-to-right shunting and tachypnea from increased pulmonary interstitial fluid. While variable, PVR usually reaches a nadir around 2 weeks postnatally. Symptoms include tachypnea and feeding difficulties with poor weight gain. The cardiac examination is almost always abnormal, usually with a pathologic systolic murmur and possible diastolic rumble. A loud, narrowly split or single S2 indicates pulmonary hypertension. Ventricular septal defects cause holosystolic, regurgitant murmurs, usually at the left mid to lower sternal border or at the apex, depending on the location of the defect. The diastolic rumble is produced by the large flow volume crossing the mitral valve. Besides simple VSD, other defects with related anatomy, pathophysiology, and auscultatory findings include complete atrioventricular canal, double outlet right ventricle, some forms or tricuspid atresia and truncus arteriosus. Patent ductus arteriosus and aortopulmonary window have continuous flow from the aorta into the pulmonary artery, resulting in a murmur that has late systolic accentuation, then crosses S2 into early diastole. Often, multiple systolic clicks like the sound of water moving over a water-wheel can be heard, probably due to increased flow in the dilated pulmonary artery or ascending aorta.

Heart Disease Presenting in Childhood or Adolescence

Since most serious congenital defects present in infancy, heart disease presenting later is typically either asymptomatic or difficult to detect, progressive in severity leading to later presentation, or acquired.

Occult Congenital Defects

Atrial septal defects often go undetected for several years, as they rarely cause symptoms in infancy but may result in decreased exercise tolerance in the adolescent. The classic findings on cardiac examination are a fixed and widely split S2, best heard at the mid to upper sternal border. There may be a grades 1–2/6 systolic ejection murmur at the left upper sternal border of increased flow across the pulmonary valve ("relative pulmonary stenosis") and a diastolic low-pitched rumble at the left lower sternal border of increased flow across the tricuspid valve. Obstructive lesions such as aortic stenosis or coarctation that present later, are nonductal dependent, progressive lesions that rarely cause symptoms until severe. Both may be associated with a bicuspid aortic valve, which usually can be detected by listening carefully at the apex, especially in the sitting position, for an early, constant systolic ejection sound (or "click"). The murmur of aortic stenosis is a harsh, throat-clearing systolic ejection murmur, best heard at the right upper sternal border. Coarctation of the aorta results in systolic hypertension in the upper extremities, decreased pulses and blood pressure in the lower extremities, and a systolic ejection murmur best heard over the left back or left axilla. Causes of acquired valve abnormalities include endocarditis and rheumatic fever.

Mitral regurgitation from leaflet infection or inflammation results in a harsh, sometimes high-frequency pan systolic, regurgitant murmur heard best at the apex. The patient should be placed in the left lateral decubitus position to detect this murmur.

Cardiomyopathy

Familial hypertrophic cardiomyopathy often presents in the 14–18-year-old age range, when it is also most likely to result in sudden death in the athlete, accounting for approximately 40–50% of sudden cardiac death in the teenaged athlete in the United States. Symptoms include shortness of breath, chest pain, dizziness, or syncope with exercise. Family history of heart disease or sudden death prior to age 40 should raise index of suspicion. In 25% of patients, there is dynamic left ventricular mid cavity obstruction that results in a systolic ejection murmur that increases in intensity in the standing position. The ECG is almost always abnormal, either with increased ventricular forces or strain (tall R wave or inverted T waves in lateral precordial leads). Dilated cardiomyopathy usually results in CHF with decreased exercise tolerance and shortness of breath. On exam, there may be increased jugular venous pressure, pulmonary rales, hepatomegaly, and possibly peripheral edema. Cardiac auscultation may reveal an S3–4 summation gallop, best heard with the bell at the left lower sternal border or apex.

Myocarditis

Myocarditis should be suspected in any child with signs of heart failure who was previous well, especially with a preceding history of a viral illness. Symptoms may include chest pain, shortness or breath, or syncope. On cardiac exam there is often unexplained tachycardia and the heart sounds are usually muffled. On ECG there are often low voltages. The presence of ventricular arrhythmias indicates fulminant presentation and should prompt immediate transfer to the intensive care unit for potential cardiopulmonary support.

- The cardiac silhouette occupies 50–55% of the chest width on an anterior–posterior chest X-ray
- When assessing the cardiovascular system on a chest X-ray, the following must be noted:
    - The size of the heart (small, normal, or large)
    - The contours of the heart reflecting various cardiovascular components which can be enlarged, absent, or displaced
    - The Pulmonary vascularity which can be diminished, normal, or increased

- Many newborn children appear to have cardiomegaly when in fact the thymus is contributing to the "cardio-thymic shadow" giving the appearance of an enlarged heart. The lateral view, where the thymus can be seen occupying the anterior portion of the chest cavity with no evidence of cardiomegaly, can separate this from true cardiomegaly
- An enlarged heart coupled with an increase in pulmonary vascular markings can be indicative of left to right shunting such as ASD, VSD, and PDA. This can also be seen in many cyanotic heart diseases where there is excessive pulmonary blood flow

An enlarged heart with no evidence of increase in pulmonary vascular markings suggests an obstructive lesion

Chapter 2
Cardiac Interpretation of Pediatric Chest X-Ray

Ra-id Abdulla and Douglas M. Luxenberg

Key Facts

- The cardiac silhouette occupies 50–55% of the chest width on an anterior–posterior chest X-ray
- When assessing the cardiovascular system on a chest X-ray, the following must be noted:

  - The size of the heart (small, normal, or large)
  - The contours of the heart reflecting various cardiovascular components which can be enlarged, absent, or displaced
  - The Pulmonary vascularity which can be diminished, normal, or increased

- Many newborn children appear to have cardiomegaly when in fact the thymus is contributing to the "cardio-thymic shadow". The lateral view of CXR can separate this from true cardiomegaly.
- An enlarged heart coupled with an increase in pulmonary vascular markings can be indicative of left to right shunting such as with ASD, VSD, and PDA.

Introduction

Chest X-ray is an important tool in evaluating heart disease in children. Noninvasive imaging such as echocardiography and cardiac MRI provide valuable and detailed assessment of the cardiovascular system; however, the cost incurred from these

Ra-id Abdulla (✉)
Center for Congenital and Structural Heart Diseases, Rush University Medical Center,
1653 West Congress Parkway, Room 763 Jones, Chicago, IL 60612, USA
e-mail: rabdulla@rush.edu

Ra-id Abdulla (ed.), *Heart Diseases in Children: A Pediatrician's Guide*,
DOI 10.1007/978-1-4419-7994-0_2, © Springer Science+Business Media, LLC 2011

diagnostic procedures is significant making their routine use difficult. Chest X-ray on the other hand is easy to perform, economical, and provides important information including heart size, pulmonary blood flow, and any associated lung disease. History of present illness coupled with physical examination provides the treating physician with a reasonable list of differential diagnoses which can be further focused with the aid of chest X-ray and electrocardiography making it possible to select a management plan or make a decision to refer the child for further evaluation and treatment by a specialist.

Approach to Chest X-Ray Interpretation

Unlike echocardiography, chest X-ray does not provide details of intracardiac structures. Instead the heart appears as a silhouette of overlapping cardiovascular chambers and vessels. Chest X-ray obtained in two perpendicular views, specifically anteroposterior (AP) and lateral, makes it possible to construct a mental three-dimensional image of the heart.

The size and shape of the heart as well as the pulmonary vascular markings, pleura and parenchymal lung markings provide helpful information regarding the heart/lung pathology.

It is easy to be overwhelmed with a prominent pathology on a chest X-ray thus overlooking more subtle changes; therefore, it is imperative to conduct interpretation of chest X-ray carefully and systematically considering the following issues.

Heart size: The size of the heart represents all that lies within the pericardial sac. This includes the volume within each cardiac chamber, cardiac wall thickness, pericardial space, and any other additional structure such as mass from a tumor or air trapped within the pericardium (pneumopericardium). Therefore, enlargement of any of these structures will lead to the appearance of cardiomegaly on chest X-ray. Dilated atria or ventricles such as that seen in heart failure will cause the cardiac silhouette to appear large, as would hypertrophy of the ventricular walls or fluid accumulation within the pericardial space (Tables 2.1 and 2.2).

Heart shape: The presence of certain subtleties in the cardiac shape may point to a particular pathology and thus help narrow the differential diagnosis. Enlargement or hypoplasia of a particular component of the heart will alter the normal shape of the cardiac silhouette. Therefore, each aspect of the heart border should be examined to assess for abnormalities. Examples of this include prominence of the aortic arch in patients with systemic hypertension or aortic stenosis (AS) due to dilation of the aorta. On the other hand, pulmonary atresia will cause the mediastinum to be narrow due to hypoplasia of the pulmonary artery.

Pulmonary blood flow: Pulmonary vasculature is normally visible in the hilar region of each lung adjacent to the borders of the cardiac silhouette. An increase in pulmonary blood flow or congestion of the pulmonary veins will cause prominence of the pulmonary blood vessels. A significant increase in pulmonary blood flow

Table 2.1 Cardiac pathology and changes of cardiac silhouette

Cardiac pathology	Features
Right atrial enlargement	AP view: fullness of the right heart border
Right ventricular enlargement	AP view: uplifting of the cardiac apex
	Lateral view: fullness of the lower retrosternal region of the cardiac silhouette
Main pulmonary artery dilation	AP view: prominence of the main pulmonary artery trunk in the midleft border of the cardiac silhouette
	Lateral view: fullness of the midretrosternal portion of the cardiac silhouette
Branch pulmonary artery dilation	AP view: prominent pulmonary arteries over the corresponding lung field, typically in the hilar region
Left atrial enlargement	AP view: double shadow in the midcardiac silhouette region as well as widening the tracheal branching (carina)
	Lateral view: prominence of the posterior border of the cardiac silhouette with posterior deviation of the esophagus
Left ventricular enlargement	AP view: enlarged cardiac silhouette with lateral and downward displacement of the cardiac apex
Aortic arch dilation	AP view: prominent aortic arch in the upper region of the left border of the cardiac silhouette
Thymus gland	AP view
	Enlarged: a sail like sign over the upper-midcardiac silhouette, in severe cases may give the impression of cardiomegaly
	Atrophy: narrowed mediastinum
	Lateral view
	Enlarged: soft tissue occupying the upper retrosternal field, typically occupied by lung tissue
	Atrophy: absence of soft tissue in the upper retrosternal region, may be normal in older children but in neonates should cause suspicion of DiGeorge syndrome

Table 2.2 Congenital heart diseases and changes in cardiac chambers

Atrial septal defect	Right atrial enlargement, right ventricular enlargement, pulmonary artery dilation
Ventricular septal defect	Left ventricular enlargement, pulmonary artery dilation, left atrial enlargement
Patent ductus arteriosus	Pulmonary artery dilation, left atrial enlargement, left ventricular enlargement
Aortic stenosis	Left ventricular enlargement
Pulmonary stenosis	Right ventricular enlargement
Coarctation of the aorta	Left ventricular enlargement, Rib notching
Atrioventricular canal defect	All cardiac chambers enlarged
Tetralogy of Fallot	Right ventricular enlargement, hypoplasia of pulmonary arteries, coeur en sabot
Double outlet right ventricle	Right ventricular enlargement
Pulmonary atresia	Right ventricular hypoplasia
Tricuspid atresia	Right ventricular hypoplasia

(continued)

Table 2.2 (continued)

Pulmonary atresia-intact ventricular septum	No tricuspid regurgitation: right ventricular hypoplasia
	Severe tricuspid regurgitation: right atrial enlargement, right ventricular enlargement
Truncus arteriosus	Right ventricular enlargement, pulmonary artery hypoplasia
Total anomalous pulmonary venous return	Dilation of veins draining anomalous pulmonary veins, such as vertical vein, innominent vein, superior vena cava, "Snowman" sign
Hypoplastic left heart syndrome	Left ventricular hypoplasia, ascending aorta and aortic arch hypoplasia
Transposition of the Great Arteries	Narrowed mediastinum, "egg on a string"

will cause dilation of peripheral pulmonary vessels, allowing their visualization in the normally dark peripheral lung fields.

Pleural space: Heart failure results in venous congestion which may lead to fluid accumulation within the pleural spaces manifesting as a pleural effusion. Pleural effusion may be noted on chest X-ray as a rim of fluid in the outer lung boundaries of the chest cavity or as haziness of the entire lung field in a recumbent patient due to layering of the fluid behind the lungs.

Normal CXR

Anteroposterior View

The cardiac silhouette occupies 50–55% of the chest width. Cardiomegaly is present when the cardiothoracic (CT) ratio is more than 55%. The right border of the cardiac silhouette consists of the following structures from top to bottom: superior vena cava, ascending aorta, right atrial appendage, and right atrium (Fig. 2.1). The left border of the cardiac silhouette is formed from top to bottom by the aortic arch (aortic knob), pulmonary trunk, left atrial appendage, and the left ventricle. Of note is that the right ventricle does not contribute to either heart border.

In the normal chest X-ray only the larger, more proximal pulmonary arteries can be visualized in the hilar regions of the lungs and the lung parenchyma should be clear with no evidence of pleural effusion (Fig. 2.2).

Lateral View

The cardiac silhouette in this view is oval in shape and occupies the anterior half of the thoracic cage. Lung tissue occupies the dorsal half of the chest cavity.

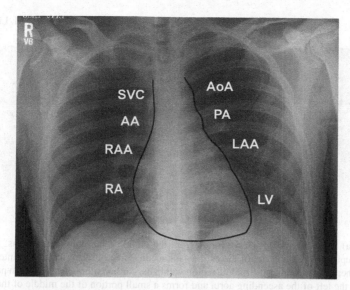

Fig. 2.1 Heart border: The cardiac silhouette is formed by a variety of cardiovascular structures. In an AP view, the right heart border is formed from top to bottom by superior vena cava, ascending aorta, right atrial appendage, and the right atrium. On the *left side*, the heart border is formed from top to bottom by the aortic arch (knob), main pulmonary artery, left atrial appendage, and the left ventricle. *AA* ascending aorta, *AoA* aortic arch, *LAA* left atrial appendage, *RAA* right atrial appendage, *RA* right atrium, *SVC* superior vena cava

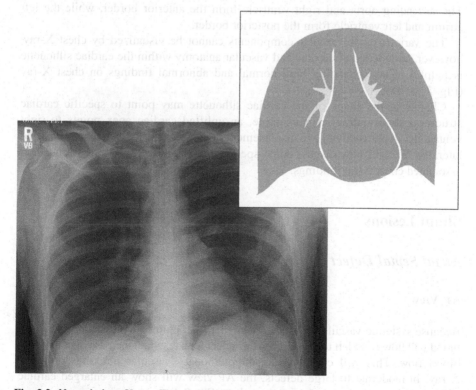

Fig. 2.2 Normal chest X-ray: The cardiac silhouette is normal in size and contour. A normal pulmonary blood flow pattern is present with no evidence of pleural disease

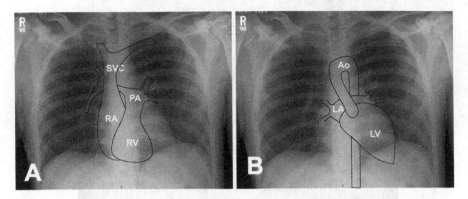

Fig. 2.3 (**a**) The superior vena cava forms from the union of the innominate veins. The right atrium occupies the right border of the cardiac silhouette. The right ventricle is the anterior most part of the heart and occupies the middle region within the cardiac silhouette. The main pulmonary artery is to the left of the ascending aorta and forms a small portion of the middle of the left cardiac silhouette border as it courses posteriorly and bifurcates into right and left pulmonary arteries. (**b**) The left atrium lies behind the left ventricle, the ascending aorta courses to the right of the pulmonary artery and then arches at the superior aspect of the mediastinum. The mediastinum is formed by the crossing of the aorta and pulmonary artery. *Ao* aorta, *LA* left atrium, *LV* left ventricle, *PA* pulmonary artery, *RA* right atrium, *RV* right ventricle, *SVC* superior vena cava

The ascending aorta and right ventricle form the anterior border, while the left atrium and left ventricle form the posterior border.

The various cardiovascular components cannot be visualized by chest X-ray, however, knowledge of cardiac and vascular anatomy within the cardiac silhouette is helpful in understanding both normal and abnormal findings on chest X-ray (Fig. 2.3a, b).

Change in the shape of the cardiac silhouette may point to specific cardiac structural abnormalities; for example, an uplifted cardiac apex points to right ventricular hypertrophy due to displacement of the left ventricular apex upward and laterally. We will now discuss some specific congenital cardiac lesions and their associated chest X-ray findings.

Shunt Lesions

Atrial Septal Defect

AP View

Because systemic vascular resistance is higher than pulmonary vascular resistance blood will flow from left to right across the defect with resultant increase in pulmonary blood flow. This will cause prominent pulmonary vascular markings on chest X-ray. In moderate to large defects, the AP view will show an enlarged cardiac silhouette due to fullness of the right atrium (Fig. 2.4).

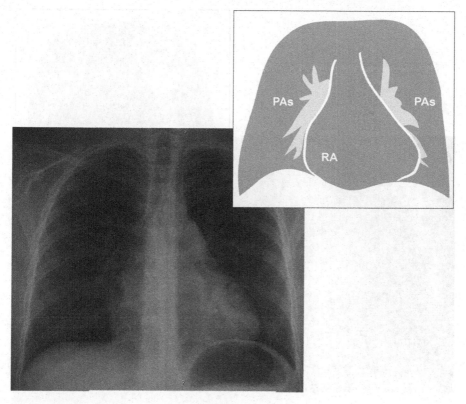

Fig. 2.4 Atrial septal defect. An atrial septal defect causes an increase in heart size with fullness of the right heart border due to right atrial enlargement. The pulmonary arteries are full and may be well visualized even in the peripheral lung fields indicating an increase in pulmonary blood flow. *PAs* pulmonary arteries, *RA* right atrium

Lateral View

Prominent pulmonary vasculature is noted, particularly in the hilar region. In severe cases, the right ventricle is dilated and is noted as fullness of the anterior most aspect of the cardiac silhouette causing obliteration of the usual space between the heart and sternum.

Ventricular Septal Defect

AP View

Left to right shunting at the ventricular level will cause an increase in pulmonary blood flow. The increase in pulmonary blood flow will manifest as engorged pulmonary vasculature. The increase in return of blood to the left atrium and ventricle may cause left atrial and left ventricular dilation (Fig. 2.5).

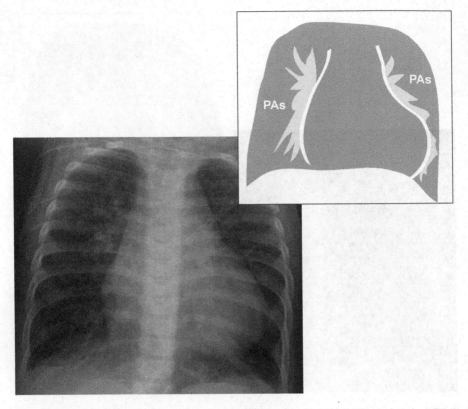

Fig. 2.5 Ventricular septal defect (VSD). Cardiomegaly is noted in most moderate to large VSDs. An increase in pulmonary blood flow results in prominent pulmonary vasculature which may be noted in the peripheral lung fields. *PAs* pulmonary arteries

Lateral View

The lateral view shows a posteriorly deviated esophagus reflective of a dilated left atrium.

Patent Ductus Arteriosus

AP View

Left to right shunting at the arterial level causes dilation of the pulmonary vasculature. The main pulmonary artery is dilated which may be noted by prominence of the main pulmonary artery segment at the left heart border just below the aortic arch on the AP view. The left atrium and ventricle become dilated due to increased

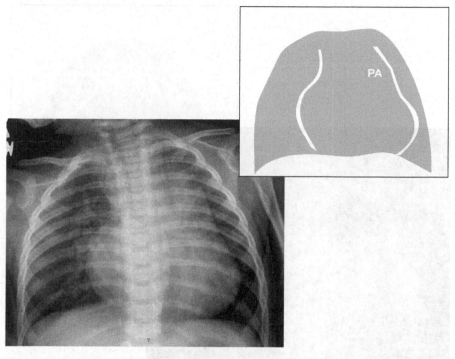

Fig. 2.6 Patent ductus arteriosus (PDA). In addition to the PDA itself, the dilated main and branch pulmonary arteries cause the middle segment of the left heart silhouette to be prominent. *PA* pulmonary artery

pulmonary venous blood return to the left atrium resulting in cardiomegaly. Left atrial dilation may cause widening of carina angle (Fig. 2.6).

Lateral View

Prominent pulmonary vasculature and a dilated left atrium are noted. Left atrial dilation may cause posterior deviation of the esophagus.

Atrioventricular Canal Defect

AP View

Large atrial and ventricular septal defects (VSDs) are common with this lesion. The resultant significant increase in pulmonary blood flow results in prominent pulmonary vasculature. This, coupled with regurgitation of the atrioventricular valve, results in cardiomegaly due to dilation of all cardiac chambers. Left atrial dilation may cause a widening of the carina angle as well (Fig. 2.7).

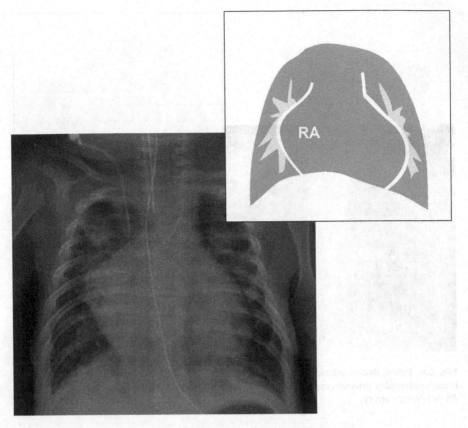

Fig. 2.7 Atrioventricular canal defect. The heart is enlarged due to dilation of all cardiac chambers from to left to right shunting and atrioventricular valve regurgitation. The pulmonary arteries are very prominent. This patient also has right upper lobe atelectasis which may be seen in patients with a significant increase in pulmonary blood flow and heart failure. *RA* right atrium

Lateral

Prominent pulmonary vasculature and cardiomegaly are noted. Left atrial dilation may cause posterior deviation of the esophagus.

Obstructive Lesions

Pulmonary Stenosis

AP View

The jet-like flow across the narrowed pulmonary valve orifice causes the main pulmonary artery to dilate. This manifests as prominence of the pulmonary artery

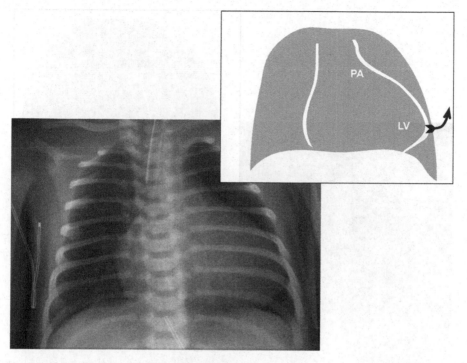

Fig. 2.8 Pulmonary stenosis. The main pulmonary artery is dilated (seen in the mid left border of the cardiac silhouette) and the left ventricular apex is uplifted secondary to right ventricular enlargement. *LV* left ventricle, *PA* pulmonary artery

segment in the midleft border of the cardiac silhouette, just below the aortic arch prominence. Right ventricular dilation and hypertrophy are present in cases of severe and prolonged pulmonary stenosis (PS). Right ventricular enlargement will manifest as uplifting of the cardiac apex (Fig. 2.8).

Lateral View

A dilated main pulmonary artery may be seen as fullness of the upper retrosternal portion of the cardiac silhouette. Right ventricular enlargement will cause fullness of the lower retrosternal portion of the cardiac silhouette.

Aortic Stenosis

AP View

The jet-like flow across the narrowed aortic valve orifice will result in the dilation of the ascending aorta which will be noted in the mid region of the right heart border.

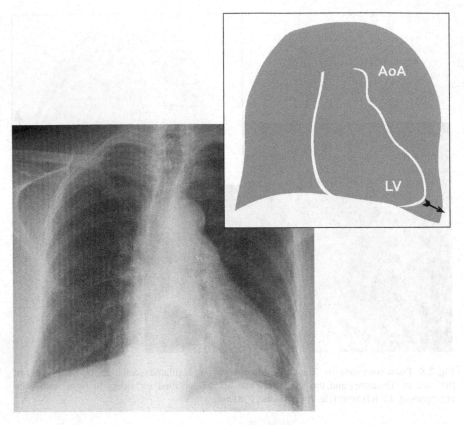

Fig. 2.9 Aortic stenosis. The aortic arch (upper left border of the cardiac silhouette) is prominent with the evidence of left ventricular dilation. Note the down and outward displacement of the cardiac apex. The heart is enlarged as well. *AOA* aortic arch, *LV* left ventricle

In severe cases, the aortic knob (the upper portion of left border of cardiac silhouette) will be prominent.

Prolonged AS will cause left ventricular failure and dilation which will manifest as a downward and lateral displacement of the cardiac apex (Fig. 2.9).

Lateral View

This is typically normal except in cases of congestive heart failure where cardiomegaly is seen.

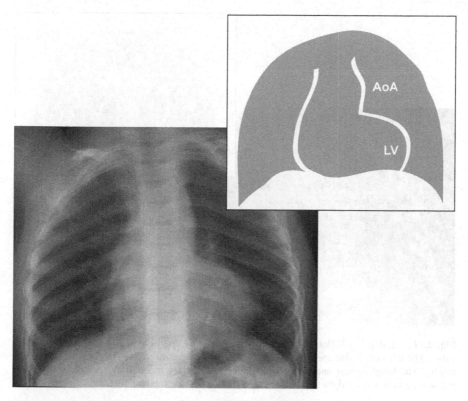

Fig. 2.10 Coarctation of the aorta. The aortic arch is hypoplastic in this patient resulting in the absence of aortic knob prominence at the upper left border of the cardiac silhouette. Cardiomegaly is present due to left ventricular failure and dilation. *AOA* aortic arch, *LV* left ventricle

Coarctation of the Aorta

AP View

While coarctation of the aorta (CoA) is most often not initially detectable by CXR, prolonged and severe disease may lead to left ventricular hypertrophy, and dilation, manifesting as cardiomegaly. Long standing CoA may cause a "reverse 3 sign" noted in the aortic knob (the upper portion of left cardiac silhouette border) and "rib notching" which is a deformation of the inferior surface of the ribs (Fig. 2.10).

Lateral View

Cardiomegaly may be noted; otherwise no significant pathology is typically present.

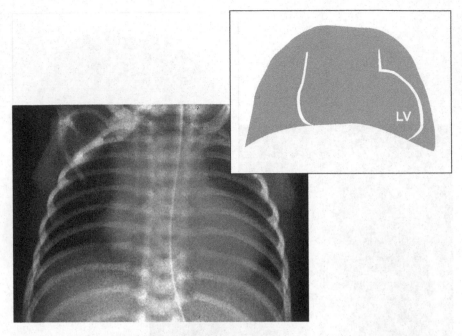

Fig. 2.11 Tetralogy of Fallot. The mediastinum is narrow due to hypoplasia of the pulmonary valve. The left ventricular apex is displaced laterally and upward due to right ventricular hypertrophy. The lungs appear anemic due to reduced pulmonary blood flow secondary to severe pulmonary stenosis and right to left shunting at the ventricular septal defect. *LV* left ventricle

Cyanotic Congenital Heart Lesions

Tetralogy of Fallot

AP View

Small, hypoplastic or atretic pulmonary arteries will cause the mediastinum to appear narrow. Right ventricular hypertrophy secondary to PS will cause an uplifting of the cardiac apex. Together, these two findings will give the classic *coeur en sabot* (boot shaped) appearance of the heart. Severe PS will restrict pulmonary blood flow, this will manifested as diminished pulmonary vascular markings (Fig. 2.11).

Lateral View

Right ventricular hypertrophy will cause fullness of the cardiac silhouette in the retrosternal region. An "anemic" lung appearance due to reduced pulmonary blood flow will be noted.

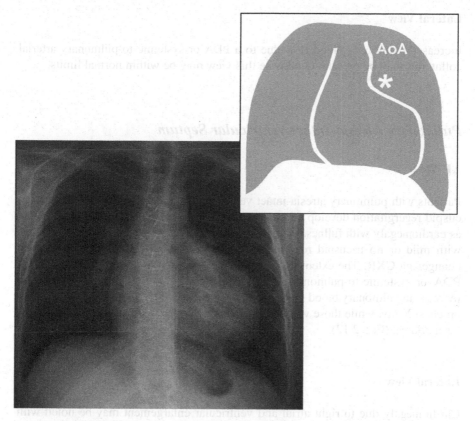

Fig. 2.12 Pulmonary atresia. Reduced pulmonary blood flow gives the appearance of "anemic lungs"; this may be seen in tricuspid as well as in pulmonary atresia when the patent ductus arteriosus is small. *AOA* aortic arch, *asterisk* (*) indicates the absence of pulmonary artery segment due to hypoplasia of the main pulmonary artery

Tricuspid Atresia

AP View

In patients with tricuspid atresia (TrA) and intact ventricular septum, the right ventricle will be hypoplastic, rendering the heart size small on chest X-ray. This can be subtle and the chest X-ray may appear normal. Because patients with TrA must have a patent ductus arteriosus (PDA) or systemic-to-pulmonary arterial collaterals to survive, the pulmonary blood flow is typically increased with resultant prominent pulmonary vasculature (Fig. 2.12).

Lateral View

Increased pulmonary blood flow due to a PDA or systemic-to-pulmonary arterial collaterals may be present. Otherwise this view may be within normal limits.

Pulmonary Atresia-Intact Ventricular Septum

AP View

Patients with pulmonary atresia-intact ventricular septum (PA-IVS) and severe tricuspid regurgitation develop dilation of the right atrium and ventricle manifesting as cardiomegaly with fullness of the right heart border. On the other hand, patients with mild or no tricuspid regurgitation will have small right ventricles and no changes on CXR. The extent of pulmonary blood flow depends upon the size of PDA or systemic-to-pulmonary arterial collaterals. Large shunts will cause an increase in pulmonary blood flow manifesting as prominent pulmonary vasculature on chest X-ray, while those with small shunts will have reduced pulmonary vascular markings (Fig. 2.12).

Lateral View

Cardiomegaly due to right atrial and ventricular enlargement may be noted with severe tricuspid regurgitation. Prominent pulmonary vasculature is noted with large shunts due to a large PDA or significant systemic-to-pulmonary arterial collaterals.

Truncus Arteriosus

AP View

The normal mediastinum is largely contributed to by the "x-like" crossing of the pulmonary artery and aorta. In truncus arteriosus (TA) there is a single great vessel (truncus) resulting in a narrow mediastinum. In addition, many patients with TA have DiGeorge syndrome, where there is small or no thymus gland, further contributing to the appearance of a narrow mediastinum. The size and origin of the pulmonary arteries can be quite variable in this lesion and may be speculated at in this view by the amount of flow noted to each lung segment (Fig. 2.13).

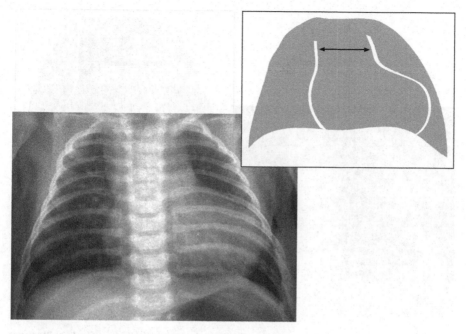

Fig. 2.13 Truncus arteriosus. Narrowed mediastinum and cardiomegaly due to biventricular enlargement as a result of increased pulmonary blood flow

Lateral View

The thymus gland is seen as soft tissue in the high retrosternal region of lateral chest X-ray. An absent thymus suggests DiGeorge syndrome.

Total Anomalous Pulmonary Venous Return

AP View

Total anomalous pulmonary venous return (TAPVR) gives a classic appearance when the anomalous pulmonary veins return through a vertical vein to the innominate vein. The dilated vertical vein, innominate vein, and superior vena cava create a round image above the cardiac silhouette giving a "snowman" appearance. The pulmonary vasculature is prominent, mainly due to pulmonary venous congestion. Other types of anomalous pulmonary venous drainage, such as those connecting to the inferior vena cava may not be noted by chest X-ray (Fig. 2.14).

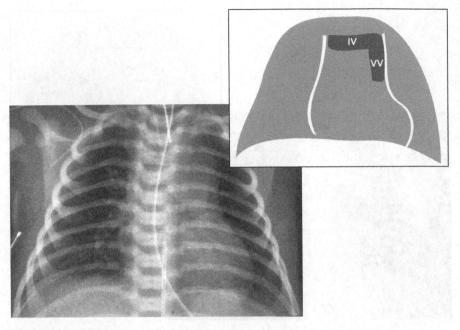

Fig. 2.14 Total anomalous pulmonary venous return to the superior vena cava. Cardiac silhouette has a "snowman" appearance formed by two round structures; the heart forms the round structure below and the dilated vertical vein, innominate vein and the superior vena cava forming the round structure above that of the heart. *IV* innominate vein, *VV* vertical vein

Lateral View

This view may demonstrate the congested pulmonary vasculature but is not otherwise helpful.

Transposition of the Great Arteries

AP View

Generally normal at birth, the oval/egg-shaped cardiac silhouette combined with the front-to-back orientation of the aorta and pulmonary artery leads to a narrowed mediastinum resulting in the classic "egg on a string" appearance. Over time, chest X-ray may demonstrate an enlarged cardiac silhouette with a marked increase in pulmonary vasculature.

Lateral View

This may show an increase in pulmonary vascularity.

Chapter 3
Electrocardiography – Approach and Interpretation

Ra-id Abdulla and Douglas M. Luxenberg

Key Facts

- The initial step in reading any ECG is to know patient's age since all parameters are age specific.
- Make sure the standardization and speed of paper are normal (10 mm/mV and 25 mm/s).
- QRS axis varies by age; newborn children have a rightward axis (60–180°), while adolescents and adults have a QRS axis of −15 to 110°.
- RAE manifests as tall P-wave, while LAE manifest as wide, notched P-wave.
- LVH manifests as deep S-wave in V1and a tall R-wave in V6.
- RVH manifests in many forms including:

  - Tall R in V1 and deep S in V6
  - rsR′ in V1 and V2
  - qR in V1 and V2
  - Pure R-wave in V1 and V2

Introduction

Electrocardiography (ECG) is a relatively simple way to assess heart rate, rhythm, and chamber size. It can also give an indication of any strain or ischemia within the heart as well as provide suspicion of electrolyte imbalance and reflect systemic diseases. Interpretation of ECG in a child is often intimidating to most practitioners especially given the variability in patient age and size encountered. The key to successful and proper interpretation is to employ a systematic methodology. Looking

Ra-id Abdulla (✉)
Center for Congenital and Structural Heart Diseases, Rush University Medical Center,
1653 West Congress Parkway, Room 763 Jones, Chicago, IL 60612, USA
e-mail: rabdulla@rush.edu

Ra-id Abdulla (ed.), *Heart Diseases in Children: A Pediatrician's Guide*,
DOI 10.1007/978-1-4419-7994-0_3, © Springer Science+Business Media, LLC 2011

at an ECG without a step by step approach can result in confusion and cause the interpreting physician to overlook some anomalies while dwelling on others. This chapter will lead you through a step by step approach to deciphering the data provided through an electrocardiogram.

Basic Components of an ECG

A typical ECG (often referred to as a "12-lead ECG") consists of six limb leads (I, II, III, aVR, aVL, and aVF) and six precordial leads (V1–V6). Leads V1–V3 sit over the right heart and are referred to as the right chest leads while leads V4–V6 are considered the left chest leads. In addition, there is often a continuous "rhythm strip" that runs along the bottom of the ECG (most often lead II) which allows for better detection of any abnormalities in rhythm (Fig. 3.1).

Each heart beat is represented on the ECG by a series of waves, referred to as P, Q, R, S, and T-waves. Atrial depolarization is represented by the P-wave on the surface ECG.

The next series of waves are collectively referred to as the QRS complex and represent ventricular depolarization. A Q-wave is any downward (negative) deflection following the P-wave. The R-wave reflects ventricular depolarization and is the first positive (upward) deflection following the P-wave. The S-wave represents continuation of depolarization of the ventricles which produces electrical changes away from leads in which they are seen. An S waves is the first downward deflection after an R-wave. In some circumstances a second R-wave may be present in the QRS complex which is denoted R' (R-prime). A typical QRS complex will have one or more of these components, but none are specifically required to be present. The T-wave follows the QRS complex and represents ventricular repolarization. Rarely, a U-wave may be seen following the T-wave.

By convention, lower case letters may be used to denote smaller voltage waves while capital letters signify larger voltage waves. For example, qR implies a small Q-wave followed by a larger R-wave while rsR' signifies small R and S-waves are followed by a larger R'-wave.

Standardization

The voltage and paper speed settings on an ECG must be determined by the operator. The standard setting in an ECG for voltage produced by limb and chest leads are traced on ECG paper such that for each 1 mV, a 10 mm deflection is produced. Normal values rely on the fact that such standardization is used. In cases where R waves are excessively tall or the S waves are excessively deep, overlapping of QRS waves from different leads can occur, leading to inability to determine magnitude of such waves. For this reason ECG machines are equipped with the ability to alter the standardization to half or even a quarter of what is normally used. In these cases, each reduced wave must be multiplied by the reducing factor to restore

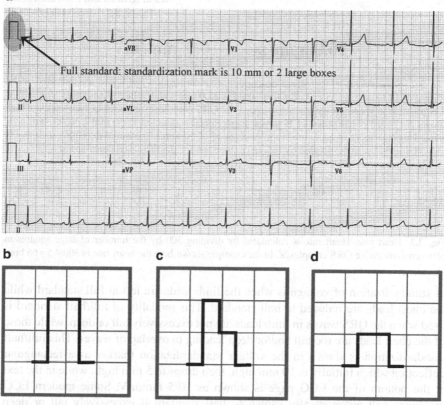

Fig. 3.1 Standardization marker: A *rectangular shaped* deflection, typically at the onset of each line within an ECG tracing to indicate the voltage standardization of the ECG tracing. Normal values of ECG deflections are based upon "full standard" mode of ECG recording. When QRS complexes are too tall or deep, overlap occurs making proper interpretation difficult. In such cases, a half standard mode is used to separate the overlapping waves. Whenever a half standard is used, the ECG deflections (such as R or S-waves) must be multiplied by two to determine if they fall within known normal parameters. (**a**) Standardization marker as shown in a 12-lead ECG tracing, a "full standard" marker is 10 mm (two large or ten small boxes) high. (**b**) Full standard: the standardization marker is 10 mm tall indicating that ECG deflections are in full standard. (**c**) Full/half standard: the standardization marker is 10 mm high, then drops to 5 mm indicating that limb leads are full standard while chest leads are half standard. All deflections in the chest leads should be multiplied by two for interpretation. (**d**) Half standard: the standardization of the ECG deflections is 5 mm high, all deflections should be multiplied by two for interpretation

to a normal standardization For example all waves should be multiplied by two if the standard was halved (5 mm/mV).

Voltage standardization is exhibited in two locations: at the beginning of each ECG tracing line (Fig. 3.1) as well as the bottom of ECG tracing page (Fig. 3.2). ECG performed in normal standard shows a rectangular deflection before each ECG tracing line of 10 mm in height and a text print at the bottom of the ECG page indicating that the voltage is 10 mm/mV. Half standard is when the rectangular standardization deflection is 5 mm in height and text print at the bottom of the ECG page indicating that the voltage is 5 mm/mV. Another common alteration

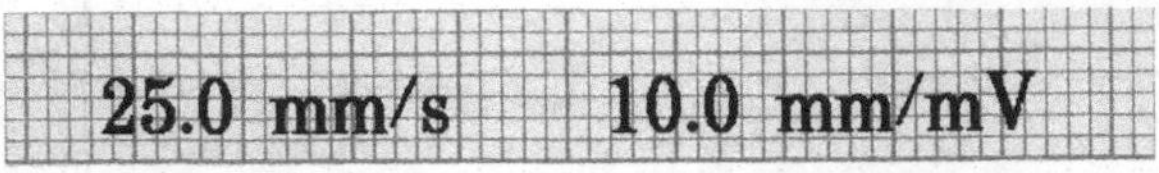

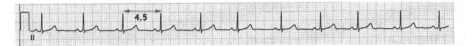

Fig. 3.2 Standardization and speed description. Standardization and speed are indicated at the bottom of ECG tracings. Standard paper speed is 25.0 mm/s and voltage standard is 10 mm/mV. It is possible to speed up the tracing to space out QRS complexes in cases of tachycardia which allows for better visualization of P-waves. Paper speed is doubled to 50 mm/s, which will alter manual measurement of ECG intervals. At a speed of 50 mm/s, measured durations such as PR and QT interval must be divided by two to compensate for the increased paper speed

Fig. 3.3 Heart rate. Heart rate is calculated by dividing 300 by the number of large squares in between consecutive QRS complexes. In the example shown here the heart rate is 300/4.5=66 bpm

in standardization of voltage is when the limb leads are left at full standard while the chest leads are reduced to half standard. This modality of full/half standard is used when the QRS waves in limb leads are not excessively tall or deep, while those of the chest leads are too tall and/or deep leading to overlap of waves. This full/half standardization is shown in the voltage standardization marker as a rectangular deflection which initially is 10 mm high, then drops to 5 mm high, while in the text at the bottom of the ECG page is shown as 10/5 mm/mV. Some modern ECG machines will automatically switch to half standard if excessively tall or deep waves are noted while others require a manual entry to override the standard.

The speed of ECG paper normally runs at 25 mm/s. Formulas used to determine heart rate (RR interval) as well as PR, QRS, and QT durations are based upon this standard speed of paper. In patients with excessive tachycardia resulting in inability to separate P waves from QRS complexes the operator can increase paper speed to 50 mm/s, thus allowing more space between ECG waves to improve clarity. In such events all durations such as RR, PR, QRS, and QT durations should be divided by 2 to enable comparison to normal values. Determination of paper speed can be done through the paper speed print at the bottom of the ECG page (Fig. 3.3) or by examining the voltage standardization at the onset of each ECG tracing line. These voltage standardization marks are five small squares (one large square) in width when paper speed is standard (25 mm/s) and become twice as wide, i.e., ten small squares (or two large squares) wide when paper speed is doubled to 50 mm/s. Machines will not change paper speed automatically, if required, it must be set by the operator.

Patient Data

Age is an important factor in determining interpretation of ECG. (Table 3.1) The heart of a neonate differs in many aspects from that of a toddler, which in turn differs from an adolescent and an adult. This cardiac maturation occurs gradually over

Table 3.1 Normal ECG values by age

Age	HR (bpm)	QRS axis (s)	PR interval (s)	QRS interval (s)	R in V1 (mm)	S in V1 (mm)	R in V6 (mm)	S in V6 (mm)
1st week	90–160	60–180	0.08–0.15	0.03–0.08	5–26	0–23	0–12	0–10
1–3 weeks	100–180	45–160	0.08–0.15	0.03–0.08	3–21	0–16	2–16	0–10
1–2 months	120–180	30–135	0.08–0.15	0.03–0.08	3–18	0–15	5–21	0–10
3–5 months	105–185	0–135	0.08–0.15	0.03–0.08	3–20	0–15	6–22	0–10
6–11 months	110–170	0–135	0.07–0.16	0.03–0.08	2–20	0.5–20	6–23	0–7
1–2 years	90–165	0–110	0.08–0.16	0.03–0.08	2–18	0.5–21	6–23	0–7
3–4 years	70–140	0–110	0.09–0.17	0.04–0.08	1–18	0.5–21	4–24	0–5
5–7 years	65–140	0–110	0.09–0.17	0.04–0.08	0.5–14	0.5–24	4–26	0–4
8–11 years	60–130	−15 to 110	0.09–0.17	0.04–0.09	0–14	0.5–25	4–25	0–4
12–15 years	65–130	−15 to 110	0.09–0.18	0.04–0.09	0–14	0.5–21	4–25	0–4
>16 years	50–120	−15 to 110	0.12–0.20	0.05–0.10	0–14	0.5–23	4–21	0–4

many years. Therefore it makes sense that heart rate, QRS axis, as well as amplitude of P and QRS waves depend upon the age of patient. Normal neonatal ECG findings, such as a heart rate of 150 bpm, or right ventricular dominance are abnormal when found in an older child or adult. Patients' sex and race play a limited factor in ECG interpretation. African American teenage boys tend to have higher left ventricular voltage than others and their ECGs may give the impression of borderline left ventricular hypertrophy when in reality they have a normal left ventricular mass.

Patient history, other laboratory data and current medications can provide valuable information for proper interpretation of findings on ECG (Tables 3.2–3.4).

Table 3.2 ECG changes with electrolyte abnormalities

Hyperkalemia
5.5–6.5 mEq/L: Tall and peaked T-wave, widening of QRS complex
7–8 mEq/L: above + wide P-wave
8–9 mEq/L: above + small or no P-wave
Higher than 9 mEq/L: above + AV block, ventricular tachycardia or fibrillation
Hypokalemia
Flattened T-wave, with or without ST depression, prominent U-wave, prolonged QT
Hypercalcemia
Short ST segment, sinus bradycardia, sinus arrest, worsening AV block caused by digoxin
Hypocalcemia
Prolonged QTc (unlike hypokalemia, QRS duration is not prolonged)
Hypermagnesemia
First degree AV block
Interventricular conduction delay
Short ST segment, therefore shorter QTc
Hypomagnesemia
Prolonged QTc, prominent U-wave
Prolonged ST segment
Hypernatremia and hyponatremia
Within possible physiological range, there are no ECG changes

Table 3.3 ECG changes in systemic diseases

CNS Injury
Increased vagal tone results in bradycardia, A-V block, and J-wave
Hypothermia
Sinus bradycardia, prolonged PR interval and QTc, J-wave
Hypothyroidism
Sinus bradycardia, absent ST segment, low P, QRS, and T-wave voltage
Hyperthyroidism
Sinus tachycardia, LVH, prolonged PR interval, nonspecific ST, and T-wave changes
Hypoglycemia
Changes secondary to hyperkalemia
Hypoxia and acidosis
Changes secondary to hyperkalemia. Atrial and ventricular arrhythmias may be noted in addition to AV block

Table 3.4 Medications and ECG changes

Digoxin
    Bradycardia, 1° AV block, ST depression, tall R-wave
    Toxicity: bradycardia, 2° or 3° AV block, PACs, SVT, PVCs, and ventricular tachycardia
Quinidine, procainamide, and disopyramide
    Prolonged QRS and QTc
    Toxicity:
    Tachycardia, wide P-wave, 1° AV block, prolonged QRS > 125%, further prolonged QTc,
        PVCs, and ventricular tachycardia
Beta-blockers
    Bradycardia, 1° AV block, and Short QTc
Anesthetic agents (halothane, methoxyflurane, teflurane, and enflurane)
    Short QTc, depressed T-wave, bradycardia, and ventricular arrhythmias
Phenothiazines
    Decreased T-wave amplitude with prominent terminal repolarization (may be mistaken for
        U-wave), prolonged QTc
Tricyclic antidepressants
    Sinus tachycardia, 1° AV block, flat T-wave, prolonged QRS, prolonged QTc, ST segment
        and T-wave changes
Imipramine
    Toxicity: atrial flutter, AV block, and ventricular tachycardia

Rate

Heart rate reflects the rate of ventricular contractions per minute, often expressed in beats per minute (bpm). Since QRS complexes reflect ventricular contraction, the rate of QRS complexes will provide the heart rate. To explain how this is done, some basic ECG facts should be explained: Each small square in an ECG represents 0.04 s of time. There are five small squares in each large square, thus making the duration of one large square 0.2 s. Therefore, 300 large squares represent 1 min (0.2 ms × 300 = 60 s) and the number of ventricular cycles (RR interval) within 300 large squares will represent the heart rate. Therefore, to measure the heart rate, simply divide 300 by the number of large squares between two consecutive QRS complexes (Fig. 3.3).

A table of normal values is useful when determining whether a given heart rate is appropriate for an individual (Table 3.1).

Rhythm

Heart rhythm is closely associated with heart rate measurement since both are caused by a common mechanism. To determine heart rhythm, the P-wave axis must be first determined. A P-wave representing origination from the sinus node with normal propagation toward the AV node has an axis of 0–60° represented by an upward (positive) deflection in leads I and aVF. An abnormal P-wave axis may indicate abnormal origination of cardiac electrical impulse, such as those seen in an ectopic atrial rhythm (Fig. 3.4).

In normal sinus rhythm the electrical impulse initiating each heartbeat originates from the sinus node and propagates through the atria down to the AV node resulting in a P-wave with a normal axis. Normal sinus rhythm is present when the heart rate is normal; P-waves originate from the sinus node and each P-wave is followed by a QRS complex, indicating synchrony between atrial and ventricular contractions (Fig. 3.5).

Sinus bradycardia is present when all the above criteria are met with the exception of a slower than expected heart rate (Fig. 3.6) and sinus tachycardia is thus the presence of a faster than normal heart rate with an otherwise normal ECG rhythm (Fig. 3.7).

A normal heart rhythm propagates from the sinus node to the AV node and then to the ventricles through the bundles of His. Normal atrioventricular conduction leads to atrioventricular synchrony. This can be determined through the ECG by examining the relationship of the P-wave to the QRS complex and the resulting PR interval (Fig. 3.8) Normal conduction is determined when each P-wave is followed by a QRS complex with a normal and constant PR interval. A normal PR interval indicates that the conduction of electrical impulses from the atria to the ventricles is neither delayed nor too rapid while constancy in duration ensures that the electrical

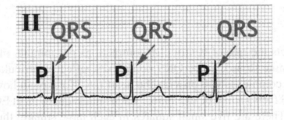

Fig. 3.4 P-wave axis. P-wave reflects atrial depolarization which originates from the sinus node. The direction of electrical flow is from the right upper portion of the right atrium toward the left lower portion of the atria. Therefore, a normal P wave axis is approximately 60° (positive deflection in leads I and aVF)

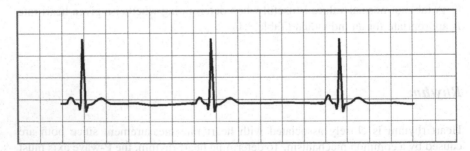

Fig. 3.5 Normal sinus rhythm. P-waves are upright in lead II and preceding each QRS complex at a constant PR interval

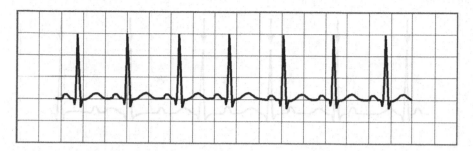

Fig. 3.6 Sinus bradycardia. Slower heart rate than expected with normal P-wave axis. QRS complexes are preceded by P-waves with normal QRS duration

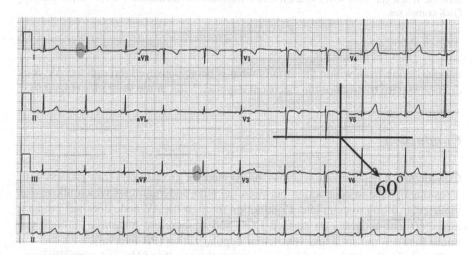

Fig. 3.7 Sinus tachycardia. Rapid heart rate for age with a normal P-wave axis. QRS complexes are preceded by P-waves with normal QRS duration

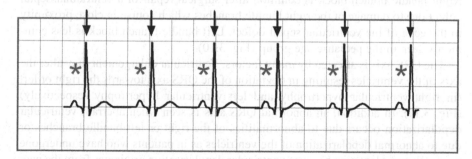

Fig. 3.8 Atrioventricular (AV) synchrony. Electrical conduction within the heart starts within the atria, then travels through the AV node and finally depolarizes the ventricles which manifests as a QRS complex. Therefore, each P-wave should be followed by a QRS complex after an appropriate pause (PR interval). AV synchrony indicates normal conduction of electrical activity from the atria to the ventricles. *Asterisk* indicate P waves, *arrow* indicate QRS complexes

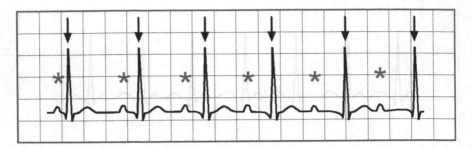

Fig. 3.9 Atrioventricular dissociation. Loss of AV synchrony indicates atrioventricular dissociation or complete heart block. In these types of arrhythmias the atrial P-waves do not consistently precede the ventricular QRS waves with a fixed PR interval. *Asterisk* indicate P waves, *arrow* indicate QRS complexes

depolarization from within the atria is what is being conveyed through the AV conduction system to produce the electrical depolarization in the ventricles (Fig. 3.9).

Conduction

Conduction of depolarization across the AV node is a (relatively) slow process with a resultant pause in contraction between the atria and ventricles which allows for ventricular filling to complete. Conduction through the AV node does not produce any electrical activities on surface ECG and is therefore measured through the pause between the atrial and ventricular depolarization (PR interval).

Depolarization of the ventricles occurs via the bundle of His and normally completes within 0.08–0.12 s. Any delay will result in a widening of the QRS complex reflected by a right or left bundle branch block (RBBB and LBBB respectively). Right bundle branch block is common after surgical repair of a ventricular septal defect due to damage of the right bundle branches which course in close proximity to the edge of the ventricular septal defect. Left bundle branch block is less commonly seen in the pediatric age group (Fig. 3.10).

The QRS axis is affected by many factors. Ventricular enlargement may alter the axis of the ventricles resulting in deviation of the QRS axis towards the right or left (in right ventricular hypertrophy and left ventricular hypertrophy respectively) (Fig. 3.11). In addition, an abnormal QRS axis is seen when aberrant ventricular depolarization occurs due to abnormalities of the right or left bundle branches or due to abnormal depolarization of the ventricles as in patients who have undergone pacemaker implantation because ventricular depolarization originates from the pacing wires, rather than the bundles of His (Fig. 3.12).

Superior axis deviation is a unique finding in patients with an atrioventricular canal defect due displacement of the bundles of His as a result of the atrial and ventricular septal defects (Fig. 3.13).

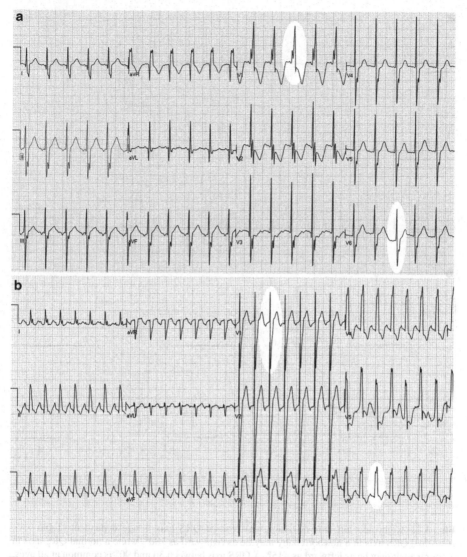

Fig. 3.10 Right and left bundle branch block. (**a**) Right bundle branch block (RBBB): Blocked conduction through the right branch of the bundle of His will cause electrical conduction through the left bundle branch to reach the left ventricle first, which then travels to the right ventricle through myocardial electrical conduction through muscle fibers. Conduction in this way will take a longer time to reach the right ventricle thus resulting in a wider QRS duration. An RSR' (M-shaped) QRS pattern will be noted in the right chest leads (V1, V2). (**b**) Left bundle branch block (LBBB): Blocked conduction through the left branch of the bundle of His will cause electrical conduction through the right bundle branch to reach the right ventricle first and then reaches the left ventricle through myocardial electrical conduction. Conduction of electrical impulses this way will take a longer time to reach the right ventricle thus resulting in a wider QRS duration. An RSR' (M-shaped) QRS pattern will be noted in the left chest leads (V5, V6)

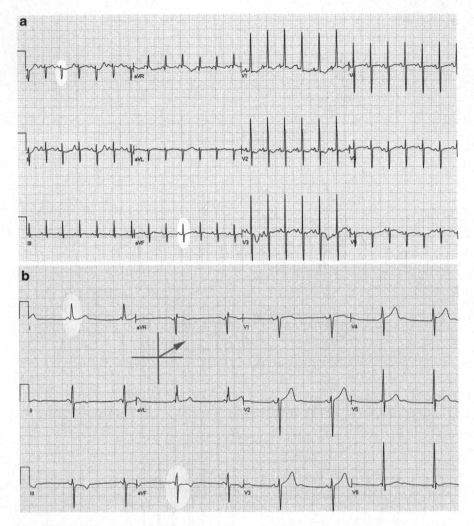

Fig. 3.11 Right and left axis deviation. (**a**) Normal QRS axis is age dependent (Table 3.1). A normal QRS axis in a newborn baby may be as rightward as 180°, while a normal QRS axis in a young adult may be as leftward as −15°. A QRS axis between 30 and 90° is common at all ages. Therefore, a positive QRS wave complex in leads I and aVF indicates normal QRS axis. While QRS axes outside of this range may still be normal depending upon age of patient. (**a**) Right axis deviation. The QRS is negative in lead I and positive in lead aVF indicating that the QRS axis is between 90 and 180°. The negative QRS deflection in lead I is more than the positive deflection in aVF indicating that the QRS axis is closer to 180 than 90° (approximately 160°). (**b**) Left axis deviation. The QRS is positive in lead I and negative in aVF indicating that the QRS axis is between 0 and −90°. The net deflection is greater in lead I than in aVF, indicating that the QRS axis is closer to 0 than −90° (approximately −30°)

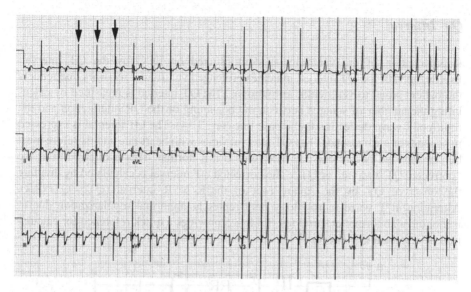

Fig. 3.12 Pacemaker. A pacemaker spike can be seen prior to all QRS complexes. The pacemaker is in DDD mode where it senses the P-wave, waits for an appropriate interval (this is programmed into the pacemaker as the PR interval), then stimulates the ventricle if no QRS is sensed. The QRS complexes are wide because pacemaker stimulation of ventricles occurs through the myocardial tissue and not through the natural conduction system

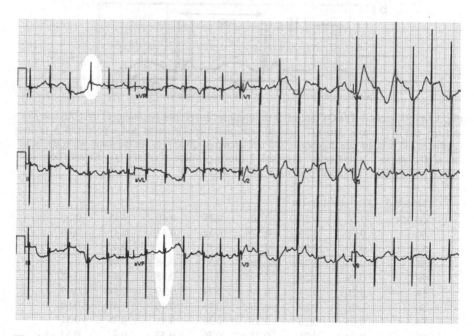

Fig. 3.13 Superior axis in AVC defect. Most children with an atrioventricular canal defect have a superior QRS axis (negative deflections in I and aVF). This is due to abnormal position of conduction pathways as they are displaced by the inlet ventricular septal defect

QT Interval

Repolarization of the ventricles is demonstrated on ECG by the QT interval. Prolongation of the QT interval indicates prolonged ventricular recovery and renders the patient prone to ventricular arrhythmias. The QT interval is measured by calculating the number of squares between the beginning of the QRS deflection and the return of T wave deflection to the base line (Fig. 3.14). The QT interval is expressed in seconds or milliseconds. The QT interval varies with heart rate and therefore must be standardized before one can determine if it is normal. This is referred to as the "corrected QT interval" or QTc. The corrected QT interval is calculated by dividing the observed QT by the square root of the R to R interval ($QTc = QT/\sqrt{RR}$). Alteration in T wave morphology may represent abnormal repolarization due to ischemia or abnormal electrolytes. Table 3.5 provides a quick reference for calculation of corrected QT intervals.

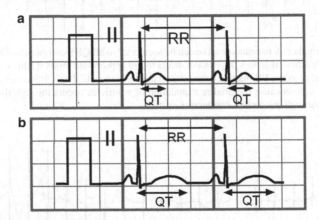

Fig. 3.14 QT interval. The QT interval is the distance between the beginning of the QRS complex and the end of T-wave. The QT interval represents depolarization and repolarization of the ventricles and is heart rate dependent. QT and corrected QT (QTc) are the same when the heart rate is 60 beats per minute (bpm). *See Table 3.1 for upper limit of normal QTc for each heart rate range). (**a**) Normal QT interval. (**b**) Prolonged QT interval

Table 3.5 QTc measurement

QT/HR	0.20	0.25	0.30	0.35	0.40	0.45	0.50
50	0.18	0.23	0.27	0.32	0.37	0.41	0.46
52	0.19	0.23	0.28	0.32	0.37	0.42	0.46
54	0.19	0.23	0.28	0.33	0.38	0.42	0.47
56	0.19	0.24	0.29	0.34	0.38	0.43	0.48
58	0.20	0.24	0.29	0.34	0.39	0.44	0.49
60	0.20	0.25	0.30	0.35	0.40	0.45	0.50
63	0.21	0.25	0.31	0.36	0.41	0.46	0.51
66	0.21	0.26	0.31	0.36	0.42	0.47	0.52
68	0.22	0.26	0.32	0.37	0.43	0.48	0.53

(continued)

Table 3.5 continued

71	0.22	0.27	0.33	0.38	0.44	0.49	0.55
75	0.23	0.27	0.34	0.39	0.45	0.51	0.56
79	0.24	0.28	0.34	0.40	0.46	0.52	0.57
83	0.24	0.29	0.35	0.41	0.47	0.53	0.69
88	0.25	0.29	0.36	0.43	0.49	0.55	0.61
94	0.26	0.30	0.38	0.44	0.50	0.56	0.63
100	0.27	0.31	0.39	0.45	0.52	0.58	0.65
107	0.28	0.32	0.40	0.47	0.53	0.60	0.67
115	0.28	0.35	0.42	0.49	0.55	0.63	0.69
125	0.29	0.36	0.43	0.51	0.58	0.65	0.72
136	0.30	0.38	0.45	0.53	0.60	0.68	0.75
150	0.32	0.40	0.47	0.56	0.63	0.71	0.79

This table provides QTc durations for QT intervals of 0.20–0.50 s for heart rates ranging from 50 to 150 bpm

Chamber Hypertrophy

Right Atrium

Right atrial enlargement causes an increase in the electrical voltage produced which is reflected by a taller than normal P-wave. Normal P-waves are 2 mm high in young children (up to 3 mm in adults) (Fig. 3.15).

Left Atrium

Left atrial enlargement leads to a larger atrial mass which requires a longer period of depolarization. This manifests as a widened P-wave. In addition, the larger than normal, atrial mass causes the depolarization to occur in different directions throughout the cycle leading to a bifid or biphasic P-wave.

Right Ventricle

The right ventricle is dominant in utero. Therefore, neonates and young children have a proportionally larger right ventricular mass (as compared to the left ventricle) than is seen in older children and adults. The large right ventricular mass is demonstrated on ECG, particularly during the first several years of life by high R-wave voltage (Table 3.1) and an RSR' QRS pattern in the right chest leads (V1–V3) (Fig. 3.16). This pattern of RSR' is accepted as normal in younger children, but can

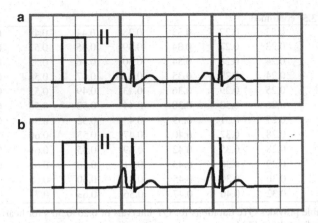

Fig 3.15 Atrial enlargement. An enlarged right atrium will cause the P-waves to be taller than normal (>2 mm in small children and >3 mm in older children and adults. (**a**) Right atrial enlargement. (**b**) Left atrial enlargement

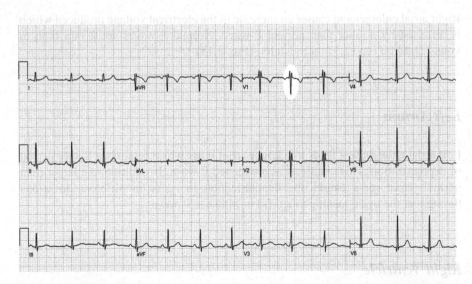

Fig 3.16 (**a**): rSr′ in V1. Children are born with dominant right ventricles; the QRS pattern during the first decade of life reflects this RV dominance. The QRS in older children and adults consists of an initial small "r"-wave reflecting the relative smaller right ventricular myocardial mass, followed by a deep "S"-wave reflecting the larger and more dominant left ventricular mass. In newborn and young children the QRS complex consists of an initial R-wave representing right ventricular contraction, followed by an S-wave representing left ventricular contraction. This is followed by a second R-wave (R′) which reflects the large right ventricular mass

reflect right ventricular hypertrophy in older children and adults. There are many ECG patterns consistent with right ventricular hypertrophy, with some of the more common described below:

- Tall R wave in lead V1 and deep S in V6:
  An increase in right ventricular mass leads to an increase in the voltage produced during depolarization manifesting as taller than usual R-wave in V1 and a deeper than normal S-wave in V6 which represent ventricular depolarization (Fig. 3.17a).
- rsR' in V1 or V2:
  An increase in the right ventricular mass may alter the normal configuration of the QRS complex in the right chest leads without increasing the voltage of QRS waves. The downward progression of the R-wave into an S-wave may be overcome by continuing right ventricular depolarization, causing a reversal in the direction of electrical charges and a second upward wave in the right chest leads, manifesting as an R'. In this pattern of right ventricular hypertrophy the R' is

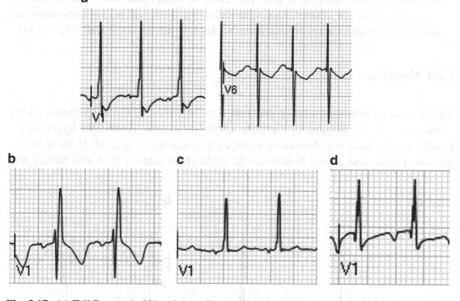

Fig. 3.17 (**a**) Tall R-wave in V1 and deep S-wave in V6. Right ventricular hypertrophy leads to a tall R-wave in V1 and a deep S-wave in V6 due to the enlarged right ventricular mass. (**b**) rsR' in V1 or V2. Although an rSr' pattern is normal in young children, if the second R-wave is taller than the initial R-wave, this reflects a larger right ventricular mass than normal. (**c**) Pure R-wave in V1 or V2. A significantly larger right than left ventricular mass will cause the right ventricular forces to completely overcome any LV effect on the QRS complex in the right chest leads with resultant "pure" R-wave in V1 and V2. (**d**) qR wave in V1 or V2. The initial depolarization of the ventricles starts in the ventricular septum in the same direction as that of the right ventricular wall mass as recorded in V1 and V2 resulting in an initial R-wave deflection in these leads without a Q-wave. In patients with right ventricular hypertrophy there may be deviation of the plane of the ventricular septum leading to a small Q-wave with resultant qR pattern in V1 and V2

typically higher in voltage than the initial small r wave, thus resulting in an rsR′ appearance of the QRS (Fig. 3.17b).

- Pure R-wave in V1 or V2:
  Ventricular depolarization in some cases of right ventricular hypertrophy may be represented in the right chest leads by a single or "pure" R-wave. Similar to changes leading to an rsR′ pattern described above, the right ventricular electrical dominance may be significant enough to completely mask any left ventricular forces in the right chest leads, resulting in a pure R-wave configuration (Fig. 3.17c).

- qR wave in V1 or V2:
  Since the bundle of His travels through the ventricular septum, the ventricular septum is the first part of the ventricle to undergo depolarization. This process occurs in a rightward and anterior direction thus contributes to the R-wave in the right chest leads on the ECG. The ventricular septum may deviate secondary to right ventricular hypertrophy thus acquiring an abnormal position within the chest. This will cause an initial downward deflection in the right chest leads, manifesting as a q-wave. This is followed by a prominent R-wave reflecting right ventricular hypertrophy, thus resulting in a qR pattern in the right chest leads. This qR pattern can be also seen in dextrocardia, ventricular inversion, and pectus excavatum, all due to abnormal location of ventricular septum within the chest wall (Fig. 3.17d).

Left Ventricle

The R-wave in left chest leads represents depolarization of the left ventricle. This is mirrored by the S-wave in the right chest leads. Left ventricular hypertrophy results in increased depolarization voltages and manifests as a tall R-wave in the left chest leads and a deep S-wave in the right chest leads (Fig. 3.18). Severe left

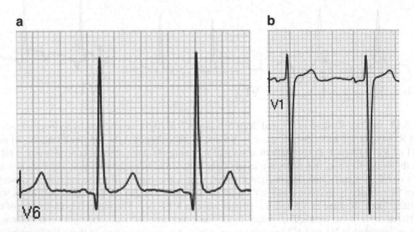

Fig. 3.18 LVH. The increase in mass of the left ventricle seen in LVH will result in increased voltages on the ECG represented as a tall R-wave in V6 and deep S-wave in V1. (**a**) Tall R-wave in V6. (**b**) Deep S-wave in V1

ventricular hypertrophy may result in myocardial ischemia due to a relative hypoxia of the left ventricular myocardium as a result of increased workload. This manifests as changes in the ST segment and T-waves known as left ventricular strain.

Ischemia

Ischemia is very rare in the pediatric age group and presents on an ECG, in much the same way as it does in an adult, specifically with ST segment elevation or depression. This is typically the result of ventricular hypertrophy or rarely, an abnormal coronary artery origin resulting in inadequate coronary perfusion and myocardial ischemia. Two of the most common coronary artery anomalies are described below.

Anomalous Left Coronary Artery from Pulmonary Artery (ALCAPA)

In this anomaly, the left main coronary artery originates from the pulmonary artery instead of the aorta. Interestingly, the low oxygen saturation from the pulmonary artery blood (70–75%) does not lead to ischemia. It is the low pressure in the pulmonary artery (typically <1/3 systemic pressure) that causes poor perfusion of the anomalous coronary artery which leads to ischemia, followed by infarction. Patients subsequently develop a dilated cardiomyopathy due to the large areas of infarcted left ventricle. ECG in these cases show left ventricular infarction pattern with deep Q waves in leads I and aVL as well as evidence of ischemia in the left chest leads.

Origin of the Left Coronary Artery from the Right Coronary Sinus of Valsalva

This lesion is typically initially silent with no symptoms or ECG changes. Events causing acute insufficiency of coronary blood flow due to mechanical changes not currently well understood lead to compression of the abnormally located left coronary artery resulting in stunning of the myocardium and manifesting as syncope or sudden death. An ECG pattern of left ventricular ischemia [ST segment and T-wave changes in the inferior (II, III, and aVF) and left chest leads] is noted during and following an episode.

Chapter 4
Pediatric Echocardiography

W. Reid Thompson, Thea Yosowitz, and Stephen Stone

Key Facts

- Echocardiography is noninvasive with no known harm to patients. However, it incurs significant cost and therefore should be used judicially.
- Pediatric echocardiography should be performed by pediatric cardiac sonographers and interpreted by pediatric cardiologists trained in this field to avoid overlooking congenital heart diseases. Imaging and interpretation by specialists outside the field of pediatric cardiology is likely to lead to errors.
- Echocardiography shows cardiac anatomy through 2D imaging.
- Blood flow, both normal and abnormal can be studied through color Doppler.
- Pressure gradient measurements is determined by Doppler flow velocity measurement.
- Echocardiography is poorly equipped to see peripheral pulmonary arteries and veins.

Introduction

Echocardiography has become the primary tool of the pediatric cardiologist for diagnosing structural heart disease. It is highly accurate when performed and interpreted in an experienced laboratory, and in most cases is sufficient for understanding the anatomy and most of the hemodynamic consequences of the most

W.R. Thompson (✉)
Department of Pediatric Cardiology, John Hopkins Medical Institutes, 600 North Wolfe Street, Brady 521, Baltimore, MD 21205, USA
e-mail: Thompson@jhmi.edu

Ra-id Abdulla (ed.), *Heart Diseases in Children: A Pediatrician's Guide*,
DOI 10.1007/978-1-4419-7994-0_4, © Springer Science+Business Media, LLC 2011

complicated congenital defects. As miniaturization of ultrasound technology and price points improve, it may eventually become feasible for noncardiologists to purchase portable ultrasound devices and incorporate imaging of the heart into their physical examination. However, due to the level of expertise involved in performing and interpreting a study to rule out congenital heart disease, screening for heart disease currently is still more appropriately done by a careful history and physical examination and will likely remain so for the foreseeable future.

Echocardiography in infants and children, performed to diagnose or follow congenital or acquired heart disease that affects this age group, is technically very different from adult echocardiography and requires specific equipment and expertise usually not found in typical adult echocardiography laboratories. This has been recognized by accreditation agencies that have developed specific requirements for quality control of pediatric studies. In addition, children under the age of three are often too uncooperative for a complete, comprehensive echocardiography, which can take up to 30–45 min, therefore in many cases sedation is required and should only be done in a laboratory with pediatric cardiologists on-site to optimize acquisition and interpretation of the study.

The pediatrician is often faced with the question of when an echocardiogram should be ordered directly versus requesting a cardiologist consultation at first. There are many indications for echocardiography that are appropriately ordered directly by the generalist, and only if abnormalities are found, would a consultation with the cardiologist be important. In other cases, consultation as the first strategy is more efficient and usually leads to more appropriate testing (Tables 4.1 and 4.2).

Table 4.1 When to order an echocardiogram versus obtaining a pediatric cardiology consult

Evaluation of suspected patent ductus arteriosus
Screening for cardiac defects in patient with known or suspected chromosomal or other genetic syndrome with cardiac involvement
Assess persistence of pulmonary hypertension (PPHN)
Assess central line placement or ECMO cannula position
Evaluate ventricular function
Monitor for thrombus formation
Monitor left ventricular hypertrophy in children with established etiology of hypertension

Table 4.2 When to consult a pediatric cardiologist rather than obtain an echocardiogram

Heart murmur which is likely to be pathologic:
• Harsh murmurs
• Murmur intensity is 4/6 or more
• Murmur associated with abnormal S1 or S2
Presence of abnormal signs suggestive of cardiac anomalies:
• Cyanosis
• Clubbing of digit
• Poor capillary refill
Stridor associated with abnormal chest X-ray or bronchoscopy findings suggestive of vascular ring

When to Order an Echocardiogram Directly

The American College of Cardiology/The American Heart Association Task Force on Practice Guidelines published guidelines for indication for echocardiography in 1997. An extensive list of situations suitable for echocardiography is included in these guidelines. The following is an outline of situations in which echocardiography is a valuable and helpful tool to the practitioner.

In the neonatal period, echocardiography is indicated in the evaluation of suspected patent ductus arteriosus (Fig. 4.1) and murmurs suspicious for a congenital heart defect. It should also be used for screening for cardiac defects in patient with known or suspected chromosomal or other genetic syndrome with cardiac involvement (Fig. 4.2). Echocardiography is commonly used to assess persistence of pulmonary hypertension (PPHN) (Fig. 4.3) to evaluate right ventricular pressure and function (Fig. 4.4) and exclude congenital heart disease, such as obstructed total anomalous pulmonary venous return. Lastly, echocardiography can be used to assess central line placement (Fig. 4.5) or ECMO cannula position, evaluate ventricular function, and monitor for thrombus formation.

Consensus recommendations for the use of echocardiography in suspected Kawasaki disease (KD) assumes that the pediatrician is able to order the study directly, and only if coronary or other abnormalities are detected is a *cardiology* consultation needed. In uncomplicated cases, an initial echocardiogram should be done at diagnosis, at 2 weeks, and at 6–8 weeks after onset of disease. If the echocardiogram is normal at 6–8 weeks, a follow-up study 1 year later is optional. If abnormalities are detected on any of the echocardiographic studies, additional studies will usually be ordered by the cardiologist, with frequency and length of

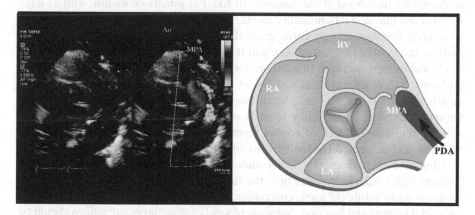

Fig. 4.1 *Ao* aorta, *LA* left atrium, *RA* right atrium, *RV* right ventricle. Color Doppler echocardiography: parasternal short axis view color Doppler shows direction of blood flow. Typically, the setting is such that *red color* indicates flow towards the probe, while *blue* is blood flow away from the probe. In this image, blood flow can be seen from aorta into the pulmonary arteries through the patent ductus arteriosus, PDA flow is represented by black arrow

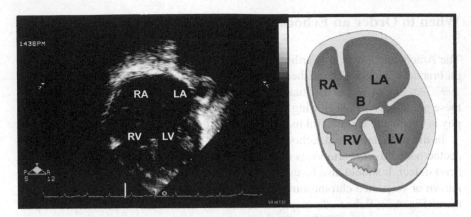

Fig. 4.2 *RA* right atrium, *RV* right ventricle, *LA* left atrium, *LV* left ventricle, *B* bridging leaflet. 2D echocardiography: four chamber view in a child with Trisomy 21 showing complete atrioventricular canal defect. The illustration on the *left hand* shows cardiac anatomy, *red* and *blue* coloring reflects well oxygenated and poorly oxygenated blood in different cardiac chambers. This coloring scheme should not be confused with the red and blue coloring of color Doppler

follow-up determined by the severity of the abnormalities. Treatment with IVIG does not need to be withheld waiting for the initial echocardiogram, as the diagnosis is not usually dependent on the imaging, which is often normal on the first study. It is important to note that it is difficult to obtain high quality coronary imaging on a fussy infant or young child, which may necessitate the use of sedatives to enable completion of echocardiography. After IVIG, irritability usually abates, though sedation may still be required. For atypical cases, the echocardiogram can be used to decide the likelihood of the diagnosis of KD. For infants <6 month, with ≥7 days of fever and elevated inflammatory markers (ESR and/or CRP), even in the absence of clinical findings, an echocardiogram should be done to look for early signs of cardiac involvement typical of KD, and if present, a presumptive diagnosis can be made and therapy initiated. In addition, for any infant or child with ≥5 days of fever and only 2–3 classic clinical criteria, or elevated inflammatory markers but <3 supplemental lab criteria, an echocardiogram can be used to help make the presumptive diagnosis. In addition to early coronary dilatation, perivascular echogenicity ("brightness"), lack of normal tapering of the coronary arteries, pericardial effusion, and decreased LV function are often seen in KD.

Routine echocardiography is recommended in patients with hypertension. In patients with systemic hypertension, the first echocardiogram should include a full anatomy study to rule out aortic coarctation, as well as an assessment of left ventricular wall thickness and function. Subsequent yearly follow-up examinations should be done to look for abnormal increases in left ventricular mass or changes in function.

The diagnosis and follow-up of pulmonary hypertension includes the use of echocardiography. In cases of obstructive sleep apnea, the extent to which hypoventilation has affected the heart can be assessed through measurement of

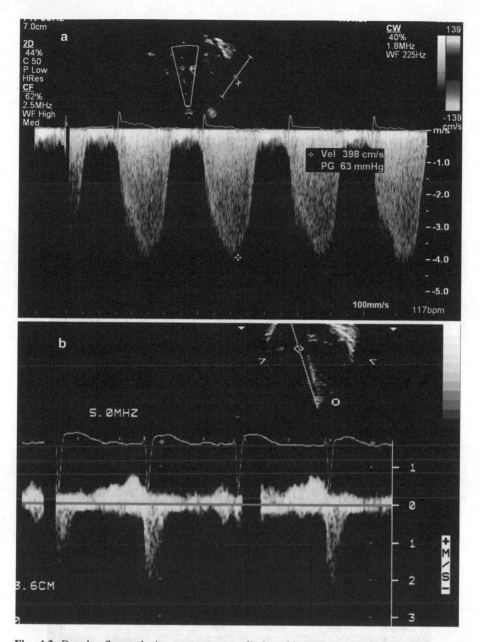

Fig. 4.3 Doppler flow velocity measurement of tricuspid regurgitation showing pulmonary hypertension. (**a**) Doppler flow velocity measurement of tricuspid regurgitation (TR) in a normal child. Mild tricuspid regurgitation is frequently noted in many individuals. The velocity of flow of the TR jet reflects the right ventricular (RV) systolic pressure over that of the right atrium (RA) (pressure = velocity^2 × 4 + RA pressure). The TR Doppler flow velocity in the child in (**a**) is 2 m/s, therefore the RV systolic pressure in this child is: 2^2 × 4 = 16 mmHg. RA pressure is typically low (2–5 mmHg) and therefore may be ignored in most circumstances. (**b**) The TR Doppler flow velocity in the patient in (**b**) is 4 m/s, therefore the RV systolic pressure in this child is: 4^2 × 4 = 64 mmHg. This reflects RV systolic hypertension, which will reflect pulmonary hypertension assuming a nonstenotic pulmonary valve

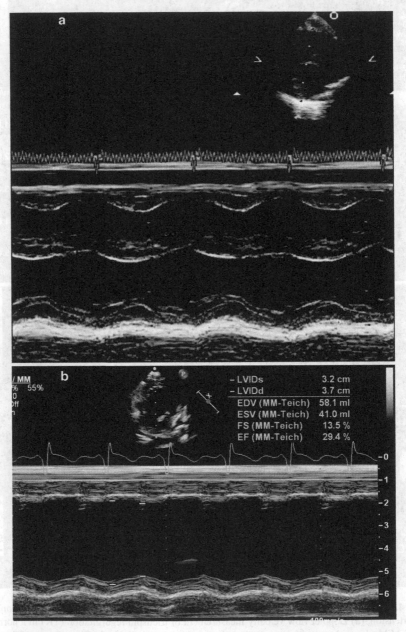

Fig. 4.4 M-mode echocardiography showing normal (**a**) and abnormal (**b**) left ventricular function. The motion of the ventricular walls is normal (**a**) reflecting brisk wall motion. On the other hand, the motion of ventricular walls in the patient in (**b**) is flat reflecting limited ventricular wall motion

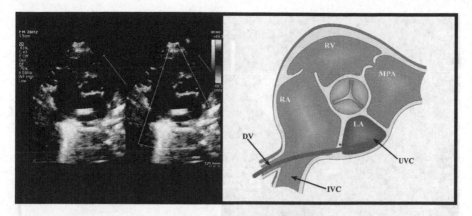

Fig. 4.5 *DV* ductus venosus, *IVC* inferior vena cava, *RA* right atrium, *RV* right ventricle, *MPA* main pulmonary artery, *LA* left atrium, *UVC* umbilical venous catheter (central line), *: PFO central line (UVC) tip noted to be placed too far in; the catheter crosses the patent foramen ovale with the tip in the left atrium. The catheter should be pulled back to rest in the right atrium just beyond the IVC-RA junction. The illustration on the *left hand* shows cardiac anatomy, *red* and *blue* coloring reflects well oxygenated and poorly oxygenated blood in different heart chambers. This coloring scheme should not be confused with the *red* and *blue* coloring of color Doppler

right ventricular pressure (using tricuspid valve Doppler or interventricular septal position), wall thickness, and function. Patients with sickle cell disease and increased pulmonary artery pressure as estimated by echocardiography have higher mortality.

Cardiomegaly or other abnormal cardiovascular findings noted on X-ray, especially if associated with other signs or symptoms of potential heart disease should prompt echocardiography. If possible, pericardial effusion is suspected, especially in the setting of hemodynamic compromise possibly representing cardiac tamponade, emergency echocardiography is indicated and may be used to assist in pericardiocentesis (Fig. 4.6).

Patients suspected of having connective tissue disease such as Marfan syndrome or Ehlers–Danlos syndrome should have echocardiography. Specifically, echocardiogram is used to evaluate the aortic root in individuals with suspected Marfan syndrome and to evaluate for Mitral Valve prolapse. These patients should be followed by a cardiologist once the diagnosis is made.

Echocardiography is indicated for surveillance in various genetic disorders (Table 4.3). Patients diagnosed with Tuberous Sclerosis should undergo echocardiography to evaluate for rhabdomyomas. Since this is an autosomal dominant disease with various organ involvements, echocardiography is useful in screening family members.

Other appropriate indications for ordering an echocardiogram include workup of possible Rheumatic fever to look for evidence of carditis, infectious endocarditis to rule out vegetation, or valve lesions associated with systemic lupus erythematosus. Saline contrast echocardiography should be requested in cases of stroke to rule out

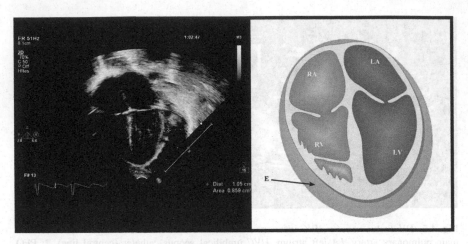

Fig. 4.6 Pericardial effusion – apical four-chamber view showing a pericardial effusion *RA* right atrium, *RV* right ventricle, *E* pericardial effusion, *LA* left atrium, *LV* left ventricle

Table 4.3 Syndromes and diseases requiring echocardiographic evaluation of the heart even in the absence of evidence of cardiac disease

Syndrome	Associated congenital heart disease
Alagille syndrome	Peripheral pulmonary stenosis, and tetralogy of Fallot
Beckwith–Wiedemann syndrome	Cardiomegaly, atrial, and ventricular septal defects, and truncus arteriosus
CATCH syndrome	Tetralogy of Fallot, ventricular septal defect, interrupted aortic arch, and pulmonary atresia, truncus arteriosus
CHARGE syndrome	Tetralogy of Fallot, atrial, ventricular and atrioventricular septal defects, aortic arch anomalies, hypoplastic left heart syndrome, and double aortic arch
Cornelia de Lange syndrome	Ventricular septal defect, pulmonary stenosis, tetralogy of Fallot, patent ductus arteriosus, and coarctation of the aorta
DiGeorge syndrome	Truncus arteriosus, double outlet right ventricle, tetralogy of Fallot, and interrupted aortic arch
Down syndrome	Congenital heart disease is seen in 40% of patients, these include: atrioventricular canal defect, ventricular septal defect, atrial septal defect, tetralogy of Fallot, and patent ductus arteriosus
Glycogen storage disease	Hypertrophic cardiomyopathy
Holt–Oram syndrome	Atrial septal defect, less common ventricular septal defect, aortic stenosis, and tetralogy of Fallot
Jervell–Lange–Nielsen syndrome	Long Q-T interval, arrhythmia
Kartagener syndrome	Situs inversus and dextrocardia (mirror image situs). Not associated with additional congenital heart disease
Marfan syndrome	Aortic root dilation, aortic dissection, mitral valve prolapse and regurgitation
Neurofibromatosis	Neurofibromata of the heart, renal artery stenosis, and renal hypertension

(continued)

Table 4.3 (continued)

Syndrome	Associated congenital heart disease
Noonan syndrome	In 50% of cases: pulmonary stenosis, conduction abnormalities (superior axis deviation), atrial septal defect, ventricular septal defect, tetralogy of Fallot, sub-aortic stenosis, complex congenital heart disease
Trisomy 13	Eighty percent of cases: ventricular septal defect, patent ductus arteriosus, atrial septal defect, coarctation of aorta, dextrocardia, and complex defects
Trisomy 18	Ventricular septal defect, polyvalvular disease
Tuberous sclerosis	Cardiac rhabdomyomas, Wolff–Parkinson–White syndrome
Turner syndrome	Coarctation of aorta, bicuspid aortic valve, aortic dilatation, dissection and rupture
VACTERL syndrome	Ventricular septal defect
Velo-cardio-facial syndrome	Ventricular septal defect, tetralogy of Fallot, and pulmonary atresia
Williams syndrome	Thickening of media (muscular layer) of systemic and pulmonary arteries resulting in supravalvar aortic and pulmonary stenosis, peripheral pulmonary stenosis, coronary artery stenosis leading to myocardial infarction, cardiomyopathy, and congestive heart failure
Factor	Associated congenital heart disease
Fetal alcohol syndrome	Ventricular septal defect, atrial septal defect, tetralogy of Fallot, coarctation of aorta
Fetal hydantoin syndrome	Ventricular septal defect, tetralogy of Fallot, pulmonary stenosis, patent ductus arteriosus, atrial septal defect, and coarctation of aorta
Fetal rubella syndrome	Pulmonary stenosis, peripheral pulmonary stenosis, and patent ductus arteriosus
Fetal thalidomide syndrome	Ventricular septal defects, pulmonary stenosis, patent ductus arteriosus, and conotruncal malformation
Fetal Warfarin syndrome	Patent ductus arteriosus and peripheral pulmonary stenosis
Maternal systemic lupus erythematosus	Complete atrioventricular block, cardiomyopathy, and l-transposition of the great vessels
Fetal rubella syndrome	Patent ductus arteriosus, peripheral pulmonary stenosis, ventricular septal defect, atrial septal defect, fibromuscular and intimal proliferation of medium and large arteries
Maternal lithium ingestion	Ebstein's malformation, Tricuspid atresia, and atrial septal defect
Maternal diabetes	Transposition of the great vessels, ventricular septal defect, coarctation of aorta, and Hypertrophic cardiomyopathy

possible right to left embolism from patent foramen ovale. Another rare indication for contrast echocardiography is in patients with Hereditary Hemorrhagic Telangiectasia, in which pulmonary arteriovenous malformations can be life-threatening. In patients exposed to potentially cardiotoxic agents, such as chemotherapy including anthracyclines, baseline and routine interval follow-up echocardiograms are used to follow left ventricular function.

When to Request a Cardiac Consultation First

In infants outside of the neonatal period, children, and adolescents with a possible pathologic murmur or other abnormal cardiac auscultation finding, it is usually most effective and efficient to start with the cardiologist's evaluation. In many cases the murmur or other finding may be determined to be innocent and echocardiography is not required. When echocardiography is indicated, the study is often assisted by having specific likely diagnoses listed based on the cardiologist's assessment, and decisions about need for sedation, timing of study, and immediate interpretation of results to patient and family is facilitated. Likewise, patients with other findings such as tachypnea, failure to thrive, or cyanosis are best referred to the cardiologist, rather that ordering an echocardiogram directly. The workup of stridor and/or difficulty in swallowing should exclude a possible vascular ring, which can be definitively diagnosed by echocardiography, but can be difficult, especially in laboratories with little experience in aortic arch anomalies in small children. The cardiologist can thus decide whether alternative imaging (barium swallow, CT, or MRI), may be required.

Chest pain is common in older children and adolescents and, unless associated with exertion, is usually not due to cardiac disease. Echocardiography is rarely needed, as careful history and physical examination, are usually all that is required to exclude heart disease. Likewise, syncope, unless during exercise, is usually not due to structural heart disease and often does not need echocardiography in the workup. An abnormal electrocardiogram should first be confirmed by a cardiologist prior to decisions about further testing such as echocardiography.

Screening for occult heart disease in patients being considered for use of stimulant medication or as part of pre sports participation evaluation requires careful and directed history and physical examination, but does not include screening echocardiography. *The American Academy of Pediatrics/American Heart Association published a statement in 2008 concerning the importance of addressing possible cardiac disease prior to starting stimulant medication for ADHD. EKG screening is suggested at the discretion of the pediatrician. If further concerns arise, the patient should then be referred to a cardiologist for further evaluation.*

What to Expect from an Echocardiogram

Echocardiography is the imaging modality of choice for defining intracardiac anatomy of congenital heart defects. The connections of major systemic veins and pulmonary veins can be defined, as well as the pulmonary arteries and the aortic arch with its major branches. In most cases, coronaries arteries, at least proximally, can also be imaged and their origins clearly defined. Doppler technology allows the detection of blood flow velocity and direction, and provides an ability to estimate pressures and pressure gradients. Color Doppler enables detection of shunting, even in cases where defects are too small to detect by imaging. 3D echocardiography is now available and is likely to enhance the ability to understand complex septal defects and valve disease. In addition, global systolic and diastolic function as well as regional wall mechanics can now be investigated in detail. Stress echocardiography can assess changes in hemodynamics and function with exertion.

Limitations of Echocardiography

Echocardiography is highly dependent on the skill, expertise, and experience of the sonographer and the interpreting physician. Important congenital defects can be missed due to incomplete or inadequate imaging or to incorrect interpretation of the images. Patient movement makes adequate imaging virtually impossible. Ultrasonography requires adequate tissue windows, without interference from air or other structures that reflect sound. In certain conditions, such as severe obesity, pneumothorax or pneumomediastinum, severe scoliosis or pectus excavatum, or when chest bandages are present, adequate windows cannot be obtained. The use of transesophageal echocardiography (TEE) can improve sensitivity of imaging of small structures and abnormalities such as vegetations. However, TEE requires deep sedation or general anesthesia, as well as possibly intubation. In some cases, distal pulmonary arteries, pulmonary or systemic venous anomalies, or aortic arch problems cannot be completely defined by echocardiography and alternative imaging modalities such as MRI, CT, or angiography may be required. Coronary artery stenoses are not reliably seen by standard transthoracic echocardiography and require intravascular ultrasound, coronary angiography, or CT to define.

Chapter 5
Cardiac Catheterization in Children: Diagnosis and Therapy

Anas Saleh Lutfi Taqatqa, Umang Gupta, Ra-id Abdulla, and Ziyad M. Hijazi

Key Facts

- Diagnostic cardiac catheterization is performed with much less frequency than the past due to advancement of other, less invasive, imaging modalities. Diagnostic cardiac catheterization may be required if other imaging modalities are not informative, hemodynamic evaluation to assess extent of shunts, cardiac output and pressure measurements are needed.
- Interventional cardiac catheterization is becoming more common as new tools allow a wider range of therapeutic intervention. Common interventional procedures include balloon dilation of stenotic valves, cardiac biopsy, closure of septal defects, and occlusion of abnormal communications and unwanted vessels.
- Complications of cardiac catheterization include cardiac wall and vascular injury, arrhythmias, hypoventilation and apnea, embolism, allergic reaction, and even death (0.3%).

Introduction

Cardiac catheterization uses intravascular catheters to access cardiac chambers and vascular structures to obtain hemodynamic information such as pressure and oxygen saturation as well as enable injection of contrast material while recording radiographic movie clips (angiogram), thus providing details of cardiac anatomy and pathology.

Pressure measurements obtained through catheters and wires during catheterization allow accurate pressure measurements of various chambers and vessels and the detection of any pressure gradients across stenotic valves or vessels. Measurement

Z.M. Hijazi (✉)
Department of Pediatrics and Internal Medicine, Rush University Medical Center,
1653 W. Congress Parkway, Suite 770 Jones, Chicago, IL 60612, USA
e-mail: Ziyad_Hijazi@rush.edu

Ra-id Abdulla (ed.), *Heart Diseases in Children: A Pediatrician's Guide*,
DOI 10.1007/978-1-4419-7994-0_5, © Springer Science+Business Media, LLC 2011

of oxygen saturation on the other hand allows for calculation of cardiac output and extent of shunts within the cardiovascular system. The combination of pressure and cardiac output measurements allow for the determination of vascular resistances (systemic and pulmonary) which are essential to determine therapeutic options in children with heart diseases.

Angiograms obtained through opacifying cardiac chambers and vascular structures through contrast injection continue to be an essential tool in diagnosis of heart diseases in children. Images obtained from angiography provide great details of specific regions of the cardiovascular system not easily accessible to echocardiography.

Indications

Cardiac catheterization is a valuable tool in diagnosis and management of heart diseases in children. It is more common nowadays to perform cardiac catheterization for therapeutic (interventional) purposes rather than for diagnosis. This is secondary to the increasing tools available for interventional pediatric cardiologists in managing heart defects in the cardiac catheterization laboratory, thus providing more indications for interventional catheterization procedures. In addition, the increasing accuracy of echocardiography and other noninvasive tools, such as CT and MRI imaging are making diagnostic cardiac catheterization an uncommon indication.

Indications for cardiac catheterization include:

- Limited echocardiographic window. This may be due to structures not accessible by echocardiography such as peripheral pulmonary vasculature or pulmonary pathology rendering echocardiographic window small such as with lung disease.
- The need for better delineation of vascular abnormalities pre and postsurgical intervention such as with systemic to pulmonary arterial collaterals.
- Hemodynamic evaluations prior to surgical interventions such as prior to the Glenn and Fontan procedures.
- Cardiac biopsy for diagnosis and followup especially in patients with cardiac transplantation.
- Interventional procedures such as closure of atrial or ventricular septal defects, occlusion of vascular structures such as patent ductus arteriosus (PDA), dilation of stenotic valves or vessels, and implantation of percutaneous valves in the pulmonic position.

Procedure

Patient Preparation

Full review of detailed history is essential, including full knowledge of the patient's diagnosis, indications, previous surgeries, previous catheterizations, previous vascular access, sedation history, medications and allergies. In addition, it is important to review previous studies such as electrocardiography and echocardiography, chronic illnesses, recent lab studies like blood count and renal function tests.

Patient should not be given solid food or milk 6 h and clear fluids 2 h prior to the procedure.

Vascular Access

Access to vascular structures is done through a needle to puncture the vessel percutaneously, followed by a wire introduced through the needle to secure vascular access. The needle is then removed and a sheath is placed over the wire. Vascular sheaths are hollow structures with a built in diaphragm to prevent bleeding. Catheters can be placed into and out of the sheath with minimal loss of blood.

Access to the Cardiovascular System

Femoral arterial and venous access (Seldinger technique) is the method of choice in the pediatric age group. The right and/or the left groins may be used. This port of access provides advantage of being away from the thoracic region for ease of catheter manipulation away from the radiographic cameras surrounding the child's thorax.

Umbilical arterial and venous access is used in newborn babies up to 7 days of age.

Internal jugular, subclavian, axillary, and transhepatic venous access is occasionally required due to lack of femoral vascular access or need to position the catheter at a particular trajectory not provided through femoral venous access. In transhepatic venous access a needle punctures the liver transcutaneously to enter hepatic vein, then a wire is introduced to reach the right atrium though the hepatic venous system.

Catheters

Large selection of catheters and wires are available for the pediatric age group. Catheters are of two categories:

- End-hole catheters used mainly for measurement of pressures, obtaining blood samples, reaching different locations, and exchanging over wires.
- Side-hole catheters used for performing angiography.

Catheter sizes are described in "French" measurements. This refers to the outer circumference of the catheter in millimeters. Each French unit equals a circumference of 1 mm and an outer diameter of 0.33 mm. Wires are also diverse including stiff and soft wires and used mainly to guide and stiffen catheters to reach different locations within the cardiovascular system. A particular type of wire (Radi wire) has a pressure transducer at its tip to allow for pressure measurements in areas where catheters are difficult to introduce.

Hemodynamic Measurements

Cardiac catheterization is the only source of reliable hemodynamic data. Echocardiography and MRI provide essential hemodynamic data, but cardiac catheterization remains the gold standard for such information because of the accuracy and diversity of data provided. Hemodynamic data obtained through catheterization include pressures and flow volumes. Pressure measurement of a vascular chamber may suggest stenosis, which can then be confirmed by pull back pressure measurement which would uncover an area of obstruction to blood flow. Measurement of oxygen saturation in different chambers and vessels can be used in formulas to calculate cardiac output (from the right or left heart chambers, referred to as Q_p and Q_s respectively). In turn, such measurement of Q_p and Q_s allows for measurements of the volume of blood shunted through a defect such as an atrial or ventricular septal defects or PDA.

In the presence of a shunt, measurement of oxygen saturations from the high superior vena cava represents the mixed venous oxygen saturation, while oxygen saturation of the pulmonary artery and aorta represent the oxygen saturation of the pulmonary and systemic circulations respectively. The pulmonary vein saturations are assumed to be similar to the aortic saturations unless there exists a right to left shunt or there are concerns about pulmonary vein pathology in which case they are measured directly.

Oxygen saturations measured are plugged into formulas to measure flows. By knowing the oxygen saturation and hemoglobin concentration of blood going out of the heart to the pulmonary or systemic circulation, the oxygen content of that blood can be determined. Similarly, by measuring the oxygen content of the blood returning back to the heart from the systemic or pulmonary circulations, the volume of blood flow returning to each circulation can be determined (please see cardiac output formulas below).

Cardiac output measurement reflects capability of the heart to generate blood flow to the body. Low cardiac output may reflect myocardial disease such as with myocarditis or dilated cardiomyopathy. On the other hand the cardiac output from the left ventricle may be different from that of the right ventricle due to intracardiac shunts, which again can be determined by comparing both cardiac outputs. A patient with an atrial septal defect with left to right shunting will have more pulmonary cardiac output than systemic. A small atrial septal defect may cause the pulmonary output to be mildly elevated (e.g., 1.5 times increase in pulmonary output, expressed as $Q_p{:}Q_s$ of 1.5:1). On the other hand, a large atrial septal defect with excessive pulmonary blood flow will cause an increase of $Q_p{:}Q_s$ to 3:1 or more. Therefore measurement of Q_p and Q_s provide valuable information regarding extent of shunts.

Fick's law uses the difference in oxygen content to measure blood volume. This is possible through measuring oxygen consumption prior to cardiac catheterization (this may be assumed using tables providing oxygen consumption values for different age groups). The difference in oxygen content of blood going out to a circulation (systemic or pulmonary) and that of blood returning from that circulation can be used to determine how much blood carried that oxygen, thus providing a cardiac output.

$$Q_p = \frac{\text{Oxygen consumption}(VO_2)}{\text{pulmonary venous oxygen content} - \text{pulmonary arterial oxygen content}}$$

$$Q_s = \frac{\text{Oxygen consumption}(VO_2)}{\text{aortic venous oxygen content} - \text{mixed venous oxygen content}}$$

Oxygen content is measured through the following formula:

$$\text{Oxygen saturation} \times \text{Hgb} \times 1.36 + 0.003 \times PaO_2$$

where, Oxygen saturation is that of the chamber or vessel examined, Hgb is the concentration of hemoglobin in mg/dl, 1.36 is a constant reflecting that each milligram of hemoglobin carries 1.36 ml of oxygen when fully saturated, 0.003 is a constant reflecting the volume of oxygen in milliliters for each PaO_2 measured through blood gas.

Measurements of Pulmonary and Systemic Vascular Resistance

The vascular resistance of the pulmonary or arterial circulation is the result of resistance offered by the arterioles at the distal end of the circulation. Elevation in vascular resistance reflects damage to that circulation such as noted in pulmonary vascular obstructive disease due to long standing excessive pulmonary blood flow leading to pulmonary hypertension.

Measurement of vascular resistance is important in determining the health of the vascular resistance and whether the blood pressure would return to normal if shunt is eliminated. Systemic and pulmonary vascular resistance can be calculated using data obtained through cardiac catheterization.

Systemic vascular resistance (SVR)

$$\text{SVR} = \frac{\text{mean pressure in aorta} - \text{mean pressure in right atrium}}{\text{Systemic blood flow}(Q_s)}$$

Normal SVR is about 24 Wood units (mmHg/L/min/M²)Pulmonary vascular resistance (PVR)

$$\text{SVR} = \frac{\text{mean pressure in pulmonary artery} - \text{mean pressure in left atrium}}{\text{Systemic blood flow}(Q_s)}$$

Normal PVR is less than 3 Wood units (mmHg/L/min/M²)

Angiography

Injection of radioopaque contrast in cardiac chambers and vascular structures while recording radiographic movie clip (30–60 frames/sec) allow clear visualization of cardiac anatomy and defects. Angiography may be performed to demonstrate cardiac anatomy that is not possible to see by less invasive imaging devices or performed in preparation for an interventional procedure. Contrast material filling a cardiovascular structure may show:

- Anatomical details of structure.
- Size of cardiac chamber or vessel.
- Presence and extent of an abnormal communication such as an atrial or ventricular septal defect.
- Thickness and motion of an abnormal valve.
- Extent of regurgitation of a valve.
- Communication of various cardiac chambers and vessels to each other as contrast material travels with blood flow.

Complications of Cardiac Catheterization

Vascular

Vascular injury is more likely in small children, when using large sheaths or catheters, when patient is using anticoagulants, after interventional procedures, and in arterial access sites.

Minor bleeding: It is expected to have minor bruising of the access site. Significant hematomas may occur and if large, may be painful and result in hemodynamic compromise.

Major bleeding: including

- Retroperitoneal bleeding after femoral access. This is suspected when there is severe back pain, unexplained drop in hematocrit or hemodynamic compromise. Abdominal ultrasound or CT scan can be used to visualize such bleeding.
- Hemothorax after subclavian approach. This is suspected when respiratory distress is noted. Chest x-ray can demonstrate this type of bleeding.

Vascular injury as a result of cardiac catheterization includes:

- Arterial occlusion: Patency of arteries should always be carefully monitored after cardiac catheterization. Signs of limb ischemia such as pallor, coldness, paresthesia, and decrease or absent peripheral pulses and delayed capillary refill should be monitored and if present treated promptly. Treatment consists of anticoagulation with heparin, thrombolysis with streptokinase or TPA, or even rarely thrombectomy.

- Venous occlusion: this presents as venous congestion and swelling. Management is typically conservative through monitoring.
- Pseudoaneurysm: This is a connection between a hematoma and the arterial lumen. It presents as a pulsatile mass, sometimes with a systolic bruit. Duplex ultrasonography is used for diagnosis. Management includes prolonged compression or thrombin injection in selected patients. If it is large, surgery is necessary.
- Arteriovenous (AV) fistula: This is a track, formed between an artery and a vein. It presents clinically as palpable thrill or continuous bruit. Many are small and resolve spontaneously. If large or persistent, surgery is required.

Arrhythmias:

- Atrial and ventricular premature beats are usually caused by catheter manipulation but are insignificant and transient.
- Atrial tachycardia may be induced by catheter manipulation. If it persists, overdrive pacing or electrical cardioversion is performed for termination.
- Ventricular tachycardias or fibrillations are rare. It occurs mainly in sick infants and responds to medical or electrical cardioversion.
- Atrioventricular conduction disturbances are rare and usually transient.

Cardiac Perforation

This is a rare occurrence due to improvement in technique. Most common sites of perforations are: atrial appendage and right ventricular outflow tract in small infants. Hemopericardium should be suspected if the patient developed hypotension, enlarged cardiac silhouette, and decreased movement of the silhouette normally generated by contractility. Echocardiogram is diagnostic. Management includes removal of the catheter, and observation. If clinically indicated, pericardiocentesis is performed.

Hypoventilation and Apnea

Depressed breathing may result from sedation used to perform cardiac catheterization. High-risk patients for respiratory depression include: Down syndrome patients, airway abnormality, borderline cardiac function, patients with gastroesophageal reflux, increased pulmonary vascular resistance, and the use of prostaglandin infusion. It is customary in many centers to have experienced anesthesiologists to be supervising anesthesia/sedation, airway patency, and effective respiration during cardiac catheterization, particularly if patients or procedure are deemed high risk.

Embolism

This may be systemic or pulmonary and include:

- Air embolism: this can be prevented by using appropriate size sheath and frequent catheter flushing.
- Thrombus: this can be prevented also by systemic heparinization of the patient.
- Fractured catheter or wires.

Neurological Complications

These are rare and transient. Most commonly related to systemic embolization or can be contrast induced.

Allergy

It may be precipitated by local anesthetics, iodinated contrast agents, or latex exposure. It ranges from mild urticaria to anaphylactic shock. Treatment includes: Diphenhydramine, H2 blockers, fluid resuscitation, and epinephrine.

Complications Related to Intervention

This includes balloon or device damages to nearby cardiac structures, heart perforations and embolization. Capture and removal of the device is attempted first, if not successful, surgical intervention is necessary to remove embolized device.

Death

Death rates have declined steeply over the past two decades reaching less than 0.3% due to improved catheterization techniques and safer anesthesia.

Interventional Catheterization

The role of interventional cardiac catheterization in managing children with heart disease continues to expand and include lesions which were, till recently, amenable only to surgical repair.

Improvement in tools available for interventional catheterization such as catheters, stents, and devices and the improvement in imaging techniques during procedures such as transesophageal echocardiography and intracardiac echocardiography in addition to fluoroscopy are allowing safe and effective therapeutic procedures in children with heart diseases.

Balloon Atrial Septostomy (Rashkind Procedure)

Catheters with inflatable balloons are used to enlarge atrial communications and allow better shunting across the atrial septum. These catheters are introduced through a venous access (femoral or umbilical veins) and into the right atrium, then across the patent foramen ovale (PFO) into the left atrium. Once the catheter tip is inside the atrium, the stiff balloon is inflated and the catheter is then yanked back. This will cause the inflated balloon to be pulled through the atrial septum and into the right atrium, thus tearing the atrial septum and enlarging the atrial communication.

Indications: lesions requiring better mixing of systemic and pulmonary blood at the atrial level, such as in:

* Transposition of the great arteries with restrictive atrial septal defect. Larger atrial communication will allow better mixing of blood and higher level of oxygen saturation till surgical repair is possible.
* Hypoplastic left heart syndrome with restrictive atrial septal defect.
* Total anomalous pulmonary venous return with restrictive atrial septal defect.
* Patients with pulmonary atresia with small atrial septal defect, mitral atresia, and tricuspid atresia.

If Rashkind atrial septostomy did not produce an effective atrial communication, then special catheters with blades embedded within an inflatable balloon can be used. The blades are exposed once the balloon is inflated, thus creating cuts in the atrial septal wall to allow for more effective enlarging of the atrial septal defect.

Balloon Valvuloplasty

Balloon dilation of stenotic valves is a well established technique to eliminate stenosis. Balloon Valvuloplasty is the first line of therapy in pulmonary stenosis. Aortic stenosis may be relieved with balloon valvuloplasty as long as aortic regurgitation is not significant since this may worsen with balloon valvuloplasty.

Pulmonary Valve Stenosis

Valvar pulmonary stenosis can respond to balloon dilation if the pulmonary annulus size is normal with no significant additional stenosis below or above the valve since supra and subvalvar stenosis do not respond well to balloon dilation. Dilating a stenotic valve results in rupture of the abnormally fused valve cusps, this will result in better opening of the valve leaflet, albeit worsening any valvular regurgitation. Pulmonary valve stenosis is performed when the pressure gradient across the valve is 50 mmHg or more.

Aortic Valve Stenosis

Valvar aortic stenosis can respond to balloon dilation. However, due to the inherent increase in valve regurgitation after balloon dilation procedure, aortic balloon dilation should not be performed if the regurgitation is already moderate or severe, since significant aortic valve regurgitation is poorly tolerated. Indications for balloon dilation of aortic valve stenosis include:

- Newborn and small infants with critical obstruction regardless of the gradient value.
- All patients with a Doppler mean systolic gradient >50 mmHg.
- Patients with left ventricular strain pattern on the ECG and a peak gradient ≥60 mmHg.
- Regardless of the gradient in all patients presenting with syncope, low cardiac output, or severe left ventricular dysfunction.

Mitral Stenosis

Balloon dilation of mitral stenosis is effective in symptomatic rheumatic mitral valve stenosis, but less effective in congenital stenosis.

Balloon Dilation of Vascular Structures

Prosthetic vessels such as systemic to pulmonary arterial shunts and vessels replacing the main pulmonary artery (MPA) (right ventricle to pulmonary artery homograft) are made of synthetic material or preserved human or animal tissue. Therefore these materials lack the ability to grow. Stenosis due to outgrowing a graft cannot be enlarged with balloon dilation since they are made from materials that are not distensible to prevent aneurysm formation. On the other hand calcification or other pathological process may cause narrowing of the lumen that can be enlarged with balloon dilation. In such circumstances, dilation has to be conducted with extreme care, since rupture of calcified homografts may occur. Dilation can be performed with balloon catheters with or without stent placement, although stents are preferred in many such cases to prevent recoil and restenosis.

Stents are usually used in older children (weight more than 20 kg) as large sheaths are needed to deliver and implant such stents. The use of stents is preferable whenever initial balloon angioplasty has failed or the lesions are known to require stent implantation to secure patency, such as compliant obstructions, stenosis due to kinking, external compression, or presence of intimal flaps.

Balloon angioplasty of coarctation of the aorta is the first choice of treatment in cases of recoarctation after previous surgical or balloon dilation procedure. This provides a very effective mode of therapy with a success rate close to 80–90%. On the other hand balloon angioplasty of native coarctation in infants less 6-months of age has higher incidence of residual or recurrent stenosis and aneurysmal formation at the dilation site. Therefore, surgical repair of coarctation of the aorta is preferred in such cases, unless not feasible due to patient instability, then balloon dilation can be attempted as a palliative procedure till more definitive repair can be performed.

Pulmonary Artery Stenosis is amenable to balloon angioplasty, this may be required when:

- There is significant pressure gradient across branch pulmonary arteries causing increase in right ventricular pressure to systemic or near systemic pressures or increase blood flow across the unaffected branch causing pulmonary artery hypertension in the unaffected lung.
- There is significant reduction of blood flow to the affected lung; this can be judged through lung perfusion scan.
- Patients are symptomatic.

Main or branch pulmonary artery stenosis is seen in patients with tetralogy of Fallot with pulmonary atresia or hypoplasia, and peripheral pulmonary stenosis such as seen in patients with Williams or Alagille syndromes.

Transcatheter Closure of Congenital Cardiac Defects

Transcatheter approach has gained wide acceptance as an alternative to open heart surgery in many congenital cardiac defects because of the accurate results and limited complications. In addition, the less invasive nature of the procedure as compared to surgery allows for a shorter hospital stay with reduced costs and a faster recovery period.

Secundum Atrial Septal Defect

Indications: Only secundum atrial septal defects can be closed using devices in the catheterization laboratory. Sinus venosus and primum atrial septal defects are not amenable to this treatment modality due to lack of circumferential atrial septal wall where the device can stay in place once deployed.

Methodology: this is typically performed through femoral venous access. A sheath is placed in the left atrium. Under intracardiac or transesophageal echocardiography guidance, the left sided disc of the occluding device is deployed first, followed by pull back of the sheath into the right atrium where the second disc (right sided disc) is deployed. Once the device is secure in place, the device is freed from its connection to the catheter. The process is visualized through x-ray and echocardiography to ensure proper deployment and effective results.

Devices available: different devices are available which have different configurations for different types of secundum atrial septal defects; these include the Amplatzer septal occluder and Gore Helex devices in the USA; other devices that are available outside the USA include the Figulla Occlutech device, CardioSeal/StarFlex, and the Cardia Atriasept devices.

Results: more than 95 % success rate with complete occlusion.

Complications: Rare, this include: device embolization/migration, cardiac arrhythmias (supraventricular arrythmias and AV conduction defects), thrombus formation, and cardiac erosion or perforation.

Patent Foramen Ovale

Indications: Device closure of PFO is still not a common practice and results of randomized clinical trials are not yet available. Some of the indications include: recurrent cerebrovascular accidents or transient ischemic attacks due to the possibility of paradoxical embolus migration through PFO to the brain. Randomized studies testing the benefit of PFO closure in patients with refractory migraine headaches is in progress.

Methodology: This is similar to ASD device closure. Imaging during the procedure is through fluoroscopy alone, however, additional imaging through echocardiography may be used. Device size is determined according to both PFO tunnel length and septal thickness.

Devices available: Amplatzer PFO occluders, CardioSEAL/STARflex occluders and Helex device, in addition, as mentioned above, outside the USA other devices are available.

Results: more than 85% complete occlusion.

Complications: rare and similar to ASD devices.

Patent Ductus Arteriosus

Indications: Hemodynamically significant ducts (moderate or large), which often cause symptoms (heart failure, recurrent respiratory infections, and failure to thrive) are usually closed during infancy. Closure of hemodynamically insignificant or small ducts with no symptoms during infancy is controversial, particularly if silent (without a murmur) and accidentally discovered during echocardiography. PDA closure is recommended when associated with continuous heart murmur.

Devices available: Amplatzer Duct Occluder devices and coil occlusion.

Coils are used in patients with small PDA (<2.5–3.0 mm). Amplatzer Duct Occluder device is used in patients with significant shunts that manifests with symptoms with left ventricular volume overload and pulmonary hypertension. Minimum patient weight amenable to this procedure is 5 kg.

Methodology: Coil occlusion: An angiogram is performed in the descending aorta to determine the site, size, and shape of the ductus arteriosus. The ductus can be crossed either anterogradely or retrogradely. For tiny ductus, a wire, followed by a catheter is advanced from aorta through PDA and into the MPA. Coils which are fed into a catheter are advanced using a wire. Pulling back the catheter and wire together causes looping of the coils at the desired site to completely occlude the ductus.

Amplatzer Duct Occluder device: Closure is anterogradely after a long sheath is advanced into the descending aorta. The device is introduced into the long sheath and the retention desk is opened in the ampulla. Withdrawing back the delivery sheath and cable, the tubular part is deployed in the ductus. Angiogram in the descending aorta can confirm device position prior to its release.

Results: more than 95% complete occlusion.

Complications: embolization (more common with coils), left pulmonary artery obstruction, and rarely hemolysis in case of incomplete closure of large PDA with coils resulting in small residual shunt causing RBC hemolysis.

Ventricular septal defect (muscular and perimembranous):

Indications

Muscular VSD: Hemodynamically significant VSD with evidence of left heart enlargement. Distance between muscular VSD and aortic, pulmonary, mitral and tricuspid valve should be at least 4 mm and the weight of the patient should be at least 5 kg.

Perimembranous VSD: moderate size VSD with evidence of left heart enlargement. There should be a tissue rim of at least 2 mm between the aortic valve and the VSD. Also weight of patient should be at least 8 kg.

Methodology: Femoral or right internal jugular veins in addition to femoral artery are accessed. The procedure is performed under transesophageal echocardiographic and fluoroscopic guidance. A catheter and then a wire are advanced into the left ventricle crossing VSD into branch pulmonary artery or SVC. Another catheter is advanced from jugular vein (if the VSD is mid muscular or apical) into the right ventricle to snare the wire in the branch pulmonary artery and get it out of the body in order to form an AV loop (one end in the femoral artery and another end in the internal jugular vein). VSD device is advanced via jugular vein into RV, crossing the defect into the ascending aorta and then deployed to close the defect.

Devices available: Amplatzer Muscular or Membranous VSD Occluder, CardioSEAL Occluder, and PFM coils.

Results: Complete occlusion is successful in up to 80–85%.

Complications: rare, but include device embolization/migration, arrhythmias (especially heart block), air embolism, hemolysis, valvular regurgitation, and pericardial effusion.

Occlusion of Vascular Communications:

Examples of vascular communications: Fistulas (systemic and pulmonary arteriovenous fistulas, and coronary AV fistula).

Devices: Coils, Amplatzer vascular plug and Amplatzer Duct Occluder.

Results: Successful occlusion in >90%.

Complications: Embolization/migration and hemolysis.

Hybrid Procedures

Definition: These procedures are performed by a team including a cardiovascular surgeon and interventional pediatric cardiologist. It involves exposing the heart through a surgical median sternotomy and introduction of interventional devices directly into the heart/blood vessels while the chest is open.

Procedures

Different types of hybrid procedures are performed and developed to perfect management of neonates and young infants with challenging cardiac lesions; procedures currently performed in this field include:

- Periventricular VSD device closure.
- Intraoperative stent placement.
- Intraoperative device occlusion of vascular structures.
- Initial palliative stage in patients with hypoplastic left heart syndrome (stent placement in the ductus arteriosus and pulmonary artery banding).

Indications: neonates and infants who are too ill to undergo the typical surgical procedure for their lesion (such as Norwood procedure for hypoplastic left heart syndrome) or inability to perform a procedure through typical approach such as with large muscular ventricular septal defects located in difficult to approach locations through surgery or conventional cardiac catheterization.

Methodology: These procedures are performed under fluoroscopy and transesophageal echocardiography. The cardiovascular surgeon opens the chest and pericardium. Catheters are advanced via a puncture through the free ventricular walls or vessels directly. The devices are then advanced to the desired location.

Case Scenarios

Case 1

History: A 4-year-old boy was known to have a ventricular septal defect. The defect was in the mid-muscular region and was moderate in size. Anticongestive heart failure medications including diuretics, digoxin, and after load reducing agents (ACE inhibitor) have been used with adequate control of symptoms. The child maintained his weight and height at the 5th percentile.

Physical examination: Heart rate was 100 bpm; regular, respiratory rate was 30/min. The Oxygen saturation while breathing room air was 95% and blood pressure in the right upper extremity was 105/55 mmHg. Mucosa was pink with good peripheral pulses and perfusion. Liver edge was palpated at 2 cm below the right costal margin. Precordium was hyperactive with increase in left and right ventricular impulses. There was no palpable thrill. On auscultation a grade 3/6 holosystolic murmur was heard over the left lower sternal border. A grade 2/4 mid-diastolic murmur was heard over the apical region.

Diagnosis: Chest x-ray showed cardiomegaly and increased pulmonary blood flow pattern, this was not significantly different than previous chest x-ray films obtained in the past.

Echocardiography showed a moderately large ventricular septal defect in the mid-muscular septum with large left to right shunt.

Management: due to the size of the ventricular septal defect and the child's failure to thrive, a decision was made to close the ventricular septal defect. Muscular ventricular septal defects may get smaller or close spontaneously. This typically occurs in the first 2 years of life. At 4 years of age, it was unlikely that this defect will close spontaneously. Muscular ventricular septal defects can be closed more effectively through percutaneous catheterization devices rather than through surgical approach due to the less invasive nature of cardiac catheterization and the difficulty to visualize these defects by the surgeon secondary to the trabecular nature of the right sided aspect of the ventricular septum.

Findings at cardiac catheterization: oxygen saturation was 80% in the high superior vena cava, 81% in right atrium, and 87% in the MPA indicating a step up of 6% in saturations between right atrium and MPA. This was indicative of a shunt at the ventricular level. An Angiogram in the left ventricle in the four-chamber view was done which showed a mid-muscular VSD (Fig. 5.1). Based on the oxygen saturations and pressures measured during catheterization the Q_p:Q_s ratio was calculated to be 2:1 with pulmonary vascular resistance of 1 WU.

In view of the size of the defect and the extent of left to right shunting, it was decided to close the defect with a 6 mm Amplatzer muscular VSD device (Fig. 5.2).

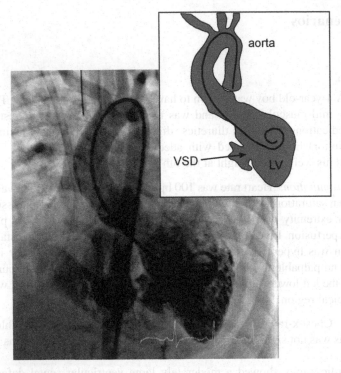

Fig. 5.1 LV angiography in four-chamber view: pigtail catheter is in the aorta and into the left ventricle. This angiogram shows the lefty ventricle (LV) and a ventricular septal defect (VSD)

Results: Next morning an echocardiogram showed device in good position with no residual shunt.

All his medications were discontinued and he was discharged home with followup scheduled in 4 weeks. Low dose Aspirin was prescribed to prevent clot formation over the newly deployed device till endothelialization completes in 6 months.

On follow up, he was found to be doing very well with no cardiovascular symptoms. Echocardiographic evaluation at that time showed no residual shunt. There was a significant improvement in the size of LA and LV.

Case 2

History: A 5-year-old girl was referred for evaluation of a heart murmur detected during routine physical examination. The child was asymptomatic with no history of significant medical problems.

Physical Examination: Heart rate was 110 bpm; regular. Respiratory rate was 28/min. Oxygen saturations while breathing room air was 98% and blood pressure

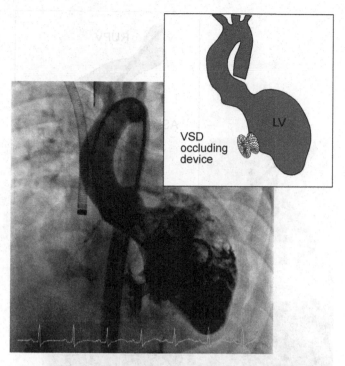

Fig. 5.2 Repeat left ventricle (LV) angiogram after a 6 mm Amplatzer muscular ventricular septal defect (VSD) device was deployed and released showing good device position and minimal foaming through the device

in right upper extremity was 108/52 mmHg. Mucosa was pink with good peripheral pulses and perfusion. Precordium was quiet with normal right and left ventricular impulses. On auscultation S1 was normal while S2 was widely split with no respiratory variation. A grade 2/6 ejection systolic murmur was heard over the left upper sternal border; in addition, a mid-diastolic grade 2/4 murmur was heard over the left lower sternal border. There was no hepatomegaly and no peripheral cyanosis or clubbing.

Diagnosis: An echocardiogram was performed showing a moderate to large secundum atrial septal defect measuring 14 mm in diameter. Shunting across the atrial septal defect was left to right. The right atrium and right ventricle were slightly enlarged.

Management: Most atrial septal defects, particularly small ones, close spontaneously in the first 2 years of life. A large number of defects close by 4–5 years of age. In this case, the child was already 5 years of age. Therefore, closure of this defect was recommended. Atrial septal defects are amenable to closure through cardiac catheterization using devices rather than through surgical approach, due to the less invasive nature of cardiac catheterization.

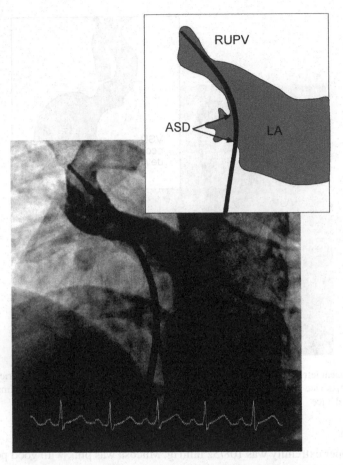

Fig. 5.3 Angiogram using a Berman angiographic catheter positioned in the right upper pulmonary vein (RUPV) in the four-chamber view. Contrast fills the left atrium (LA) with evidence of left to right shunting across the atrial septal defect and into the right atrium

Findings at Cardiac Catheterization: Oxygen saturation of 75% was measured in the high superior vena cava and 80% in the right atrium thus showing a step up of 5% in saturations. This was indicative of atrial level shunt. Angiography in the right upper pulmonary vein in the four-chamber view was performed, confirming the location and size of atrial septal defect (Fig. 5.3). An intracardiac echocardiogram (ICE) provided information regarding the rims of the defect and its size. The defect was then closed with an Amplatzer septal occluder under ICE guidance (Fig. 5.4).

Results: Echocardiogram performed next day showed the device in good position with no residual shunt. The child was discharged home with followup scheduled after 4 weeks.

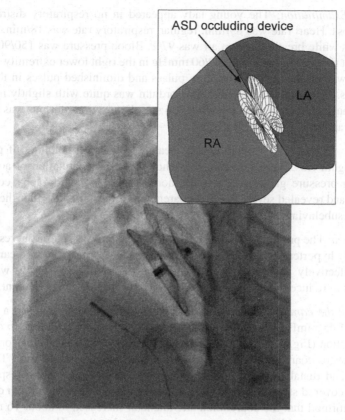

Fig. 5.4 Amplatzer atrial septal occluder (20 mm) well positioned across the atrial septum

On follow up she was found to be doing well with no cardiovascular symptoms. Echocardiography showed that the device was well situated across the atrial septum with no compromise to surrounding structures and no residual shunt. In addition, there was normalization of right atrial and ventricular size.

Case 3

History: A 17-year-old girl was referred for evaluation by pediatric cardiology secondary to high blood pressure. Blood pressure measurements obtained from the right upper extremity at the primary care physician's office at three separate occasions were higher than the 95th percentile for age and height. The child was not active and complained of claudication in the lower extremities, particularly during walking.

Physical Examination: The young lady appeared in no respiratory distress with pink mucosa. Heart rate was 89/min; regular, respiratory rate was 18/min. Oxygen saturations while breathing room air was 97%. Blood pressure was 150/90 mmHg in the right upper extremity and 100/60 mmHg in the right lower extremity. Mucosa was pink with normal upper extremity pulses and diminished pulses in the lower extremities. Liver was not palpable. Precordium was quite with slightly increased apical impulse. On auscultation a grade 2/6 systolic ejection murmur was heard in the interscapular region over the back.

Diagnosis: Chest x-ray showed normal heart size with rib notching of posterior third to eighth ribs. An echocardiogram showed severe coarctation of aorta with 50 mmHg pressure gradient across the aortic arch. CT angiography confirmed diagnosis and revealed severe discrete coarctation of the aorta just after the take off of the left subclavian artery.

Management: The pressure gradient across the aortic arch was significant resulting in upper body hypertension. Relief of coarctation of the aorta at this age can be performed effectively and safely through balloon dilation and typically with stent placement to reduce the possibility of restenosis after initial improvement.

Findings at the cardiac catheterization: Cardiac catheterization revealed a pressure gradient of 45 mmHg across the aortic arch. An angiogram was done to delineate the coarctation (Fig. 5.5). Intravascular ultrasound (IVUS) was also performed and showed severe coarctation with the narrowest diameter being 10 mm. The areas proximal and distal to the site of coarctation were 22 and 23 mm respectively. A 36 mm covered stent was deployed and then balloon dilated to 18 mm diameter. IVUS confirmed that the coarctation site diameter increased to about 16 mm. The systolic pressure gradient across coarctation dropped to 8 mmHg post stenting and angioplasty. Angiography after the balloon dilation showed good position of stent with adequate aortic arch patency (Fig. 5.6).

Results: Echocardiography performed the next morning showed stent in good position with no significant pressure gradient across the aortic arch. Blood pressure in right arm was 118/70 and right leg was 120/70 mmHg.

On follow up 3 months after the procedure, she was found to be doing very well with no cardiovascular symptoms and no claudication. Her blood pressures were 110/62 in right arm and 108/62 in right leg. An echocardiogram showed no residual pressure gradient across the aortic arch.

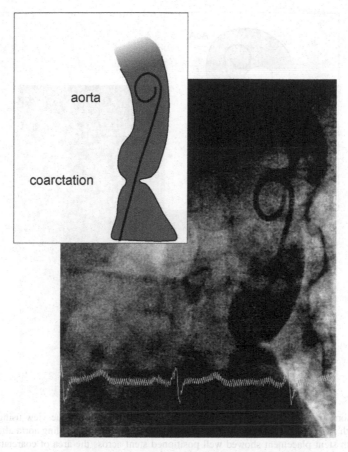

Fig. 5.5 Descending aortogram in left anterior oblique view with the pigtail catheter positioned in the high descending aorta. Contrast injection delineated the area of coarctation of the aorta

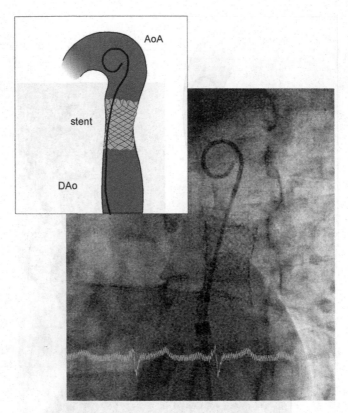

Fig. 5.6 Aortogram of the descending aorta (Dao) in left anterior oblique view using a pigtail catheter with its tip in the aortic arch (AoA). Contrast injection in descending aorta after balloon dilation with stent placement showed well positioned stent across the area of coarctation of the aorta with no residual narrowing

Part II
Congenital Heart Diseases

Chapter 6
Atrial Septal Defect

Ra-id Abdulla and Austin Hanrahan

Key Facts

- Patients with Holt–Oram syndrome frequently have atrial septal defect.
- Sinus venosus atrial septal defect is frequently associated with partial anomalous pulmonary venous return.
- Primum atrial septal defect is frequently associated with cleft mitral valve.
- Systolic ejection murmur not proceeded by ejection click plus fixed splitting of the second heart sound with or without middiastolic murmur over the left lower sternal border is pathognomonic of atrial septal defect.
- Heart size may be normal by chest X-ray in patients with atrial septal defect.
- Increase in pulmonary vascular markings on chest X-ray is frequent in patients with moderate and large atrial septal defects.
- Pulmonary vascular obstructive disease occurs in some patients with unrepaired atrial septal defect during the fourth decade of life or later.

Definition

Atrial septal defect (ASD) is a deficiency in the atrial septum leading to an abnormal communication between the right and left atria. Normally, the atrial septum forms a wall completely separating the 2 atria. ASD is different than a patent foramen ovale (PFO). The latter is a communication between the 2 atria due to patency of a normal in-utero structure caused by the space between the 2 membranes forming the atrial septum. The flaps of the atrial septum fuse later in life to seal the atrial septal wall. PFO may remain patent in older children and adults providing a small communication, this may be regarded as a normal variant.

Ra-id Abdulla (✉)
Center for Congenital and Structural Heart Diseases, Rush University Medical Center, 1653 West Congress Parkway, Room 763 Jones, Chicago, IL 60612, USA
e-mail: rabdulla@rush.edu

Ra-id Abdulla (ed.), *Heart Diseases in Children: A Pediatrician's Guide*,
DOI 10.1007/978-1-4419-7994-0_6, © Springer Science+Business Media, LLC 2011

Incidence

Defects in the interatrial septum are a common congenital heart defect. As an isolated
anomaly, atrial septal defects are the fifth most common congenital heart defect, comprising 6% of all lesions. It is also seen in 33–50% of other congenital heart defects.

Pathology

There are many types of atrial septal defects, classified according to location of
defect. These include:

- Secundum atrial septal defect: the defect is in the foramen ovale membrane, which
  is the central portion of the atrial septum (Fig. 6.1). These are the most common
  type of atrial septal defects and most likely to close spontaneously. Secundum
  atrial septal defects are more common in females who tend to be tall and thin.
- Sinus venosus atrial defect: these involve the atrial septum between the sinus
  venosus component of the two atria. The sinus venosus is the dorsal most part
  of the atria. Two subtypes of this defect are recognized. The first and more common is when the defect is close to the superior vena cava junction with the right
  atrium. This is frequently associated with abnormal drainage of right upper pulmonary vein to the right atrium (partial anomalous pulmonary venous return).
  The second type is when the sinus venosus atrial septal defect is close to the
  inferior vena cava junction with the right atrium.

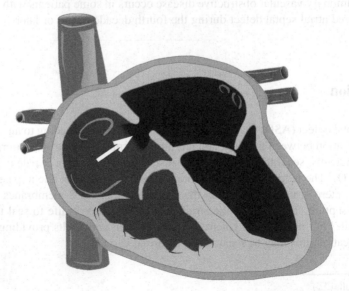

Fig. 6.1 Diagram: secundum ASD. The foramen ovale membrane is the central portion of the
atrial septum. Defect in this region results in secundum atrial septal defect (*white arrow*) which is
the most common type of atrial septal defect. Patent foramen ovale is at the same location, however, is due to lack of fusion of the two overlapping membranes (septum primum and septum
secundum), rather than lack of septum secundum tissue covering the interatrial communication

- Primum atrial septal defect (ASD): this occurs when the atrial septum does not attach to the atrioventricular valve apparatus leading to an interatrial communication just above the atrioventricular valve. Primum defects are associated with cleft of the mitral valve. Primum ASD is also a component of common atrioventricular valve defect (Chap. 9).
- Common atrium: this is when the entire atrial septum is missing. Mixing of well-saturated blood from the pulmonary veins with that of the desaturated blood from the systemic veins occurs in this anomaly leading to mild cyanosis. This is typically associated with mitral valve prolapse (MVP).

Pathophysiology

Abnormal communications between the right and left cardiac chambers or vessels create an opportunity for blood to move from one side to the other. Blood will go where resistance is least, since the pulmonary vascular resistance (PVR < 3 Wood units) is significantly less than the systemic vascular resistance (SVR≈24 Wood units), blood will shunt left to right toward the pulmonary circulation. Left to right shunting of blood will result in the reduction of cardiac output to the body (Qs) and increase in cardiac output to the pulmonary circulation (Qp) (Fig. 6.2).

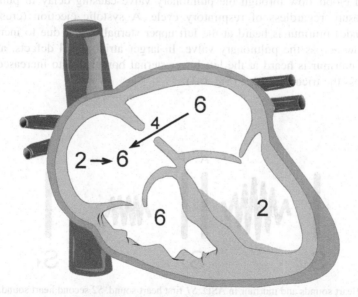

Fig. 6.2 Left to right shunting. Numbers represent volume of blood flow in liters/minute/m² (l/min/m²). The pulmonary vascular resistance is significantly less than the systemic vascular resistance, therefore, any abnormal communication between the left and right sides of the heart will result in left to right shunting. In this diagram, 6 l/min/m² of blood return from the pulmonary circulation, 4 l/min/m² cross the atrial septal defect to go to the pulmonary circulation while the remaining 2 l/min/m² go to the systemic circulation. In this scenario, the pulmonary blood flow to systemic blood flow ratio is 6:2 or 3:1. The greater this ratio, the more is the pulmonary blood flow and consequently, the worse is the extent of congestive heart failure

Increase in blood flow to the lungs will eventually lead to pulmonary edema. Drop in systemic cardiac output tends to be marginal since it is minimized by increasing the blood volume through water retention. Most of the symptoms noted in atrial septal defect, such as shortness of breath and easy fatigability are a result of pulmonary edema. Increased pulmonary blood flow over several decades will eventually cause progressive damage to the pulmonary vasculature wall resulting in pulmonary vascular obstructive disease in the third or fourth decades of life. This occurs in 5–10% of adults with unrepaired atrial septal defects.

Clinical Manifestations

Small and moderate size atrial septal defects are typically asymptomatic. Larger defects result in pulmonary edema manifesting as easy fatigability and shortness of breath. Only very large defects result in significant congestive heart failure and failure to thrive.

On examination there is a hyperactive precordium with a prominent right ventricular impulse due to right ventricular dilation. Auscultation reveals a prominent first heart sound. Second heart splitting is fixed throughout respiration due to increased blood flow through the pulmonary valve causing delay in pulmonary valve closure regardless of respiratory cycle. A systolic ejection (crescendo–decrescendo) murmur is heard at the left upper sternal border due to increase in blood flow across the pulmonary valve. In larger atrial septal defects, an early diastolic murmur is heard at the left lower sternal border due to increased blood flow across the tricuspid valve (Fig. 6.3).

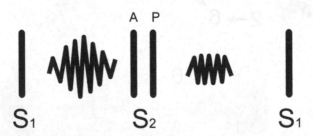

Fig. 6.3 Heart sounds and murmur in ASD. *S1* first heart sound, *S2* second heart sound, *A* aortic valve closure, *P* pulmonary valve closure. Increase in blood flow across the pulmonary valve results in a systolic ejection murmur, while the increase in blood flow across the tricuspid valve causes a middiastolic murmur. Unlike pulmonary stenosis, the systolic murmur is not preceded by a systolic click. The second heart sound is fixed in its splitting (through respiration) due to the excessive pulmonary blood flow and the need for the pulmonary valve to stay open longer throughout respiration

Diagnosis

Chest X-Ray

Prominent pulmonary vasculature due to left to right shunting is present. In addition, increase in blood flow through the right heart will cause right atrial and right ventricular dilation manifesting as cardiomegaly on chest X-ray; however, this is noted only when there is significant extent of left to right shunting. Excessive pulmonary blood flow may cause dilation of the main pulmonary artery manifested as prominent pulmonary artery at the midleft cardiac silhouette border (Fig. 6.4).

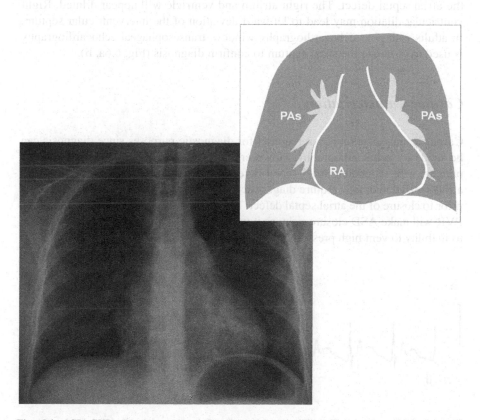

Fig. 6.4 ASD CXR. *RA* right atrium, *PAs* pulmonary arteries. Left to right shunting causes increase in blood volume in the right heart resulting in cardiomegaly. The engorged pulmonary vasculature could be seen on chest X-ray as prominent pulmonary vessels in the hilar region as well as being able to see pulmonary vessels in the peripheral lung fields

Electrocardiograph

Right atrial and right ventricular dilation/hypertrophy may be noted. Right atrial enlargement manifests as tall P waves (taller than 2 mm in children and 3 mm in adolescents and adults). Right ventricular dilation/hypertrophy manifests as tall R wave in V1 and deep S wave in V6 or as rsR′ configuration of the QRS complex in right chest leads (V1, V2). Right axis deviation of the QRS axis may also be noted (Fig. 6.5a, b).

Echocardiography

The atrial septal defect is seen by 2D echocardiography. This is best seen in the subcostal views of the heart. Color Doppler shows left to right shunting across the atrial septal defect. The right atrium and ventricle will appear dilated. Right ventricular dilation may lead to leftward deviation of the interventricular septum. In adults with poor echocardiography window, transesophageal echocardiography is used to visualize the atrial septum to confirm diagnosis (Fig. 6.6a, b).

Cardiac Catheterization

Cardiac catheterization is not required for diagnostic purposes since diagnosis can be made by echocardiography. However, cardiac catheterization is performed in patients with secundum atrial septal defect for therapeutic purposes. Adults with atrial septal defect may require diagnostic cardiac catheterization to determine PVR prior to closure of the atrial septal defect. This is because significant elevation of the PVR will make ASD closure risky as it will precipitate acute right heart failure due to inability to vent high pressure in right heart through the newly closed ASD.

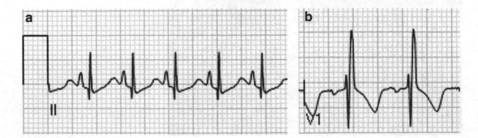

Fig. 6.5 ECG (a) lead II. Tall "P" wave (more than 2 mm) represent right atrial enlargement. (b) QRS pattern in right chest leads (V1, V2) may reflect right ventricular hypertrophy (RVH). rSR′ (where R′ is taller than r) reflect right ventricular hypertrophy. Please see Chap. 3 for different representations of RVH on ECG

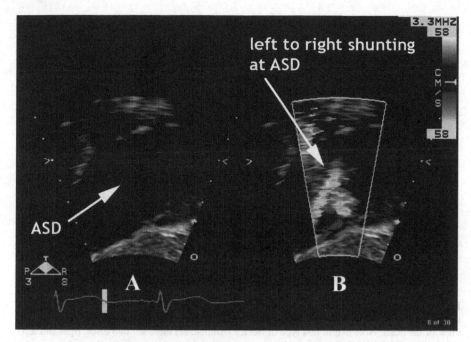

Fig. 6.6 Echocardiography (**a**) 2D echocardiography showing defect in the atrial septum (*white arrow*), this view is obtained from the subcostal region. (**b**) Color Doppler shows blood flow and its direction, *red* is the color of blood flowing toward the probe and *blue* represents the flow of blood away from the probe. In this figure, blood is shunting across the atrial septal defect from left atrium to right atrium toward the probe, therefore, *red* in color

Treatment

Most patients with atrial septal defect do not require medical treatment for congestive heart failure due to the limited impact of small to moderate increase in pulmonary blood flow. On the other hand, patients with larger defects and excessive pulmonary blood flow may benefit from anticongestive heart failure medications such as diuretics. Inotropic agents, such as digoxin and afterload reducing agents, are rarely required.

Closure of atrial septal defect is determined by the type of the defect and its size. Small (less than 5 mm in diameter) and medium (5–8 mm in diameter)-sized secundum defects diagnosed during early infancy tend to close spontaneously, often in the first 2 years of life. If at 2 years of life the defect is still present, closure could be considered through the use of occluding devices in the cardiac catheterization laboratory (Fig. 6.7). Sinus venosus and primum atrial septal defects do not close spontaneously and will require surgical repair which could be performed around 1 year of age. Surgical repair is the only modality of treatment for sinus venosus and primum atrial septal defects since they are not amenable to device

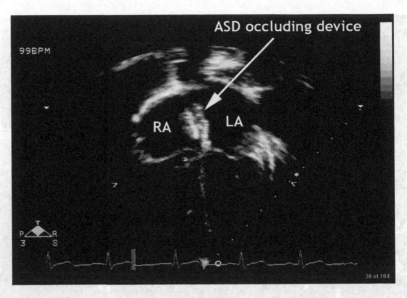

Fig. 6.7 ASD device occlusion. *RA* right atrium, *LA* left atrium, *ASD* atrial septal defect. An ASD occluding device is noted across the atrial septum in this four-chamber apical echocardiographic view of the heart. Note that in this type of device (Amplatzer) there are two discs, right and left-sided discs which hold the device in place across the atrial septal defect

closure due to lack of circumferential atrial septal wall which are used to anchor devices after deployment. This anchoring is necessary for devices to remain in position after deployment (Fig. 6.8a, b).

Prognosis

Patients with atrial septal defect typically do well with minimal symptoms relating to increase in pulmonary blood flow. If complications of unrepaired atrial septal defects are to occur, it does so later in adult life, typically in the fourth decade. These include:

- Pulmonary vascular obstructive disease: it occurs due to significant increase in pulmonary blood flow causing damage to the pulmonary vasculature. This results in elevation of the PVR. Patients with elevated PVR lead to right to left shunting at the atrial septal defect resulting in cyanosis.
- Atrial dilation and fibrosis will eventually lead to arrhythmias, such as atrial flutter and fibrillation: atrial arrhythmias occur after decades with unrepaired defects due to dilation and eventual fibrosis of right atrial walls.
- Paradoxical embolization: small clots which naturally occur in the right heart and are filtered by the lungs may find their way across the atrial septal defect due to right to left shunting (due to pulmonary vascular obstructive disease) or paradoxical embolization. This is an extremely rare complication.

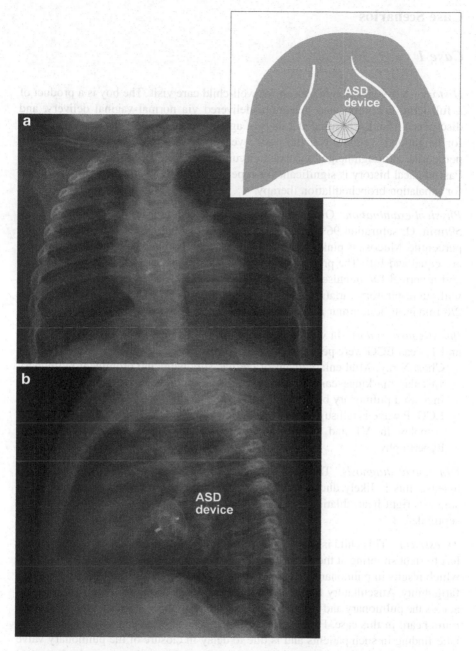

Fig. 6.8 ASD device placement. (**a**) Anterior–posterior projection of chest X-ray. The ASD occluding device is noted in the region of the atrial septum. (**b**) ASD occluding device (Amplatzer) is shown in the lateral view of chest X-ray

Case Scenarios

Case 1

History. A 3-year-old boy is seen for well-child care visit. The boy is a product of a full-term, uncomplicated gestation, delivered via normal vaginal delivery, and discharged from the hospital at 2 days of age. At birth, he was at the 50th percentile for height and weight. Over the past 2 years his weight has dropped to the 25th percentile, although height and head circumference remain in the 50th percentile. Past medical history is significant for repeated respiratory infections and the need for inhalation bronchodilation therapy.

Physical examination. On examination the child is afebrile; HR is 100 bpm, RR 50/min, O_2 saturation 96%, weight at the 25th percentile, and height at the 50th percentile. Mucosa is pink, capillary refill 2 s. Femoral and brachial arterial pulses are equal and full. The precordium is hyperactive with an increase in RV impulse and a normal LV impulse. Lungs are clear to auscultation. S1 is loud; S2 is split without respiratory variation. A 3/6 systolic murmur heard best at the LUSB and a 2/6 middiastolic murmur at the LLSB.

Investigative studies. In view of the findings on physical examination chest X-ray and 12-lead ECG were performed.
 Chest X-ray: Mild enlargement of cardiac silhouette and prominent pulmonary vascular markings can be seen. Prominent pulmonary vasculature suggests increased pulmonary blood flow.
 ECG: P wave is tall suggesting right atrial enlargement. rsR′ pattern of the QRS complex in V1 and right axis deviation (250°) suggest right ventricular hypertrophy.

Differential diagnosis. This child exhibits findings consistent with chronic lung disease, this is likely due to excessive pulmonary blood flow. In addition, ECG suggests right heart dilation and hypertrophy. Auscultation findings suggest atrial septal defect.

Assessment. This child is likely to have an atrial septal defect. These defects cause left to right shunting at the atrial level resulting in increased pulmonary blood flow which results in pulmonary congestion manifesting as shortness of breath and easy fatigability. Auscultatory findings in such patients are due to increase in blood flow across the pulmonary and tricuspid valves leading to the systolic and diastolic murmurs heard in this case. Fixed splitting of the second heart sound is the characteristic finding in such patients and is due to delay in closure of the pulmonary valve due to increased pulmonary blood flow throughout the respiratory cycle. Increased blood flow across the right heart will cause right atrial and ventricular dilation as noted from the chest X-ray and ECG findings. After the initial evaluation, chest X-ray and ECG, this patient should be referred to a pediatric cardiologist for an echocardiogram and further management.

Echocardiography provides accurate assessment regarding type and size of these defects. The atrial septal defect in this patient is secundum in type and appears to be large in size. Shunting across the atrial septum is left to right.

Management. Providing anticongestive heart failure medications is typically not warranted. In view of the signs noted in this child and evidence of failure to thrive, closure of the ASD is indicated and would resolve the child's symptoms. Secundum atrial septal defects can be closed using occlusive devices deployed through cardiac catheterization. This would not have been possible if the defect was of the sinus venosus or primum atrial septal defect types, where surgical closure would be indicated.

Case 2

History. A 45-year-old man complains of easy fatigability with minimal physical activity as well as mild bluish discoloration of lips and nail beds. The patient is otherwise healthy. Past medical history is significant for a diagnosis of reactive airway disease as a child with multiple chest infections in childhood. The patient states that the respiratory symptoms resolved in his 20s with increasing ability to perform physical activities and he was able to participate more effectively in sports. However, this has again declined over the past few years and now he fatigues after walking half a mile or ascending one flight of stairs.

Physical examination. On examination, his heart rate is 70 bpm, regular, respiratory rate is 25/min, blood pressure is 110/75 mmHg, and oxygen saturation is 85%. Mild cyanosis is noted in oral mucosa and nail beds. Mild clubbing of digits is present. Good peripheral pulses and perfusion are detected. No hepatomegaly, precordium is quiet with increased right ventricular impulse and normal apical impulse. Auscultation reveals normal first heart sound, pulmonary component of second heart sound is loud, no systolic or diastolic murmurs detected. Lungs are clear to auscultation.

Differential diagnosis. The presence of long history of respiratory disease suggests chronic lung disease. On the other hand, developing cyanosis without exacerbation of respiratory symptoms suggests etiologies other than lung disease. Long-standing congenital heart disease causing increase in pulmonary blood flow with eventual damage to the pulmonary vasculature is a likely cause of this patient's symptoms and signs.

Investigative studies. Echocardiography shows large secundum ASD with bidirectional shunting, although predominantly right to left shunting. Right atrium and ventricle are dilated and hypertrophied. Pulmonary arterial systolic pressure was measured through a tricuspid regurgitation jet which indicates a right ventricular/pulmonary arterial systolic pressure of about 100 mmHg.

Assessment. This gentleman has a large atrial septal defect with pulmonary vascular obstructive disease due to long standing increase in pulmonary blood flow. The high pulmonary blood flow caused pulmonary congestion during childhood manifesting as reactive airway disease like illness. As the patient became older the damaged pulmonary vasculature resulting in increasing PVR caused less pulmonary blood flow allowing him to have more physical stamina. However, with unrepaired lesions, there is likelihood that pulmonary vascular obstructive disease progress causing the pulmonary vascular disease to be significantly elevated, leading to right to left shunting at the atrial septal defect resulting in cyanosis.

Management. Cardiac catheterization is indicated in this case to assess PVR and its reversibility by using pulmonary vasodilators such as oxygen, nitric oxide, and pharmacological agents. If reversible, then closure with ongoing management of pulmonary vascular obstructive disease can be considered. Otherwise, the only alternative available is the chronic use of pulmonary vascular dilation therapy such as oxygen, sildenafil, bosentan, and intravenous agents such as continuous prostacyclin infusion. This may reverse the elevation of PVR and allow eventual closure of atrial septal defects. As a last resort possible heart/lung transplantation may be performed.

Chapter 7
Ventricular Septal Defect

Omar M. Khalid and Ra-id Abdulla

Key Facts

- Children with ventricular septal defects are typically asymptomatic. The murmur however tends to be harsh and easily noticeable.
- Holosystolic murmur at the left lower sternal border indicate ventricular septal defect (VSD), while at the apex reflect mitral regurgitation.
- Small VSD cause mild increase in pulmonary blood flow (PBF) and are therefore not a cause of congestive heart failure. Large defects cause significant increase in PBF resulting in congestive heart failure.
- Closure of VSD is typically done at 4–6 months of age if children are symptomatic, closure can be delayed with smaller defects.
- Closure of VSD through interventional cardiac catheterization using occluding devices is possible in muscular and perimembrenous defects, but not in outflow or inlet type VSD.

Definition

Ventricular septal defect (VSD) is an abnormal communication between the right and left ventricles. The ventricular septum is normally a solid wall completely separating the 2 ventricles. Presentation of patients with VSD vary depending on size of defect and consequently extent of left to right shunting of blood. Patients with VSD are typically recognized early in life due to the loud murmur it produces.

O.M. Khalid (✉)
Children's Heart Institute, Mary Washington Hospital, 1101 Sam Perry Blvd.,
Suite # 415, Fredericksburg, VA 22401, USA
e-mail: omarmkhalid@hotmail.com

Ra-id Abdulla (ed.), *Heart Diseases in Children: A Pediatrician's Guide*,
DOI 10.1007/978-1-4419-7994-0_7, © Springer Science+Business Media, LLC 2011

Incidence

Ventricular septal defect is the most common cardiac defect, and it accounts for 15–20% of all cardiac defects. The incidence of ventricular septal defect is slightly more common in females (56%).

Pathology

The ventricular septum can be divided into a small membranous region and a much larger muscular septum; the latter makes up the bulk of the ventricular septum and can be further divided into an inlet, trabecular, and outlet regions. Ventricular septal defects may occur in any part of the ventricular septum, it may be single or multiple, and it may also be associated with other forms of congenital heart defects. The ventricular septal defect is usually classified by its location in the ventricular septum.

Membranous ventricular septal defect is the most common type (70%). The defect occurs in the membranous septum and involves some of the surrounding tissue, thus sometimes called perimembrenous or paramembrenous defect (Fig. 7.1).

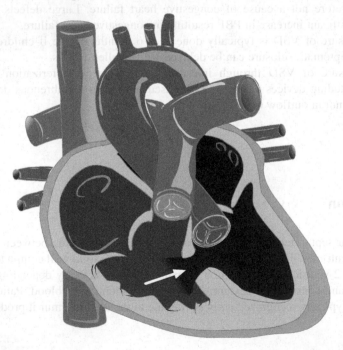

Fig. 7.1 Ventricular septal defect (VSD). A defect in and around the membranous region of the ventricular septum is known as perimembrenous ventricular septal defect (sometimes referred to as paramembrenous). This diagram depicts a perimembrenous ventricular septal defect (*white arrow*). This defect is located beneath the aortic valve, close to the tricuspid valve. Defects in the muscular region are closer to the apex than perimembrenous VSD, while outlet defects are closer to the pulmonary valve. Inlet defects are posterior, close to the tricuspid and mitral valves and away from the anteriorly positioned aortic and pulmonary valves

   Inlet (AV canal type) ventricular septal defect accounts for 5–8% of all ventricular septal defects. It is located beneath the tricuspid valve, posterior, and inferior of the membranous septum.

   Muscular ventricular septal defect accounts for 5–20% of all ventricular septal defects. It is located in the muscular septum. These defects may be anterior (marginal), mid-muscular, posterior, or apical.

   Outlet (infundibular, conal, and supracristal) ventricular septal defect account for 5–7% of all types of defects. The defect is located in the outlet septum, beneath both semilunar (pulmonary and aortic) valves.

Pathophysiology

The magnitude of shunting from one chamber to the other depends on the size of the defect and the difference between the systemic and pulmonary vascular resistance.

   In small ventricular septal defects the defect is restrictive and the amount of shunting will be hemodynamically insignificant. If the defect is large there will be significant shunting to the right side depending primarily on the difference between the systemic and pulmonary vascular resistance (Fig. 7.2), this will cause dilatation

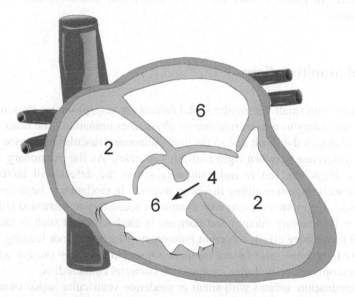

Fig. 7.2 Left to right shunting numbers represent the volume of blood flow in liters/minute/M^2 (l/m/M^2). The pulmonary vascular resistance is significantly less than the systemic vascular resistance, therefore, any abnormal communication between the left and right sides of the heart will result in left to right shunting. In this diagram, 6 l/m/M^2 of blood return from the lungs. Since the pulmonary vascular resistance is significantly less than the systemic vascular resistance, blood shunts left to right across the VSD, thus increasing blood flow to the lungs. In the scenario depicted in this diagram, 4 l/m/M^2 shunts across the VSD, thus leaving only 2 l/m/M^2 of cardiac output to the systemic circulation. Blood flow to the lungs versus that to the body (Qp:Qs ratio) in this scenario is 6:2 or 3:1

of the pulmonary arteries, left atrium, and left ventricle. The excessive shunting will also cause increase in pulmonary blood flow and congestive heart failure secondary to volume overload. Pulmonary congestion will lead to respiratory symptoms, recurrent respiratory infections, and feeding difficulties. Significant left to right shunting will cause decrease in the systemic cardiac output manifested by exercise intolerance, diaphoresis, poor feeding, and failure to thrive. The pulmonary vascular resistance is high in the newborn period, and the left to right shunting will not be significant, therefore the infant is typically asymptomatic in the first 2 months of life, with no significant heart murmur in the first few days of life. This may make diagnosis difficult during the newborn exam. With a large (unrestrictive) ventricular septal defect, the right ventricle and the pulmonary vascular bed will be facing systemic pressures; if left untreated, this may cause an irreversible change in the pulmonary arterioles causing pulmonary vascular obstructive disease (Eisenmenger's syndrome) with subsequent right to left shunting and cyanosis. This complication is delayed according to the size of the defect; large defects may cause irreversible changes in the pulmonary vasculature during early childhood. Smaller defects cause Eisenmenger's syndrome later in life.

Blood shunting in a turbulent fashion across the ventricular septal defect may affect adjacent structures such as the aortic valve leading to prolapse of the aortic cusp closer to the defect and this may progress to aortic valve regurgitation. If left untreated, it may cause left ventricular dilatation and worsening heart failure.

Clinical Manifestations

Most infants with small ventricular septal defects are asymptomatic. Presentation is typically secondary to a heart murmur on physical examination. The heart murmur may not be detected at birth due to the high pulmonary vascular resistance and low pressure difference between right and left ventricles. As the pulmonary vascular resistance drops, the left to right shunting across the defect will increase and become more turbulent resulting in a heart murmur. In moderate to large ventricular septal defect, the infants present with symptoms secondary to increased pulmonary blood flow (pulmonary edema) and decrease in cardiac output such as tachypnea, increased respiratory effort, recurrent pulmonary infections, poor feeding, diaphoresis, easy fatigability, and failure to thrive. Older patients may present with heart failure, hemoptysis, arrhythmia, cyanosis, or bacterial endocarditis.

On examination, infants with small or moderate ventricular septal defects usually present only with holosystolic murmur (Fig. 7.3). In large ventricular septal defects, infants are often tachypneic with failure to thrive and show signs of congestive heart failure such as respiratory distress (respiratory retraction and nasal flaring), and an enlarged liver. The precordium is hyperactive sometimes with a precordial bulge. A systolic thrill may be palpable in small or medium ventricular

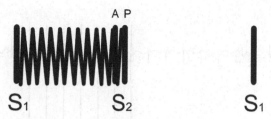

Fig. 7.3 Heart sounds and murmur in patients with VSD S1: first heart sound, S2: second heart sound, A: aortic valve closure, P: pulmonary valve closure. Once the ventricles contract, blood shunting across the VSD flows in a turbulent fashion, thus creating a murmur. Since blood shunts across a VSD throughout systole, the murmur produced is holosystolic

septal defects. The intensity of S1 is diminished by the onset of the heart murmur; S2 is normal in small ventricular septal defects, but it increases in intensity in moderate ventricular septal defect; S2 is loud and single in patients with pulmonary hypertension. Frequently, secondary to the holosystolic murmur, S1 and S2 are masked by the murmur spanning the entire duration of systole.

Ventricular septal defect murmurs may be 2–5/6 in intensity and harsh in quality, it is best heard over the left lower sternal border. A mid-diastolic rumble at the apical region is often heard in large ventricular septal defects due to the increased flow across the mitral valve.

Chest Radiography

The chest X-ray is normal in small ventricular septal defects. In moderate and large ventricular septal defects (Fig. 2.5), there is usually cardiac enlargement with increased pulmonary vascular markings. The degree of cardiomegaly and increased vascular markings is proportional to the amount of left to right shunting. In pulmonary vascular obstructive disease, the cardiac size is normal with no evidence of increase in pulmonary vascular markings, but the pulmonary artery segment at the mid left border of the cardiac silhouette may be more prominent.

Electrocardiography

Electrocardiogram (ECG) is usually normal in small ventricular septal defect. Left atrial dilatation and left ventricular hypertrophy may be seen in moderate ventricular septal defect. With a large defect, the ECG shows biventricular hypertrophy (Fig. 7.4). The ECG may show right ventricular hypertrophy only with high right ventricular pressure secondary to pulmonary obstructive disease in advanced cases of ventricular septal defect complicated by pulmonary vascular obstructive disease (Eisenmenger's syndrome).

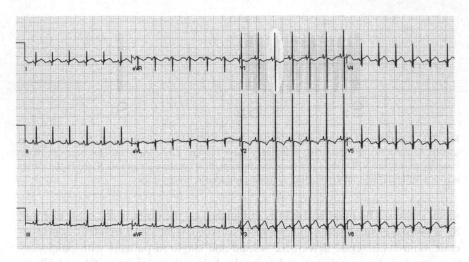

Fig. 7.4 ECG in patients with VSD Volume overload of the right and left ventricles causes biventricular hypertrophy. Most chest leads, particularly the right chest leads in this tracing show increase in anterior (tall R waves) and posterior (deep S waves) forces indicating right and left ventricular hypertrophy. This ECG may suggest more prominent right ventricular hypertrophy

Echocardiography

The echocardiogram is the gold standard tool to diagnose ventricular septal defect. It can identify the size, location, and number of ventricular septal defects. Echocardiography can measure the right ventricular and pulmonary pressures by assessing the pressure gradient across the defect as well as assess the degree of shunting. Echocardiography can also identify associated lesions such as aortic valve prolapse and regurgitation, coarctation of the aorta, or double-chambered right ventricle.

Cardiac Catheterization

Cardiac catheterization is typically not required for diagnosis since echocardiography can provide all details required to plan management. Cardiac catheterization is indicated in older children with pulmonary hypertension to assess the pulmonary vascular resistance prior to surgical repair.

Therapeutic interventional cardiac catheterization has been increasing in recent years. Device closure of muscular ventricular septal defect is now performed in many centers due to the difficulty accessing these defects surgically and the ability to close such defects effectively without the need for surgery. Device closure of the membranous ventricular septal defect is still under investigation, but soon will become more widely used.

Treatment

Medical management is indicated in presence of signs and symptoms of congestive heart failure, respiratory distress, and failure to thrive, Symptomatic patients may receive diuretics, after load reducing agents or digoxin.

Small ventricular septal defects can be managed conservatively in patients with no history of congestive heart failure or pulmonary hypertension. Surgical closure is indicated in symptomatic infants including congestive heart failure, failure to thrive or recurrent respiratory infections and those who fail medical management. Surgery is also indicated in children with significant left to right shunting and ventricular dilatation prior to 2 years of age. Infants with large ventricular septal defect and pulmonary hypertension should have surgical repair between 3 and 12 months of age. The surgical mortality is less than 3%. Mortality is higher in the presence of multiple ventricular septal defects, other associated defects, and in young infants less than 2 months of age. Surgical complications may include: residual ventricular septal defect, right bundle branch block or complete heart block, or injuries to the tricuspid or aortic valve. If the repair was performed through the ventricle (ventriculotomy), this will cause a ventricular scar that might affect its function and may also cause ventricular arrhythmias. Indications for closure of ventricular septal defects of the muscular type using interventional cardiac catheterization approach are similar to that of surgical approach.

Maintaining a good dental hygiene is important, but endocarditis prophylaxis is not indicated based on the most recent recommendations of the American Heart Association.

Case Scenarios

Case 1

A 3-month-old male infant presented with a 2-week history of decreased feeding, shortness of breath, cough, and wheezing. The diagnosis of bronchiolitis was made by the primary care physician and he was admitted to the general pediatric floor for further management. On physical examination, the infant was in respiratory distress, his heart rate was 142 bpm, respiratory rate was 66 breaths per minute, blood pressure was 90/50 mmHg, and oxygen saturation was 98% while breathing room air. Chest examination revealed moderate retractions with bilateral crackles. The precordium was hyperactive, there was 3/6 holosystolic murmur at the left sternal border and no diastolic murmur. The abdomen was soft, the liver was palpable (3 cm below costal margin), the peripheral perfusion was normal, and there was no peripheral edema noted.

Chest X-rays shows cardiomegaly with increase in pulmonary vascular markings. The 12-lead ECG revealed a heart rate of 145 bpm, left axis deviation, and voltage criteria of left ventricular hypertrophy.

The respiratory distress in this child is most likely secondary to a congestive heart failure rather than simple bronchiolitis. The presence of an active precordium, heart murmur, and a palpable liver are signs of left to right shunt, pulmonary over-circulation, and volume overload. The murmur is typical for a ventricular septal defect. The murmur and the respiratory distress did not develop earlier in life due the high pulmonary vascular resistance at birth that prevents significant left to right shunting. This usually drops in the first few weeks of life causing an increase in pulmonary circulation and volume overload. This emphasizes the importance of followup in young infants as a normal newborn exam may not exclude the presence of a congenital heart disease.

Echocardiography provides an accurate assessment regarding the type and size of the ventricular septal defect. Treatment with anti-congestive heart failure medications is warranted in this patient. This may include diuretics, such as furosemide (Lasix); inotropic agent, such as digoxin; and after load reducing agent, such as captopril. Indication of surgical closure depends on the size of the defect and response to medical therapy. If the infants continue to be symptomatic in spite of medical management then surgery is recommended. Interventional cardiac catheter closure of defect is recommended if they are of the muscular type.

Case 2

A 1-year-old female presented for a well-check visit. She is currently asymptomatic. Past medical history is remarkable for recurrent chest infections. She was born at term with no perinatal complications. On physical examination she was alert, her weight was 7.2 kg, which is below the 5th percentile, and height was 73 cm on the 25th percentile. Heart rate was 110 bpm and respiratory rate was 55 breaths per minute. Chest examination shows minimal retractions, there is normal vesicular breath sounds bilaterally with no wheezing or crackles, cardiac examination revealed an active precordium, and there is normal upper and lower extremity pulses. Cardiac auscultation showed a grade 2/6 holosystolic murmur at the lower left sternal border, the abdomen was soft with no hepatomegaly. Peripheral pulses and perfusion were normal.

Twelve-lead ECG shows tall R waves in V6 and deep S waves in V1 indicating left ventricular hypertrophy.

Echocardiography revealed a moderate apical muscular ventricular septal defect with left to right shunting; there is mild right ventricular dilatation.

Cardiac catheterization was performed and hemodynamic data showed a significant left to right shunt with a Qp: Qs ratio of 2.5:1. The pulmonary vascular resistance was normal. The angiogram confirmed the diagnosis of a moderate size apical ventricular septal defect. Ventricular septal defect device closure was performed during the catheterization procedure with no adverse effect and effective elimination of left to right shunting.

The ventricular septal defect in this patient was moderate in size with significant left to right shunt. Therefore closure of the defect is indicated. Defects in the apical region of the ventricular septum are difficult to close surgically due to their location. Device closure of muscular ventricular defects is now possible using specially made devices. The proximity of the aortic and atrioventricular valves and the conduction pathways to the membranous, inlet, or outlet ventricular defects, makes it more difficult to close these defects with a device, although experimental attempts are underway to develop such devices and methodologies, particularly those for perimembrenous ventricular septal defects. On the other hand, muscular defects are remotely situated from any vital structures and thus more amenable to device closure.

Chapter 8
Patent Ductus Arteriosus

Omar M. Khalid and Jacquelyn Busse

Key Facts

- The incidence of PDA is inversely related to gestational age in premature infants.
- Clinical presentation of PDA in premature infants is different than in older children. They present with increased work of breathing or an increasing need for mechanical ventilatory support. The murmur in these premature infants tends to be systolic rather than continuous.
- Older children are typically asymptomatic and develop a continuous, harsh murmur heard best over the left subclavicular region.
- Treatment of PDA in premature infants is different than in older children. Pharmacological agents such as indomethacin and ibuprofen are the first line of management in this age group. Failure of pharmacological therapy necessitates surgical closure.
- Management in older children consists of device closure via interventional cardiac catheterization. In the rare instances where this is not possible, surgical ligation is performed.

Definition

The ductus arteriosus is a vascular structure connecting the left main pulmonary artery to the upper part of the descending aorta just distal to the left subclavian artery. The ductus arteriosus is an important structure in fetal circulation, allowing the right ventricle to pump blood directly to the descending aorta thus bypassing the pulmonary circulation. In normal newborns, the ductus is mostly closed by the second or third day of life and is fully sealed by 2–3 weeks of life.

O.M. Khalid (✉)
Children's Heart Institute, Mary Washington Hospital, 1101 Sam Perry Blvd.,
Suite # 415, Fredericksburg, VA 22401, USA
e-mail: omarmkhalid@hotmail.com

Ra-id Abdulla (ed.), *Heart Diseases in Children: A Pediatrician's Guide*,
DOI 10.1007/978-1-4419-7994-0_8, © Springer Science+Business Media, LLC 2011

Incidence

The incidence of patent ductus arteriosus (PDA) in term infants is about 0.138–0.8 per 1,000 live term births. The frequency is much higher in premature infants and infants with congenital rubella syndrome and Trisomy 21. In addition, it occurs in 5–10% of all congenital heart disease. It is twice as common in females than males.

Pathology

The ductus arteriosus remains patent in utero due to low oxygen tension in the blood and a high level of circulating prostaglandins. With the baby's first few breaths, the oxygen tension rises. Simultaneously, there is a drop in the prostaglandin level due to metabolism in the infant's lungs and elimination of the placental source.

Closure of the ductus is initiated by smooth muscle contraction a few hours after birth. This is followed by enfolding of the endothelium, subintimal disruption and proliferation. The lumen is thus obliterated and the closed ductus is transformed into a fibrous ligament known as the ligamentum arteriosum. Failure of the ductus arteriosus to close results in maintenance of patency and therefore a channel for blood to shunt from the aorta to the pulmonary circulation (Fig. 8.1).

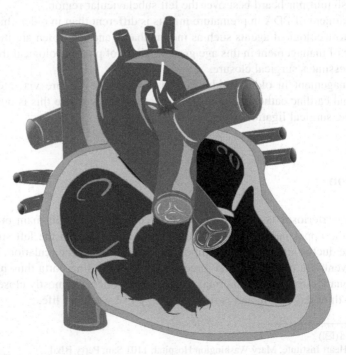

Fig. 8.1 PDA diagram. The patent ductus arteriosus connects the aortic arch to the main pulmonary artery at the take-off of the left pulmonary artery. The aortic end of the PDA is just before, at or just after the take-off of the left subclavian artery

Pathophysiology

After birth, the pulmonary vascular resistance begins to drop. If the ductus arteriosus fails to close, there will be shunting of blood from the high pressure aorta to the pulmonary circulation. This increased blood volume then returns to the left atrium, left ventricle, and ascending aorta and can cause volume overload and dilatation of these structures (Fig. 8.2). The degree of the dilatation is proportional to the degree of shunting, which is dependent on the size of the PDA and the pulmonary vascular resistance. With prolonged exposure to high pressure and increased flow, the pulmonary vasculature undergoes progressive morphological changes which can lead to pulmonary vascular obstructive disease.

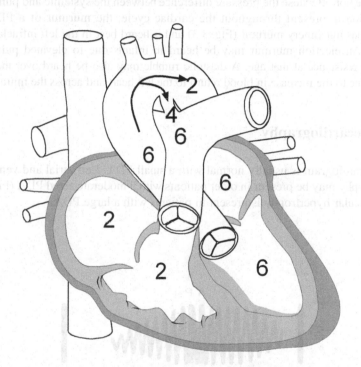

Fig. 8.2 Left to right shunting at the PDA. Numbers represent volume of blood flow in liters/minute/M^2 (l/min/M^2). The pulmonary vascular resistance is significantly less than the systemic vascular resistance, Any abnormal communication between the left and right sides of the heart will result in left to right shunting. In this diagram, 6 l/min/M^2 of blood returns from the lungs. Since the pulmonary vascular resistance is significantly less than the systemic vascular resistance, blood shunts left to right across the PDA, thus increasing blood flow to the lungs. In the scenario depicted in this diagram, 4 l/min/M^2 shunts across the PDA, thus leaving only 2 l/min/M^2 of cardiac output to the systemic circulation. Blood flow to the lungs versus that to the body (Qp:Qs ratio) in this scenario is 6:2 or 3:1. In patients with PDA there is volume overload of the left atria and left ventricle due to increase blood flow through these chambers

Clinical Manifestations

If the PDA is small, patients are typically asymptomatic. A large PDA will allow a significant volume of left to right shunting. The resulting pulmonary edema can manifest clinically as tachypnea, poor feeding, failure to thrive, recurrent respiratory infections, or congestive heart failure.

Physical findings depend on the degree of increase in pulmonary blood flow. Patients with a large PDA will develop tachycardia and tachypnea. Blood shunting from the aorta to the pulmonary arterial circulation will cause a drop in the diastolic pressure. The increase in blood return from the pulmonary veins into the left heart and aorta will cause elevation in systolic pressure. The result is an increased difference between systolic and diastolic pressures or a widened pulse pressure. The precordium is hyperactive and a systolic thrill may be palpable in the left upper sternal region. Because the pressure difference between the systemic and pulmonary circulation is present throughout the cardiac cycle, the murmur of a PDA is a continuous machinery murmur (Fig. 8.3) and is heard best in the left infraclavicular region. An ejection murmur may be heard in infants due to elevated pulmonary vascular resistance at that age. A diastolic rumble may also be heard over the apical region due to the increase in blood return to the left heart and across the mitral valve.

Electrocardiography

Electrocardiogram is usually normal with a small PDA. Left atrial and ventricular hypertrophy may be present in older patients with a moderate sized PDA (Fig. 8.4). Biventricular hypertrophy is present in patients with a large PDA.

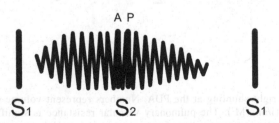

Fig. 8.3 Heart sounds and murmur in PDA. S1: first heart sound, S2: second heart sound, A: aortic valve closure, P: pulmonary valve closure. The pressure in the aorta is higher than that of the pulmonary artery during both systole and diastole, therefore, the murmur produced secondary to a PDA is continuous through systole and diastole. Due to the reduced blood volume in great vessels towards the end of diastole, blood flow is reduced just before the first heart sound and the murmur is not audible during late diastole. PDA murmur is best heard over the left infraclavicular region and tends to be harsh

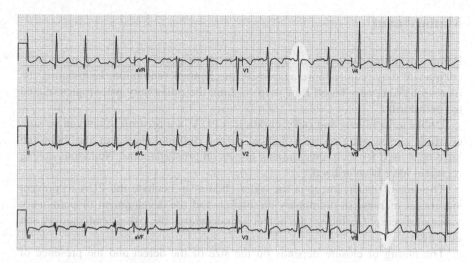

Fig. 8.4 ECG in PDA. Tall R in V6 and deep S in V1 indicate left ventricular hypertrophy. Patient with PDA may also have left atrial enlargement. The P wave in this ECG is within normal limits, though the borderline is widened

Chest Radiography

Chest X-ray is normal with a small PDA. Patients with a large shunt will develop left atrial and ventricular dilatation causing an enlargement in the cardiac silhouette (Chap. 2, Fig. 2.6). A dilated left atrium should be suspected if there is a wide angle of bronchial bifurcation at the carina and posterior deviation of the esophagus on lateral chest X-ray. Increased pulmonary vascular markings can also be seen with a large shunt.

Echocardiography

Echocardiography is the procedure of choice to confirm the diagnosis. Echocardiogram can define the size of the PDA as well as indirectly assess the degree of shunting by measuring left atrial and ventricular dilation. Echocardiography is also employed to rule out associated cardiac lesions (Chap. 4, Fig. 4.1).

Cardiac Catheterization

Cardiac catheterization is no longer necessary for diagnostic purposes. However, interventional cardiac catheterization is performed in most patients for therapeutic purposes. Occasionally, diagnostic catheterization is performed in older patients with a large PDA and pulmonary hypertension to assess the pulmonary vascular resistance and its response to vasodilators.

Management

Premature infants with a hemodynamically significant PDA develop pulmonary edema and may require more aggressive mechanical ventilation. Eliminating the increased pulmonary blood flow helps to limit the pulmonary pathologies related to prematurity.

Unlike term infants and older children, a PDA in a preterm infant can be successfully closed using pharmacological agents. Both indomethacin and ibuprofen have been used for their antagonizing effects on prostaglandins. Numerous dosing regimens have been utilized.

The aim of management in the older child is to occlude the PDA to prevent significant increase in pulmonary circulation and the development of pulmonary vascular disease. Occluding the defect also decreases the risk of endocarditis and endarteritis.

The timing of closure depends on the size of the defect and the presence of symptoms. In asymptomatic infants, conservative management is possible to allow time for spontaneous closure. In patients with a large PDA and congestive heart failure, the defect must be closed urgently.

Transcatheter occlusion has become the treatment of choice for most patients. Device closure is usually performed around 6–12 months of age. Placement of one or more coils in the ductus is usually sufficient to close small defects. In larger defects, an Amplatzer device, a cylindrical-shaped wire mesh plug, may be placed. The advantage of device closure is to avoid surgical thoracotomy; children can be discharged home the same day of procedure with good recovery. The complications may include residual leaks, coil embolization, hemolysis, pulmonary artery stenosis, or femoral vessel occlusion.

Surgical closure is performed in cases not amenable to a percutaneous approach, such as young infants with congestive heart failure or pulmonary hypertension. Ligation and division of the ductus is usually performed through left thoracotomy. More recently, some centers are using video-assisted thoracoscopic surgery (VATS) or robotic surgery to assist with the closure. Complications may include bleeding, pneumothorax, infection and rarely, ligation of the left pulmonary artery or aorta.

Long-Term Follow Up

The natural history of a PDA depends on the size of the lesion, the degree of left to right shunting and the status of the pulmonary vasculature. Patients with small defects have a normal prognosis apart from a small risk of developing endarteritis. In cases with a significant increase in pulmonary circulation and volume overload, there is a risk of congestive heart failure or irreversible pulmonary vascular disease. Rarely, marked dilatation of the PDA and possible rupture may occur in adults.

Ductus Arteriosus in Premature Infants

The increased incidence of PDA in premature infants is due to the physiological effects of prematurity rather than any abnormality of the ductus arteriosus structure itself. The incidence of PDA in preterm infants is about 8 per 1,000 live births. About 45% of newborns less than 1,750 g birth weight and about 80% of infants with a birth weight less than 1,200 g have clinical evidence of a PDA. The presence of respiratory distress syndrome may cause hypoxia and further promote ductal patency. Surfactant must be used cautiously in this population as it may rapidly lower pulmonary resistance causing an increase in left to right shunting. This is further complicated by an immature myocardium that may be unable to handle the volume overload.

Premature infants with PDA typically present at 3–7 days of age with an increase in respiratory distress, apnea and bradycardia or an inability to wean from ventilatory support. The physical examination reveals tachycardia, bounding peripheral pulses, a hyperactive precordium, and possibly a gallop rhythm on auscultation. The typical continuous PDA murmur may not be present; a systolic murmur is more likely to be heard in this age group.

Electrocardiography is usually not diagnostic, but can show tachycardia and sometimes left ventricular hypertrophy. Chest X-ray usually shows evidence of hyaline membrane disease which may obscure cardiac abnormalities. Echocardiography is diagnostic; it shows the presence and size of the defect and the amount of shunting.

Initial management usually includes fluid restriction, administration of diuretics, maintenance of a good hematocrit level, and ventilatory support as needed. The PDA can be closed pharmacologically or surgically. Pharmacologic closure can usually be achieved by a single course of indomethacin or ibuprofen. A second course may be given in case of persistence of patency. Pharmacologic closure is contraindicated in infants with thrombocytopenia, bleeding tendency (intracranial hemorrhage), necrotizing enterocolitis, renal failure (high creatinine or blood urea nitrogen), or hyperbilirubinemia. Surgical closure of PDA is utilized when medical management fails or is contraindicated. The PDA is usually ligated through a posterolateral thoracotomy. Surgical mortality is about 0–3%. Recently, the Video Assisted Thoracoscopic Surgery (VATS) has been used successfully in PDA closure.

Clinical Scenarios

Case 1

A 6-year-old boy was seen for a routine well-check visit. There was no history of shortness of breath, chest pain, palpitation, or easy fatigability. Past medical history was unremarkable. Mother reported that a heart murmur was heard on a physical examination 2 years prior. On physical examination, he was alert and in no distress. His heart rate was 84 bpm, blood pressure 100/58 mmHg, and oxygen saturation 98%. Cardiac examination revealed normal peripheral pulses, normal S1 and S2, and a grade 3/6 continuous murmur with clicking machinery sounds throughout. Electrocardiography showed normal sinus rhythm with no evidence of chamber enlargement.

The symptoms and signs noted here are suggestive of PDA. Therefore echocardiography was performed which revealed a small PDA with left to right shunting and no evidence of volume overload.

Discussion

Physical examination in this patient revealed an incidental finding of a heart murmur that is typical of a PDA murmur and should not be confused with an innocent heart murmur. Innocent heart murmurs are systolic only. The only type of innocent murmur which is continuous in nature is that of a venous hum. Those murmurs are soft, heard over the supraclavicular region, and disappear when pressure is applied over the jugular vein.

Echocardiogram confirmed the diagnosis. In a small PDA, there is no significant increase in pulmonary blood flow and patients are usually asymptomatic. However, due to the increased risk of endocarditis, closure is still recommended.

Management

The patient was referred for closure of the PDA via interventional cardiac catheterization. The defect was successfully closed using an occluding device to obstruct the small lumen of the ductus. It is recommended that such patients receive subacute bacterial endocarditis prophylaxis when indicated for 6 months after the procedure until the foreign bodies used are sealed from the circulation by a layer of endothelial tissue.

Case 2

A newborn male infant, delivered at 28 weeks gestation, with a birth weight of 900 g and APGAR scores of 6 and 8 at 1 and 5 min developed respiratory distress requiring intubation and mechanical ventilation. Surfactant was administered. The respiratory distress gradually improved and the ventilatory support was weaned. During the fourth day of life, the infant required increasing ventilatory support. Physical examination at the time showed a heart rate of 160 bpm, respiratory rate of 72/min, BP 60/20 mmHg, and Oxygen saturation 92%. Peripheral pulses were bounding. On auscultation, there were bilateral crackles and normal heart sounds with a 2–3/6 systolic murmur.

Chest X-ray showed a mildly enlarged cardiothymic silhouette with a prominent left atrium and ventricle and increased pulmonary vascular markings. An echocardiogram confirmed the diagnosis of a large PDA with left atrial and ventricular dilatation. Fluid restriction was initiated, and three doses of indomethacin were administered.

Discussion

As the pulmonary vascular resistance drops in the first few days of life, there is an increase in volume of left to right shunting. Surfactant therapy also lowers pulmonary vascular resistance, adding to the left to right shunting and worsening pulmonary overcirculation and symptoms of respiratory distress. Left to right shunting decreases systemic output and causes a widened pulse pressure due to the blood steal through the defect. The typical continuous murmur of PDA is usually not heard in premature infants; instead a short systolic murmur may be present.

Management

Patent ductus arteriosus in premature infants can be closed pharmacologically if there is no contraindication to the use of indomethacin or ibuprofen. Surgical ligation is indicated in cases where pharmacological treatment fails or is contraindicated. In many centers, the procedure is performed at the bedside in the neonatal intensive care unit avoiding the need to move the premature infant to the operating room.

Chapter 9
Atrioventricular Canal Defect

Omar M. Khalid and Surabhi Mona Mehrotra

Key Facts

- The majority of patients with complete AVC defect are children with trisomy 21 syndrome.
- AVC defect may be partial, manifesting as ASD and mitral valve cleft or complete, manifesting with ASD, VSD and a common AV valve. Many patients with AVC defect manifest with lesions in between partial and complete AVC defect.
- Combination of right ventricular hypertrophy and left axis deviation (rather than right axis deviation as one would expect secondary to right ventricular hypertrophy) on an electrocardiogram should alert to the possibility of AVC defect.
- Surgical repair in children with complete AVC defect depends on the balance of the common AV over the two ventricles. Straddling or hypoplasia of one side of the common AV valve will lead to hypoplasia of the corresponding ventricle which would prohibit biventricular repair.
- Children with hypoplasia of one of the ventricles will require univentricular repair (Glenn shunt followed by Fontan procedure).

Definition

Atrioventricular canal defects (AVCD) involve cardiac structures which develop through the embryologic endocardial cushion tissue. These anomalies may include a variety of defects such as: an ostium primum atrial septal defect (ASD), inlet type ventricular septal defect (VSD), and defects in mitral and tricuspid valves. In its extreme form, there is a single, common atrioventricular (AV) valve with adjacent

O.M. Khalid(✉)
Children's Heart Institute, Mary Washington Hospital, 1101 Sam Perry Blvd.,
Suite # 415, Fredericksburg, VA 22401, USA
e-mail: omarmkhalid@hotmail.com

Ra-id Abdulla (ed.), *Heart Diseases in Children: A Pediatrician's Guide*,
DOI 10.1007/978-1-4419-7994-0_9, © Springer Science+Business Media, LLC 2011

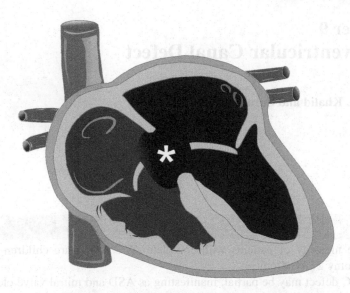

Fig. 9.1 Atrioventricular canal (AVC) defect. AVC defect includes adjacent atrial and ventricular septal defects with a common atrioventricular valve instead of separate tricuspid and mitral valve orifices

primum ASD, and inlet VSD (Fig. 9.1). This defect is also known as endocardial cushion defect, or AV septal defect.

Incidence

Atrioventricular canal defects accounts for 4% of all congenital heart diseases. About 70% of all patient of AVCD have Trisomy 21 syndrome. Children with Trsisomy 21 syndrome are commonly affected with congenital heart disease (40%) and 40% of these patients have AV canal defect.

Pathology

The degree of involvement of the endocardial cushion structures is variable. In complete AVCD there is usually a septum primum ASD, an inlet type VSD, and a common AV canal. The combination of these defects forms a large interatrial and interventricular communication. A single AV orifice spans the defect. The AV valve is usually composed of five leaflets with variable attachment to the septum. In balanced, common AVCD, the AV valve orifice is committed equally to both ventricles, i.e. sits equally over both ventricles. When the valve commitment is unbalanced, favoring one ventricle over the other, there will be discrepancy in the size of AV valves and ventricles. In severe cases, the small ventricle may be hypoplastic. The aortic valve is displaced anterosuperiorly due to the bridging leaf-lets of the common AV valve causing elongation of the left ventricular outflow tract, giving the "goose-neck" like deformity on angiographic images. Partial AV canal defect consists of a septum primum ASD with a cleft in the anterior leaflet of the mitral valve with no VSD. Transitional AV canal consists of an inlet VSD and primum ASD with a fusion of the anterior and posterior AV valve leaflets. Associated cardiac anomalies might include pulmonary valve stenosis, tetralogy of Fallot, double-outlet right ventricle, or transposition of the great arteries.

Pathophysiology

The pathophysiology of AVCD is similar to that of atrial and VSDs. There is left to right shunt across the atrial and ventricular defects in addition to the possibility of AV valve regurgitation (Fig. 9.2). Left to right shunting is usually

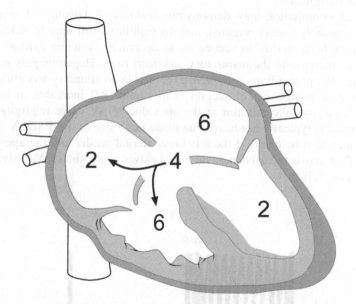

Fig. 9.2 Left to right shunting. Numbers represent volume of blood flow in liters/minute/M^2 (l/m/M^2). The pulmonary vascular resistance is significantly less than the systemic vascular resistance, therefore, any abnormal communication between the left and right sides of the heart will result in left to right shunting. In the case depicted in this diagram, 6 l/m/M^2 of blood return from the pulmonary circulation. Since the pulmonary vascular resistance is significantly less than the sys-temic vascular resistance, blood shunts left to right across the ASD and VSD, thus increasing blood flow to the lungs. In the scenario depicted in this diagram, 4 l/m/M^2 shunts across the VSD, thus leaving only 2 l/m/M^2 of cardiac output to the systemic circulation. Blood flow to the lungs versus that to the body (Qp:Qs ratio) in this scenario is 6:2 or 3:1. The increase in blood flow across the ventricles will cause biventricular enlargement. Atrioventricular valve regurgitation may also be present causing volume overload of either or both atria

significant, causing pulmonary overcirculation and decrease in left ventricular output, leading to dyspnea, easy fatigability, and failure to thrive. If left untreated, long-standing pulmonary hypertension will lead to changes in pulmonary vasculature and resistance that will eventually cause permanent pulmonary vascular obstructive disease. Children with Trisomy 21 syndrome tend to develop high pulmonary vascular resistance earlier than children without this syndrome.

Clinical Manifestations

Patients with AVCD present with symptoms of congestive heart failure due to the left to right shunting at the ASDs and VSDs, resulting in increase in pulmonary blood flow. This may include tachypnea, respiratory distress, recurrent respiratory infections, easy fatigability, and failure to thrive. When AVCD is associated with tetralogy of Fallot, there will also be cyanosis due to severe stenosis of the right ventricular outflow tract.

Physical examination may demonstrate features of Trisomy 21 syndrome. Infants are usually undernourished, and the capillary refill may be delayed due to poor peripheral perfusion secondary to decreased systemic cardiac output. There is an increase in the respiratory and heart rates. Hepatomegaly may also be present. The precordium is hyperactive. First heart sound is accentuated and the pulmonary component of second heart sound (P2) increases in intensity. There is a holosystolic murmur at the apex due to AV valve regurgitation. A VSD murmur is typically not heard due to the large size of the VSD. A diastolic murmur may also be heard at the left lower sternal border and the apex due to increase flow across the tricuspid and mitral valves as a result of AV valve regurgitation (Fig. 9.3).

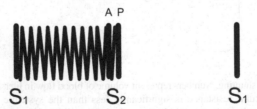

Fig. 9.3 Heart sounds and murmur in AVC defect. S1: first heart sound, S2: second heart sound, A: aortic valve closure, P: pulmonary valve closure. The VSD in AVC defect tends to be large with equal pressures in both ventricles, therefore, flow across the VSD, even though large in volume may not be turbulent and as such silent. Smaller VSDs may cause holosystolic murmur. The holosystolic murmur heard in most patients with AVC defect may be the result of AV valve regurgitation, rather than ventricular septal defect

Electrocardiography

The inlet VSD causes displacement of the normal pathway of the bundle of His and its branches resulting in abnormal direction ventricular depolarization. Depolarization of the ventricles assumes an inferior-superior direction resulting in superior axis deviation of the QRS (between −60° and −150°). In addition, electrical conduction across the abnormal bundle AV node and bundle branches will result in prolonged PR interval. ASD and VSD, together with AV valve regurgitation cause volume overload for both ventricles manifesting as right and left ventricular hypertrophy. Right ventricular hypertrophy is manifested as tall R waves in V1 and V2, or possibly through a pure R or qR wave patterns in these leads. Left ventricular hypertrophy manifests as tall R wave in V5 and V6 and deep S waves in leads V1 and V2. If severe mitral valve regurgitation is present, left atrial enlargement is also noted, this manifests as wide P waves, with or without bifid or biphasic P wave (Fig. 9.4).

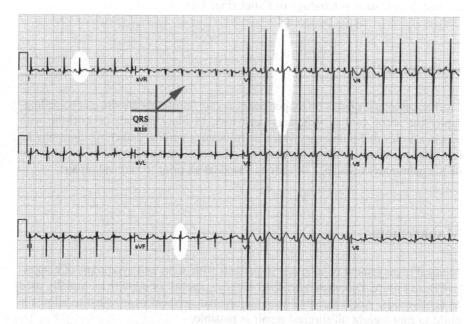

Fig. 9.4 Volume overload of right and left ventricles manifest as right and/or left ventricular hypertrophy. Displacement of the atrioventricular conduction system results in superior axis deviation seen as negative QRS axis on ECG. In the ECG shown here, the QRS axis is abnormal (−45) with RVH (tall R in V1)

Chest X-Ray

The degree of cardiomegaly and increased pulmonary vascular markings is proportional to the size of the left to right shunt and the amount of AV valve regurgitation. There is generalized enlargement of the cardiac silhouette due to enlargement of all cardiac chambers. The pulmonary vasculature is prominent, reflecting an increase in pulmonary blood flow. Left atrial enlargement may cause the carina angle to be widened since the tracheal bifurcation is anatomically just above the left atrium (Fig. 2.7).

Echocardiogram

Echocardiography allows imaging of the AVCD. The size of the atrial and ventricular defects, the anatomy of the AV valve leaflets, and the alignment to the ventricles can be clearly visualized. In addition, the AV valve chordal attachments, papillary muscles orientation, and the size of the ventricles can be accurately assessed with echocardiography. Regurgitation of the atrioventricular valve can be assessed through color Doppler. Echocardiography is also useful in assessing an associated cardiac defect, such as tetralogy of Fallot (Fig. 4.2).

Catheterization

Cardiac catheterization is no longer necessary for most patients since echocardiography can show cardiac structures very well. In older patients or in those with suspected elevated pulmonary vascular resistance, cardiac catheterization may be indicated to determine the pulmonary vascular resistance and to assess the response of the pulmonary resistance to various vasodilators prior to surgical repair.

Management

Medical management is indicated in patients with signs and symptoms of congestive heart failure. Diuretics, after-load reducing agents, or digoxin are usually used to achieve this. Anticongestive heart failure management is provided to allow the child to gain weight till surgical repair is possible.

Surgery is indicated in all patients with AVCD since this lesion is incompatible with life due to the excessive pulmonary blood flow it causes and development of pulmonary vascular obstructive disease leading to Eisenmenger's syndrome in most patients during the second or third decades of life. Surgery is best performed between 6 and 12 weeks of age since morbidity and mortality from this procedure plateaus at that age, rendering further delay unnecessary. In balanced AV canal defect, one or two patches are used to close the ASDs and VSDs. The common atrioventricular valve is reconstructed into two separate AV valves: mitral and tricuspid. Surgical mortality is approximately 3–10%. Postoperative complications may include arrhythmia, such as supraventricular tachycardia, heart block, or sinus node dysfunction; it may also include significant valve regurgitation, residual septal defect, and subaortic stenosis.

In unbalanced atrioventricular canal defect, patients usually undergo staged Fontan procedure. The Fontan procedure allows single or both ventricles to pump blood into the systemic circulation. Examples of a single ventricle within common AVCD include hypoplasia of one of the ventricles and examples of two ventricles without the possibility of complete biventricular repair is in the event of straddling of the chordal attachments of one of the atrioventricular valves into the opposite ventricle preventing closure of the VSD by surgical patch, or in the event of hypoplasia, or atresia of one of the AV valves preventing access to its ventricle. Dedicating all functional ventricles to the systemic circualtion leaves the pulmonary circulation without a pumping ventricle which is overcome by direct connection of the superior vena cava to pulmonary arteries (Glenn shunt) and subsequently the inferior vena cava to the pulmonary circulation (completion of Fontan). Glenn shunt is typically performed at 4–8 months of age and the completion of Fontan at 12–24 months of age.

Complications of unrepaired AVCD may include recurrent chest infections and congestive heart failures. Increase pulmonary blood flow will cause pulmonary vascular obstructive disease, eventually leading to irreversible changes in the pulmonary vasculature, thus leading to cyanosis and death. Irreversible pulmonary obstructive vascular disease can only be treated through heart–lung transplant.

Case 1

A 4-week-old female infant presents with a 1-week history of increased work of breathing, nasal flaring, coughing, feeding difficulties, and excessive diaphoresis.

Her past medical history is unremarkable. She was born at full term with no perinatal complications.

Physical exam reveals heart rate of 166 bpm, blood pressure of 88/56 mmHg, respiratory rate of 66 breaths per minute, and oxygen saturation of 94% on room air. The infant is in mild respiratory distress with occasional subcostal retractions. The chest examination reveals normal vesicular breath sounds bilaterally with fine crackles at the bases. Auscultation reveals holosystolic murmur at the cardiac apex. The liver edge is palpated at 2 cm below the right costal margin. The capillary refill is prolonged.

Electrocardiography shows sinus rhythm with superior QRS axis (–90°) and RVH voltage criteria. Chest X-ray shows a prominent cardiac silhouette and an increase in pulmonary vascular markings, suggestive of increased pulmonary blood flow.

Discussion

The symptoms encountered in this child are consistent with congestive heart failure due to excessive pulmonary blood flow and pulmonary edema, however, not exclusive of heart diseases, since pulmonary diseases such as pneumonia due to infectious or aspiration etiologies may result in similar presentation. The signs on physical examination on the other hand seem to suggest a cardiac etiology, particularly the holosystolic murmur. This type of murmur is seen secondary to mitral regurgitation and VSDs since blood shunting starts with the beginning of ventricular contraction and lasts throughout systole. Tricuspid valve regurgitation is typically not audible since the pulmonary and right ventricular pressures are much lower than that of the left ventricle with the exception of the immediate neonatal period or when pulmonary hypertension is present.

Chest X-ray confirms the likelihood of cardiac etiology in view of cardiomegaly and increased blood flow pattern. Electrocardiography is highly suggestive of AV canal defect in view of the superior axis deviation and right ventricular hypertrophy. Superior axis deviation is not a feature of VSD, unless it is a component of AV canal defect.

An echocardiogram is performed and shows a large primum ASD, inlet type VSD, and a balanced common AV canal defect with dilated right atrium and ventricle with moderate left AV valve regurgitation. This is consistent with common AV canal defect.

Management

Treatment is initiated with furosemide to reduce blood volume (decrease preload), as well as Captopril or enalapril to reduce the after-load and control congestive heart failure symptoms. Caloric intake is increased by increasing caloric concentration of formula to promote weight gain. Due to the increased risk of respiratory infections, the child is also placed on respiratory syncytial virus (RSV) prophylaxis, until cardiac repair can be performed, typically at 4–8 months of age.

Case 2

A 3-day-old male infant is recently diagnosed with Down syndrome. He is tolerating feeds with no difficulty, but the mother reports blue discoloration of the lips and tongue when he is crying. His past medical history is unremarkable. He was born at full term with no perinatal complications.

Physical examination reveals heart rate of 135 bpm, respiratory rate of 42 breaths per minute, and oxygen saturation of 92% on room air. The infant is alert with no respiratory distress and lungs are clear to auscultation bilaterally. Cardiovascular examination reveals a normal precordium with normal upper and lower extremity pulses. Cardiac auscultation indicates normal first heart sound and single second heart sound. There is grade 3/6 harsh systolic ejection murmur at the left upper sternal border and no diastolic murmur. The abdomen is soft, without hepatosplenomegaly.

Electrocardiogram shows sinus rhythm with a northwest QRS axis (superior axis: 100°) and RVH voltage criteria.

Discussion

History is suggestive of cyanotic congenital heart disease versus episodes of aspiration during feeding, although the latter should be accompanied by coughing and evidence of acute respiratory event. Cardiac examination provides more evidence that this child has cyanotic congenital heart disease. The oxygen saturation baseline is slightly depressed (92%) and the harsh systolic murmur is indicative of cardiac pathology, particularly that of pulmonary stenosis. Superior axis deviation in ECG suggests AVC defect, however, this is not typically associated with cyanosis unless there is tetralogy of Fallot in addition to the AVC defect, a combination of lesions typically noted in patients with Trisomy 21 syndrome.

Echocardiogram shows a common AV canal with large primum ASD, common AV valve, and mild regurgitation. In addition, the inlet VSD extends to the perimembranous region of the ventricular septum with overriding of the aorta. The right ventricular outflow tract is narrow and there is pulmonary valve stenosis, confluent but small pulmonary arteries, and no evidence of coarctation of the aorta.

There is a relatively high incidence of congenital heart disease in Down syndrome. A combination of AVCD and tetralogy of Fallot may occur. The inlet VSD extends towards the perimembranous area with anterior deviation of the infundibular septum causing right ventricular outflow tract obstruction and overriding of the aorta.

The clinical presentation depends on the degree of pulmonary stenosis. The pulmonary valve stenosis may protect the lung from pulmonary overcirculation and symptoms of congestive heart failure; the patient will be asymptomatic. But if the stenosis is severe, the patient will be cyanotic with further exacerbation of cyanosis with crying or increasing effort.

Management

Surgical repair is indicated in this child, the timing of this is determined by symptomotalogy. If the extent of pulmonary stenosis is significant, but not severe, it will prevent excessive pulmonary blood flow and surgical repair can be delayed to 6–10 months of age when morbidity and mortality for surgical repair plateaus. On the other hand, if pulmonary stenosis is severe, there will be limitation to pulmonary blood flow resulting in increasing right to left shunting at the VSD and worsening cyanosis, in this event; earlier surgical repair may be indicated. In the rare cases when pulmonary stenosis is critical with extremely depressed pulmonary blood flow, a systemic to pulmonary arterial shunt may be needed in the neonatal period to provide adequate pulmonary blood flow until more definitive repair can be preformed.

Chapter 10
Pulmonary Stenosis

Joan F. Hoffman, Surabhi Mona Mehrotra, and Shannon M. Buckvold

Key Facts

- Noonan syndrome is associated with valvular pulmonary stenosis, Williams syndrome is associated with supravalvular pulmonary (and aortic) stenosis, while Allagile and congenital Rubella are associated with peripheral pulmonary stenosis.
- Pulmonary stenosis, even when severe is typically asymptomatic. Right heart failure develops in critical or long-standing pulmonary stenosis.
- Valvular pulmonary stenosis is almost always associated with systolic click preceding the systolic ejection murmur.
- Soft P2 may indicate abnormal pulmonary valve due to pulmonary stenosis.
- Mild pulmonary stenosis rarely worsens in intensity.
- SBE prophylaxis is not required in pulmonary stenosis, regardless of severity.

Definition

Congenital obstruction to right ventricular outflow can occur at the level of pulmonary valve leaflets (valvular, 90%), in the muscular region below the valve (subvalvular, infundibular), or above the valve in the pulmonary artery (supravalvular) (Fig. 10.1). Branch pulmonary artery stenosis affecting the branch and peripheral pulmonary arteries may be present with or without valvular pulmonary stenosis.

J.F. Hoffman (✉)
Department of Pediatrics, Rush University Medical Center, 1653 W. Congress Parkway, Suite 770 Jones, Chicago, IL 60612, USA
e-mail: joan_hoffman@rush.edu

Ra-id Abdulla (ed.), *Heart Diseases in Children: A Pediatrician's Guide*,
DOI 10.1007/978-1-4419-7994-0_10, © Springer Science+Business Media, LLC 2011

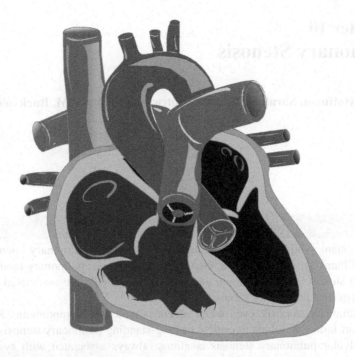

Fig. 10.1 Pulmonary stenosis (PS). The pulmonary valve orifice is small; this may be a result of thickening of valve cusps, adhesion of cusp edges rendering separation between cusps during systole limited and/or due to small valve annulus

Prevalence

As an isolated lesion, valvular pulmonary stenosis is the second most common CHD (8% of all CHDs). Pulmonary stenosis at some level, whether valvular, subvalvular, or supravalvular, occurs in 30–50% of other congenital heart diseases. Pulmonary stenosis occurs more frequently in females.

Pulmonary stenosis also occurs with greater frequency in certain genetic disorders:

- In Noonan syndrome, pulmonary stenosis occurs in 39% of patients, and can be associated with stenosis of the peripheral pulmonary arteries as well as with hypertrophic cardiomyopathy.
- In Williams syndrome, patients often develop diffuse arteriopathy, with supravalvular and peripheral pulmonary stenosis occurring in 41%.
- In Alagille syndrome, 53% of patients have stenosis at some level of the pulmonary vasculature.

Supravalvular pulmonary stenosis also occurs as a result of intrauterine (congenital) rubella infection.

Pathology

In the most common form of pulmonary stenosis, the pulmonary valve is dome-shaped, with thickened, and/or fused leaflets. The pulmonary annulus is often hypoplastic.

As a result of the small valve orifice, the right ventricle is hypertrophied. This includes the collar of muscle (the infundibulum) below the pulmonary valve, which causes subpulmonary (infundibular) stenosis. The hypertrophied right ventricle often exhibits a small chamber size, and the thick myocardium may be ischemic, particularly in the subendocardial region. On the other side of the stenotic pulmonary valve, post-stenotic dilation of the main pulmonary artery commonly occurs. Subpulmonary stenosis without valvular stenosis is unusual, except when there is an associated ventricular septal defect. In this case, poststenotic dilation of the pulmonary artery does not occur.

Supravalvular pulmonary stenosis, branch pulmonary artery stenosis, and peripheral pulmonary artery stenosis may occur in isolation, multiples, or diffusely throughout the pulmonary vasculature. The lesions are characterized by fibrous intimal proliferation, medial hypoplasia, and elastic fiber degeneration and disorganization. These ultrastructural changes within the pulmonary vasculature make the vessels small and stiff. In some cases, these changes can be progressive and severe, and when diffuse, are frequently associated with a genetic disorder. The peripheral pulmonary stenosis described in this chapter should be distinguished from normal small branch pulmonary arteries noted during the first 6 weeks of life producing an innocent heart murmur and eventually resolves spontaneously at about 6–8 weeks of life.

Pathophysiology

Pulmonary stenosis can be mild, moderate, or severe. The severity of the stenosis results in a proportional rise in right ventricular pressure so as to maintain cardiac output. A sustained increase in right ventricular pressure causes a progressive increase in right ventricular wall thickness, myocardial oxygen demand, and myocardial ischemia. These changes significantly reduce right ventricular compliance, and when combined with the small chamber size that occurs as a consequence of right ventricular hypertrophy (RVH), lead to reduced right ventricular preload and increased right atrial pressure. In the absence of an associated atrial septal defect, right ventricular failure occurs in infancy. Left ventricular failure also ensues from leftward shift of the interventricular septum, reduced preload, outflow obstruction, increased myocardial oxygen demand, and myocardial ischemia.

On the other hand, the presence of a patent foramen ovale or atrial septal defect facilitates decompression of the right atrium though a right-to-left shunt across the atrial septum, with resulting cyanosis. Cyanosis will be intensified by any increase in oxygen demand, such as with crying in a neonate or exercise in an older child, since increased tissue oxygen demands are met by increased tissue oxygen extraction. The resulting lower saturation of hemoglobin in blood that returns to the heart and is shunted across the atrial septum contributes to the appearance of frank cyanosis.

Critical pulmonary stenosis produces cyanosis secondary to increased right-to-left shunt at the atrial level, which occurs as a consequence of severe fetal pulmonary stenosis and a severely hypertensive, hypoplastic, noncompliant right ventricle. In this case, neonatal pulmonary blood flow is provided by the ductus arteriosus, so that when the ductus constricts, cyanosis is intensified.

Branch and peripheral pulmonary stenoses lead to the redistribution of blood flow to normal or less affected lung segments. As a result, some lung segments are under-perfused and subject to ischemic injury, while others are overperfused, and subject to injury from flow-related shear forces. Right ventricular hypertension and hyper-trophy occurs when branch and peripheral pulmonary stenosis is diffuse and severe.

Clinical Manifestations

As with all other obstructive lesions, the severity of obstruction predicts the clinical manifestations. Infants and children exhibit normal growth and development, even when stenosis is severe.

- Mild pulmonary stenosis is asymptomatic. The diagnosis is commonly made by the detection of a pathologic murmur. Cardiac examination is significant for a normoactive precordium, without a right ventricular heave or thrill. The first heart sound is normal, followed by a widely split S2. An ejection click at the upper left sternal border can often be detected, and corresponds to the opening of the doming pulmonary valve. The murmur is of an ejection quality and of medium intensity, usually grade 3 or less, and is best appreciated at the left upper sternal border, with radiation to the back (Fig. 10.2). The P2 intensity can be

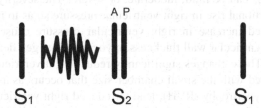

A P

S_1 S_2 S_1

Fig. 10.2 Heart sounds and murmur in PS. *S1* first heart sound, *S2* second heart sound, *A* aortic valve closure, *P* pulmonary valve closure. Obstruction to blood flow across the pulmonary valve results in the elevation of right ventricular pressure over pulmonary arterial pressure. This pressure gradient causes blood flow across the pulmonary valve to be turbulent and consequently noisy (murmur). The murmur starts with a systolic click as a result of opening of thickened valve cusps and followed by systolic ejection murmur as blood crosses the stenotic valve. The murmur's harshness increases with severity of stenosis, although in extreme cases due to resulting heart failure, the murmur may become softer. A systolic ejection murmur not preceded by a systolic click may suggest diagnosis other than pulmonary valve stenosis. Stenosis of the right ventricular outflow tract, below or above the valve with a normal valve present with a murmur similar to pulmonary stenosis, however, without the click. Pulmonary stenosis murmur is best heard over the left upper sternal border

either slightly diminished, secondary to decreased pulmonary artery pressure, or slightly increased, secondary to poststenotic pulmonary artery dilation.

- Moderate to severe pulmonary artery stenosis may result in fatigue and reduced exercise tolerance. Moderate valvular stenosis is often well tolerated in children, but produces clinical symptoms with advancing age. Severe valvular stenosis can lead to exercise-related chest pain, syncope, or sudden death. Cardiac examination is often significant for increased precordial activity, with a right ventricular heave and a palpable thrill in the area of the pulmonary valve at the left upper sternal border. The first heart sound is normal, followed by a widely split S2. The earlier the ejection click is detected at the upper left sternal border, the more severe is the stenosis. The murmur is of an ejection quality and of high intensity, usually grade 4 or more, and is best appreciated at the left upper sternal border, with radiation to the back. The louder and longer the murmur, the more severe is the stenosis. The P2 intensity is often diminished, secondary to decreased pulmonary artery pressure.
- Critical pulmonary stenosis is manifest by cyanosis in neonates shortly after birth. Since the pulmonary valve in most cases does not open, an ejection click and P2 will not be present. As very little or no flow across the pulmonary valve occurs, the murmur will be quite soft. A ductal murmur may be audible.
- Branch pulmonary artery stenosis and peripheral pulmonary stenosis may produce fatigue and exercise intolerance, but also may produce very few symptoms until either stenosis is severe and diffuse, or until a pulmonary air space disease such as infection or atelectasis occurs in the lung segments receiving the redistributed flow. Murmurs of branch pulmonary stenoses are appreciated in the back, with radiation to the axillae. A continuous murmur in the back and axillae suggests significant bilateral branch pulmonary artery stenosis. Peripheral pulmonary stenosis may produce no murmurs at all. A right ventricular systolic impulse may also be appreciated.

Chest Radiography

The heart size is often normal, except in critical pulmonary stenosis, when the heart size may be increased secondary to right atrial enlargement. A prominent main pulmonary artery notch from poststenotic dilation of the pulmonary artery can often be appreciated in older infants and children. Lung fields appear variably void of pulmonary vascular markings (black or anemic), reflecting reduced pulmonary blood flow from increasing stenosis. Cardiomegaly develops when heart failure ensues (Fig. 2.8).

Chest radiography in children with branch and peripheral pulmonary artery stenoses is commonly normal, but there may be a difference in vascularity between the two lung fields. Right ventricular and right atrial enlargement occurs when stenosis is severe and complicated by right ventricular failure.

Electrocardiography

Mild pulmonary stenosis produces a normal ECG. Moderate to severe pulmonary stenosis is reflected by right axis deviation (QRS axis 120–180 or greater) and RVH (a qR or rsR' in V1 and V3R, often with tall R waves and upright T waves). Severe pulmonary stenosis is reflected by a right ventricular strain pattern (tall R waves in V1 with depressed ST segment and inverted T waves) and sometimes by right atrial enlargement (peaked P waves >2 mm in II and V1) (Fig. 10.3).

Left axis deviation (QRS 0 to −90) is frequently demonstrated in infants with peripheral pulmonary artery stenosis – particularly with stenosis resulting from Rubella syndrome – and in infants with Noonan syndrome.

Echocardiography

Two-dimensional echocardiography demonstrates the abnormal pulmonary valve with restricted motion, and poststenotic dilation of the pulmonary artery. Measurements can be made of the pulmonary valve annulus and the branch pulmonary arteries and compared with normative data. Color Doppler demonstrates turbulent flow through the valve, and spectral Doppler produces a pulse wave from which the pressure gradient across the valve is estimated:

- Mild stenosis – Doppler pressure gradient of 35 mmHg or less, or estimated right ventricular pressure less than half the left ventricular pressure.

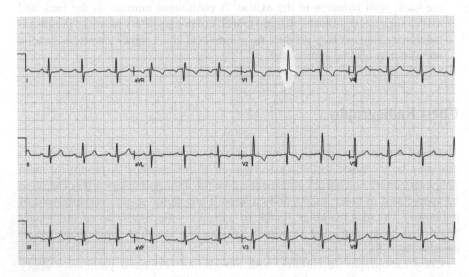

Fig. 10.3 ECG in PS. Right ventricular hypertrophy (RVH) is present. This may manifest in many different ways (see Chap. 3). In this ECG, the QRS complex pattern in the right chest leads (V1) is consistent with RVH: rsR' where the R' wave is taller than the r wave

- Moderate stenosis – Doppler pressure gradient of 36–60 mmHg or estimated right ventricular pressure 50–75% of left ventricular pressure.
- Severe stenosis – Doppler pressure gradient of greater than 60 mmHg or estimated right ventricular pressure greater than 75% of left ventricular pressure.

Two-dimensional echocardiography also demonstrates areas of supravalvular and branch pulmonary artery stenosis. Color and spectral Doppler can be similarly used to evaluate the flow and pressure gradients across the areas of obstruction. The entire right ventricular outflow must be sequentially examined, as multiple levels of obstruction may occur and impact the estimated pressure gradient across the pulmonary valve.

Right ventricular development, hypertrophy, and systolic and diastolic function can be assessed. Tricuspid valve measurements and functional assessment can be evaluated. Right atrial size, presence of an interatrial communication, and direction of atrial septal flow can be demonstrated. In neonates with concern for critical pulmonary stenosis, patency of the ductus arteriosus can be determined.

Cardiac Catheterization

Cardiac catheterization is reserved for therapeutic intervention. For valvular pulmonary stenosis, hemodynamic data are recorded, and angiography is performed for functional assessment and annular measurement of the pulmonary valve. Balloon valvuloplasty successfully provides valve patency, and has supplanted surgical valvotomy as the choice treatment for this lesion. Varying degrees of pulmonary insufficiency result from this intervention, which is typically well tolerated by the hypertrophied right ventricle.

Cardiac catheterization for supravalvular, branch, and peripheral pulmonary stenosis deserves special mention. Diagnostic cardiac catheterization is performed to provide a hemodynamic understanding of often multiple levels of obstruction, and also to provide angiographic pictures of the peripheral pulmonary vasculature. Because these lesions are characterized by ultrastructural changes such as fibrous intimal proliferation, they can be resistant to standard balloon angioplasty, and require the use of specialized equipment such as cutting balloons and stents, which provide variable results.

Following successful balloon angioplasty of severely stenotic peripheral pulmonary arteries, reperfusion injury to the distal lung segment sometimes occurs, and is clinically characterized by cough, low-grade fever, hypoxemia, and corresponding segmental air space disease on chest radiograph.

Other Diagnostic Modalities

Magnetic resonance imaging can be useful in defining peripheral pulmonary vascular anatomy and pathology, while radionuclide lung perfusion scans can be useful for quantifying blood flow to each lung.

Treatment

Mild pulmonary stenosis produces no symptoms and no difference in life expectancy. Symptoms should not be attributed to mild pulmonary stenosis if stenosis is indeed mild. Serial medical observation by a cardiologist is often advised every 3 years.

Moderate pulmonary stenosis is often treated with medical observation, and is typically well tolerated by infants and young children. Indications for catheter intervention include symptoms of fatigue and exercise intolerance, symptoms which often are experienced with increased age, even with stable stenosis.

Severe pulmonary stenosis can be successfully treated by catheter-based balloon angioplasty. Surgical valvotomy is reserved for patients in whom balloon valvuloplasty has been unsuccessful or for patients in whom multiple levels of obstruction are demonstrated.

Critical pulmonary stenosis requires prompt initiation of prostaglandin infusion to maintain ductal patency and provide pulmonary blood flow. Following complete echocardiographic assessment, most neonates proceed to the cardiac catheterization laboratory for balloon valvuloplasty, after which the prostaglandin infusion is discontinued. Occasionally, infundibular stenosis becomes apparent following balloon valvuloplasty, and a surgical Gore-tex shunt is required to maintain pulmonary blood flow. Though pulmonary valve patency has been established, many neonates continue to demonstrate moderate cyanosis, with SpO_2 of 70–80%, which improves slowly over several months as the right ventricular compliance improves and decreases the degree of right to left atrial level shunt. An infant with a history of critical or severe pulmonary stenosis and pulmonary valvuloplasty requires pulse oximetry assessment at each visit. Worsening saturations should prompt cardiology consultation.

In the rare instance of isolated infundibular stenosis, patch widening of the right ventricular outflow tract and resection of the infundibular muscle are required.

Treatment for supravalvular and branch pulmonary artery stenosis includes frequent medical observation. Catheter intervention is indicated following the onset and/or progression of symptoms. Surgical pericardial or prosthetic patch augmentation is indicated for severe stenosis not amenable to catheter-based interventions.

Treatment options for patients with diffuse peripheral pulmonary arterial obstruction syndromes (Noonan, Williams, Alagille, and Rubella) are limited and outcome is generally poor, particularly because lesions tend to be progressive. However, most patients undergo serial balloon angioplasty catheter interventions with the hope of modifying disease progression. Since the obstructions are fixed, pulmonary vasodilators such as nitric oxide, sildenafil, epoprostenol, or bosentan are ineffective.

Patients with diffuse arteriopathy are at increased risk for sudden death with procedural sedation and anesthesia, and should therefore be referred for cardiology evaluation before any procedures or surgeries.

In accordance with the most recent recommendations by the American Heart Association, subacute bacterial endocarditis prophylaxis is no longer indicated for isolated pulmonary stenosis. If pulmonary stenosis is associated with a right-to-left atrial shunt, or if associated with surgical or transcatheter prosthetic material, then subacute bacterial endocarditis prophylaxis should be provided as long as there is a residual lesion.

Case Scenarios

Case 1A

A 1-day-old infant born at 40 2/7 weeks' gestation develops cyanosis without respiratory distress at 24 h of life. On examination, she is awake, cyanotic, and tachypneic with a respiratory rate in the 60's. SpO_2 is 53% on room air. Precordium feels normal. On auscultation, lung sounds are clear and heart tones are normal, without a click or a distinct P2 component. A soft systolic murmur is appreciated at the left upper sternal border. Brachial and femoral pulses are normal on simultaneous palpation. Liver edge is palpable at the right costal margin. When provided 100% oxygen by mask, the SpO_2 changes very little.

Discussion

This history is typical of an infant with ductal-dependent pulmonary blood flow. The infant requires prompt initiation of prostaglandin infusion to maintain ductal patency. Oxygen administration does not improve the saturation because blood delivery to the lungs is compromised in the setting of obstructed pulmonary outflow and a closing ductus arteriosus. A chest radiograph, electrocardiogram, and echocardiogram can be performed to establish the diagnosis of critical pulmonary stenosis, following initiation of prostaglandin infusion. The differential diagnosis includes a variety of congenital heart lesions which include severe or critical pulmonary stenosis such as tetralogy of Fallow with severe pulmonary stenosis. On the other hand, lesions with tricuspid or pulmonary atresia are unlikely to present in this fashion since these are ductal-dependent lesions, which would provide increase in pulmonary blood flow and restriction or closure of the ductus arteriosus would result in severe and life-threatening deterioration due to acute drop in blood flow to the lungs.

Chest X-ray: In this infant, the cardiac silhouette is normal, without evidence of cardiac enlargement (Fig. 10.4). Though many infants with critical pulmonary stenosis have right atrial enlargement and cardiomegaly on chest radiograph, the diagnosis can still be suggested in infants without cardiomegaly by noting the dark lung fields which occur as a result of reduced pulmonary blood flow.

Echocardiography: An echocardiogram confirms the diagnosis of critical pulmonary stenosis with a patent ductus arteriosus supplying pulmonary blood flow to good-sized branch pulmonary arteries. The pulmonary valve annulus is reasonably sized. The pulmonary valve leaflets are thickened, doming, and minimally mobile,

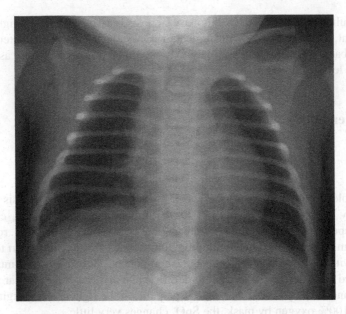

Fig. 10.4 AP Chest X-ray: The cardiac silhouette is normal, without evidence of cardiac enlargement. The pulmonary vasculature is reduced suggestive of reduced pulmonary blood flow

with no demonstrable flow across the valve. The right ventricle is hypertrophied with a small chamber size, and it contracts poorly. The interventricular septum bows into the left ventricle, suggesting the right ventricular pressure is greater than the left. The tricuspid valve is normal-sized. A patent foramen ovale is present with mostly right-to-left flow.

Cardiac catheterization: The infant is taken to the cardiac catheterization laboratory, where a catheter is advanced from the right femoral vein to the right atrium and then manipulated into the right ventricle. The measured right ventricular systolic pressure is 123 mmHg, compared with a systolic blood pressure of 74 mmHg. An angiogram is performed, which demonstrates a tiny "blow-hole" in the pulmonary valve, thereby distinguishing pulmonary valve stenosis from atresia.

The anterior–posterior view (Fig. 10.5a) and lateral view (Fig. 10.5b) of the right ventricular angiogram demonstrate a small, trabeculated right ventricle with a well-developed right ventricular outflow tract, and a narrow orifice through which contrast passes into the well-developed main pulmonary artery.

Balloon valvuloplasty of the pulmonary valve (Fig. 10.6a, b). A guidewire is advanced from the femoral vein to the right atrium, and then manipulated across the tricuspid valve and the pulmonary valve, to the ductus arteriosus and down the descending aorta. The balloon is tracked over the guidewire and positioned across the pulmonary valve. Note that as the balloon is inflated (Fig. 10.6a), the "waist" of the balloon disappears as it opens the valve and relieves the stenosis (Fig. 10.6b).

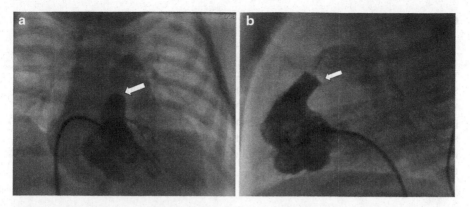

Fig. 10.5 Right ventricular angiogram: The anterior–posterior view (**a**) and lateral view (**b**) of the right ventricular angiogram demonstrate a small, trabeculated right ventricle with a well-developed right ventricular outflow tract and a narrow orifice through which contrast (*white arrows*) passes into the well developed main pulmonary artery

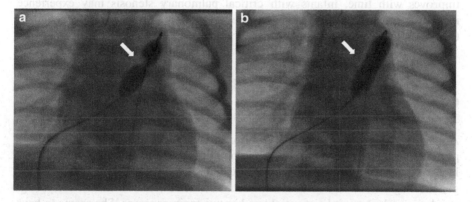

Fig. 10.6 (**a, b**) Balloon valvuloplasty of the pulmonary valve. A guidewire is advanced from the femoral vein to the right atrium, and then manipulated across the tricuspid valve and the pulmonary valve, to the ductus arteriosus and down the descending aorta. The balloon is tracked over the guidewire and positioned across the pulmonary valve. Note that as the balloon is inflated (**a**), the "waist" of the balloon disappears (*white arrows*) as it opens the valve and relieves the stenosis (**b**)

Pulse oximetry at the start of the procedure was 80% in room air, with continuous prostaglandin infusion. Following the balloon valvuloplasty, the pulse oximetry improved to 87%. The right ventricular systolic pressure is now down to 45 mmHg, compared with a systolic blood pressure of 68 mmHg. Because RVH and diastolic dysfunction persist, the patent foramen ovale still shunts blood right-to-left, decreasing the systemic SpO_2. However, as the RVH resolves and the diastolic pressure improves, the saturation will improve because the patent foramen ovale will shunt less right-to-left and more left-to-right.

Case 1B

The same infant presents to the office at 2 months of age for follow-up. Since the last visit at 1 month of age, the infant has been feeding and acting normally. The parents state that the infant still turns blue when she cries. On examination, the infant appears vigorous, but is pale and dusky. The precordium is hyperdynamic, and a thrill is palpable at the left upper sternal border. An audible click is present at the left upper sternal border, along with a 4/6 harsh ejection-quality (crescendo–decrescendo) murmur which radiates to the back and bilateral axillae. Pulse is 147. SpO_2 is 68% in room air.

Discussion

The pulmonary stenosis in this infant has progressed following the initial valvuloplasty, and requires repeat valvuloplasty. Though valvular pulmonary stenosis usually improves with time, infants with critical pulmonary stenosis may experience initially progressive disease and require reintervention. The SpO_2 is low secondary to right-to-left flow through the patent foramen ovale.

Case 2

A 15-year-old girl with Williams syndrome has relocated from another city and presents for a required routine examination prior to enrollment at her new school. Her medical history is significant for a cardiology evaluation at the time of her genetic diagnosis as an infant, which was normal. Her mother identifies the youngster being sedentary and overweight as her two main concerns. She seems to have reasonable exercise tolerance and has no complaints of shortness of breath, syncope, chest pain, or abnormal skin coloring.

On examination, the patient is polite and pleasant, demonstrating the typical features of Williams syndrome. She is above the 95th percentile for body mass index. Her skin color is normal. She exhibits no jugular venous distention. On cardiac examination, increase in the right ventricular impulse at the left lower sternal border is noted. The second heart sound is narrowly split, with a loud P2 component. No murmurs are audible in the chest or back, though the exam may be compromised by the patient's body habitus. The liver edge is not palpable and the pulses are normal.

ECG (Fig. 10.7): A 12-lead ECG demonstrates RVH, with right axis deviation (QRS axis of +120), and a qR pattern with tall R waves in V1. The other right precordial leads (V2 and V3) also have tall R waves. The Q waves and biphasic T waves in leads III and AVF suggest septal hypertrophy, which is common with RVH.

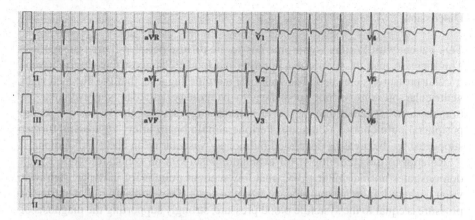

Fig. 10.7 Twleve-lead ECG demonstrates RVH, with right axis deviation (QRS axis of +120), and a qR pattern with tall R waves in V1. The other right precordial leads (V2 and V3) also have tall R waves. The Q waves and biphasic T waves in leads III and AVF suggest septal hypertrophy, which is common with RVH

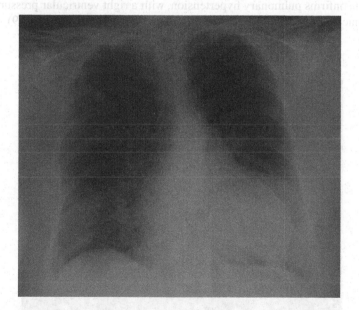

Fig. 10.8 AP chest X-ray. Left convex scoliosis is demonstrated. Mild cardiomegaly is present with mild uplifting of the cardiac apex, consistent with RVH. The upper lung fields are dark, suggesting decreased pulmonary blood flow. Bibasilar interstitial and patchy air space disease is present

Chest X-ray: A chest radiograph is performed (Fig. 10.8) to evaluate the heart size and pulmonary vascularity. Left convex scoliosis is demonstrated. Mild cardiomegaly is present with mild uplifting of the cardiac apex, consistent with RVH. The upper lung fields are dark, suggesting decreased pulmonary blood flow. Bibasilar interstitial and patchy air space disease is present.

Discussion

This patient with William syndrome has severe diffuse peripheral arterial stenosis. The increase in right ventricular impulse and loud P2 suggest that the right ventricular pressure is elevated. The lack of a murmur suggests that the elevated right ventricular pressure is not secondary to pulmonary valvular, supravalvular, or branch stenosis; rather, the lack of a murmur suggests that the stenosis is in the peripheral pulmonary vasculature. Peripheral pulmonary artery stenosis is further supported by the areas of decreased pulmonary vascularity on chest radiograph.

Referral to the cardiologist for evaluation results in an echocardiogram which demonstrates normal intracardiac anatomy without pulmonary valvular, supravalvular, right or left branch pulmonary artery stenosis. The estimated right ventricular pressure is equal to the systemic blood pressure, strongly supporting the diagnosis of peripheral pulmonary artery stenosis. The severe stenosis of the peripheral pulmonary arteries is only demonstrated on cardiac catheterization through a pulmonary angiogram.

Cardiac catheterization: In the cardiac catheterization laboratory, pressure measurement confirms pulmonary hypertension, with a right ventricular pressure equal to systemic systolic blood pressure. Pulmonary angiography (Fig. 10.9) demon-

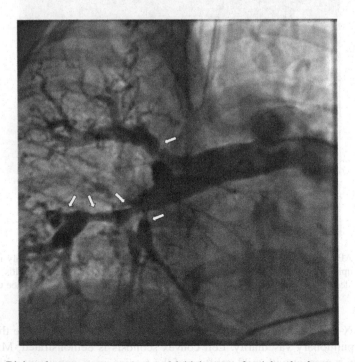

Fig. 10.9 Right pulmonary artery angiogram. Multiple areas of peripheral pulmonary stenosis are noted (*white arrows*), along with abnormal arborization of the pulmonary vasculature

strates multiple areas of peripheral pulmonary stenosis, along with abnormal arborization of the pulmonary vasculature. Since the pulmonary hypertension is severe, the patient undergoes balloon dilation of multiple areas of stenosis in the peripheral pulmonary vasculature. She also has a stent placed in right lower pulmonary artery. She is discharged after an uneventful overnight observation. The SpO_2 is 96% in room air.

Chapter 11
Aortic Stenosis

Kathryn W. Holmes and Megan A. McCarville

Key Facts

- The incidence of bicuspid aortic valve is common, however, only small percentage of such individuals develop aortic stenosis during childhood years.
- Bicuspid aortic valve may have associated ascending aortic dilation, regardless of the level of valve disease.
- Aortic stenosis may occur in association with other left heart lesions, such as mitral stenosis and coarctation of the aorta.
- Aortic stenosis is typically asymptomatic unless the stenosis is severe or critical causing compromise of cardiac output.
- Ejection systolic murmur in aortic stenosis is preceded by a click and is best heard over the right upper sternal border, radiating into the suprasternal region and neck.
- Second heart sound may be narrowly split due to delay in aortic valve closure or even paradoxically split (splitting in expiration and single in inspiration).

Definition

Congenital aortic stenosis results from abnormalities in the formation of the valve leaflets. These abnormalities include fusion of one or more valve leaflets, leading to bicuspid or unicuspid aortic valves, respectively, or malformation of the leaflets of a trileaflet aortic valve. While bicuspid aortic valve is common, comprising up to 2% of the general population, the vast majority of these valves are not obstructive during childhood. There is a heritable component to the bicuspid valve. Current evidence points to a heritable aspect to the development of congenital bicuspid valves with an

K.W. Holmes (✉)
Department of Pediatric Cardiology, John Hopkins Medical Institutes,
600 N. Wolfe Street, Brady 5, Baltimore, MD 21287, USA
e-mail: kwholmes@jhmi.edu

Ra-id Abdulla (ed.), *Heart Diseases in Children: A Pediatrician's Guide*,
DOI 10.1007/978-1-4419-7994-0_11, © Springer Science+Business Media, LLC 2011

autosomal dominant pattern of inheritance with incomplete penetrance. Of note, a bicuspid aortic valve may also have associated ascending aortic dilation that may be present, with or without evidence of valve pathology.

Acquired valvular aortic stenosis results from acute rheumatic fever or age-related degeneration secondary to valve sclerosis and calcification. The incidence of rheumatic valve disease varies dramatically worldwide. Age-related aortic stenosis is prevalent and has been recognized in up to 2% of adults over 65 population.

Incidence

Occurring in approximately 10% of cases of congenital heart disease, aortic stenosis refers to obstruction to outflow from the left ventricle due to narrowing at above, below, or at the level of the aortic valve. Narrowing at the aortic valve (valvular aortic stenosis) accounts for 71% of cases of aortic stenosis, 23% of aortic stenosis are due to narrowing below the valve (subvalvular aortic stenosis), and 6% due to narrowing above the level of the valve (supravalvular aortic stenosis). This chapter focuses on valvular aortic stenosis, which may be either congenital or acquired (Fig. 11.1).

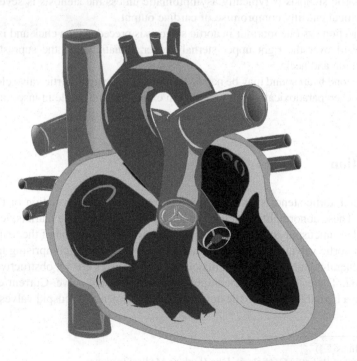

Fig. 11.1 Aortic stenosis (AS). The aortic valve orifice is small; this may be a result of thickening of valve cusps, adhesion of cusp edges rendering separation between cusps during systole limited and/or due to small valve annulus

Pathology

Pathology of aortic stenosis varies with etiology of the disease; however, obstruction develops as a result of reduced effective valve orifice.

In a bicuspid or unicuspid aortic valve, the fusion of individual valve cusps changes and reduces the normal motion of the valve. Unicuspid valves are more likely to result in stenosis in infancy and young childhood as the effective valve orifice is markedly reduced. Thickening of valve cusps over time leads to restricted cusp motion. Some valves become not only stenotic but also regurgitant as reduced coaptation of these thickened, abnormal coaptation of the valve leaflets in diastole leads to valve incompetence. In cases of critical aortic stenosis presenting in the newborn period, the valve is usually markedly abnormal and thickened, often with reduced diameter of the aortic annulus.

Congenital aortic stenosis is frequently associated with other congenital heart defects. Most typically associated are other left-sided obstructive lesions including, hypoplastic left heart syndrome, coarctation of the aorta, subvalvular aortic stenosis, supravalvular aortic stenosis, and mitral stenosis. Bicuspid aortic valves, including normally functioning, nonstenotic valves, are frequently associated with aneurysm of the ascending aorta , leading to increased risk of aortic dissection.

Pathophysiology

Regardless of the precipitating cause of aortic valve obstruction, clinical manifestations of aortic stenosis are usually progressive over time. The left ventricle gradually hypertrophies in order to accommodate the increased force necessary for aortic valve opening. As hypertrophy eventually gives way to left ventricular failure, the left ventricle and left atrium dilate and changes related to increased left ventricular end-diastolic pressure and left atrial hypertension occur.

Clinical Manifestations

Patients usually remain asymptomatic until there is a mean gradient across the valve of more than 40 mmHg by echocardiography or peak-to-peak gradient by catheterization. Newborn children with critical aortic stenosis present in shock-like state within the first hours to 1 month of life as ductal closure leads to reduced antegrade flow blood flow across the aortic valve. These patients cannot maintain adequate cardiac output and present in a shock-like state with tachycardia, tachypnea, and decreased distal perfusion. The high left ventricular end-diastolic pressure that occurs with critical aortic stenosis may also lead to mitral regurgitation and subsequent signs of heart failure and pulmonary edema.

In less critical cases, patients present with symptoms of syncope, chest pain, and dyspnea, typically with exertion. Stenosis may progress during periods of rapid

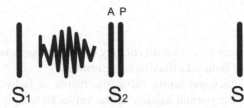

Fig. 11.2 Heart sounds and murmur in AS. *S1* first heart sound, *S2* second heart sound, *A* aortic valve closure, *P* pulmonary valve closure. Obstruction to blood flow across the aortic valve results in the elevation of left ventricular pressure over aortic pressure. This pressure gradient causes blood flow across the aortic valve to be turbulent and consequently noisy (murmur). The murmur starts with a systolic click as a result of opening of thickened valve cusps and followed by systolic ejection murmur as blood crosses the stenotic valve. The murmur's harshness increases with severity of stenosis, although in extreme cases due to resulting heart failure, the murmur may become softer. A systolic ejection murmur not preceded by a systolic click may suggest diagnosis other than aoritc valve stenosis. Stenosis of the left ventricular outflow tract, below or above the valve with a normal valve present with a murmur similar to aortic stenosis, however, without the click. Aortic stenosis murmur is best heard over the right upper sternal border

growth as the valve orifice does not grow at a rate comparable to the child. Sudden death may occur, even without a significant past history of cardiac symptoms.

On examination, patients with aortic stenosis usually presents with a midsystolic ejection murmur at the right upper sternal border that radiates to the neck or apex. The murmur varies little with positioning or maneuvers. S2 is usually narrowly split but may be paradoxically split in severe stenosis. If patients also have aortic regurgitation, a soft diastolic murmur will also be heard (Fig. 11.2).

Diagnosis

Chest Radiography

Chest radiographs are generally normal. However, in cases of heart failure, the cardiac silhouette may be enlarged due to left ventricular failure manifesting as lateral and downward displacement of cardiac apex. Pulmonary vascular congestion may also be present (Fig. 2.9).

Electrocardiography

Electrocardiograms (ECGs) may show evidence of left ventricular hypertrophy including left axis deviation, increased left-sided forces, and evidence of ischemia with ST elevation or depression (Fig. 11.3).

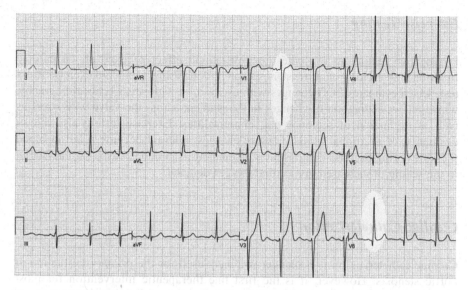

Fig. 11.3 ECG in AS. Increased pressure load of the left ventricle results in left ventricular hypertrophy manifesting as tall R wave in left chest leads (V6) and deep S wave in right chest leads (V1)

Echocardiography

Although direct pressure measurements obtained by cardiac catheterization remain the gold standard for evaluating the severity of aortic stenosis, noninvasive echocardiography has largely replaced the need for diagnostic catheterization. Echocardiography is used in the assessment of aortic stenosis to assess the pressure gradient across the aortic valve and to measure left ventricular function and wall thickness. The severity of the stenosis is estimated using the peak or mean gradient across the aortic valve as measured by pulse or continuous wave Doppler. Pulse Doppler measures velocity of blood flow at a specific location, while continuous wave measures along the entire left ventricular outflow tract and hence, may incorporate multiple levels of obstruction.

Gradients are generally categorized as mild, moderate, or severe.

Mild: mean gradient <25 mmHg
Moderate: mean gradient between 25 and 40 mmHg
Severe: mean gradient >40 mmHg.

Note that if the left ventricular function is abnormal, a significant pressure gradient may not be generated secondary to left ventricular failure. This will give the false impression that stenosis is less severe. Therefore, taking into consideration left ventricular function and effective aortic valve orifice in combination with the pressure gradient is crucial to provide an accurate assessment of such cases.

Exercise Testing

Provocative testing to evaluate the physiologic effect of exertion on cardiac function in the setting of aortic stenosis can be done using a standard exercise stress test, which evaluates ECG changes with exertion, or with stress echocardiography, which allows estimation of changes in the gradient across the valve with stress as well as evaluation of regional wall abnormalities. Exercise testing also allows evaluation of exertional blood pressure changes, relevant because a fall in blood pressure during exercise demonstrates an ominous sign of decreased cardiac output in the setting of increased myocardial oxygen demand.

Cardiac Catheterization

Cardiac catheterization is no longer routinely used for the primary evaluation of aortic stenosis. However, it is the first line therapeutic intervention for most children with aortic stenosis and will be discussed below.

Management

Management depends on the degree of stenosis and the patient's clinical status. For critically ill newborns with heart failure and shock, patients are stabilized and undergo either an emergent balloon valvuloplasty via cardiac catheterization or surgical relief of stenosis. Prostaglandins may be used to maintain patency of the ductus arteriosus to allow at decompression of the right side of the heart and preserve some cardiac output.

Patients with mild to moderate stenosis are followed-up with a careful interval history, examination, ECG, and echocardiograms as needed between 3 month and 2 year intervals depending on their age and degree of stenosis. Periodic exercise testing is indicated in children who develop symptoms, ECG changes, increasing gradient, or the desire to become pregnant or participate in sports.

Sports participation should be limited in patients with aortic stenosis based on the degree of the gradient. Assessments should be made yearly prior to participation. The 2006 American Heart Association guidelines recommend that athletes with:

1. Mild stenosis (mean gradient <25 mmHg) and normal aortic dimensions have no restrictions on participation.
2. Moderate stenosis (mean gradient between 24 and 40 mmHg) may participate in low intensity competitive sports. In addition, some athletes may participate in low and moderate static or low and moderate dynamic activities if exercise testing is normal to the level of that activity.
3. Patients with severe disease may not participate in competitive sports.

Patients who have undergone balloon valvuloplasty, valve repair, or surgical replacement also have specific participation guidelines outlined for their conditions.

Percutaneous balloon valvuloplasty is the first-line interventional method for patients with congenital aortic stenosis. In contrast, patients with acquired valve disease from rheumatic fever or age-related calcification do not have an acceptable response. Guidelines from the ACC/AHA for intervention in adolescence and young adulthood in patients with congenital aortic stenosis as follows:

1. Symptomatic patients with peak-to-peak gradient >50 mmHg by catheterization.
2. Asymptomatic patients with peak aortic gradient >60 mmHg or mean gradient >40 mmHg by echocardiographic Doppler.
3. Asymptomatic patients with aortic stenosis who develop ST or T-wave changes over the left side as rest or with exercise and have a peak gradient of >50 mmHg by catheterization.

Surgical management is reserved for adults and patients with either aortic stenosis refractory to balloon dilation or those with significant aortic regurgitation. Aortic stenosis may either be managed with valvuloplasty, valve replacement with a Ross procedure (native pulmonary valve moved to the aortic position), or valve replacement with a bioprosthetic or mechanical valve.

Follow-up is life-long. The interval depends on the severity of disease: AHA guidelines recommend follow-up yearly for patients with moderate disease and at 2 year intervals for patients with mild disease. More frequent follow-up is indicated for patients with severe disease, patients who are undergoing rapid growth (first 3–5 years of life and adolescence), athletes, and pregnant individuals.

Prognosis

Prognosis of aortic stenosis is generally good for patients with mild disease. However, gradients tend to increase with patient age as the aortic valve calcifies, as do the risks of intervention. Most patients who require an intervention in childhood will require additional interventions in adulthood including valve replacement.

Females of childbearing age require particular counseling since aortic stenosis increases the risk of pregnancy to both mother and fetus. Furthermore, anticoagulation therapy is required following mechanical valve replacement, which is often necessary in adulthood presents significant problems to both mother and fetus because of the teratogenic effects of warfarin and the increased risk of maternal hemorrhage.

Case Scenarios

Case 1

History. During a preparticipation sports physical, a previously healthy 14-year old with short stature is noted to have a murmur. During tryouts for the high school soccer team, he has a brief syncopal episode at the end of the practice. He is responsive quickly upon awakening but is sent to the emergency room for evaluation. Past medical history initially seems to be unremarkable. However, on further questioning, his mother notes that he has had a murmur since 4 years of age when he contracted rheumatic fever. Social history is notable for the fact that he was born in Nigeria.

Physical examination. Physical examination reveals a well-appearing, well-nourished African-American male. Heart rate is 80, blood pressure is 125/80, and oxygen saturation is 97% on room air. He is in the 20th percentile for height and weight. His face is symmetric and nondysmorphic. Lungs are clear to auscultation bilaterally. On cardiac exam, his precordium is mildly hyperdynamic with maximal impulse slightly leftward. There is a systolic ejection click best heard in the fourth intercostal space at the right sternal border followed by a harsh 3/6 ejection murmur with radiation to the neck and apex. There is a short 1/4 diastolic murmur best heard with the patient leaning forward. His abdomen is soft, nontender, and without the evidence of hepatomegaly. Extremities are warm and well perfused without the evidence of edema and pulses are 2+ in the right arm and right femoral regions.

Investigative studies. Chest radiographs and ECG may be helpful in assessing for cardiomegaly and specific chamber hypertrophy.

- ECG: evidence of increased leftward forces with LV strain pattern (Fig. 11.4).
- Chest X-ray: unremarkable.

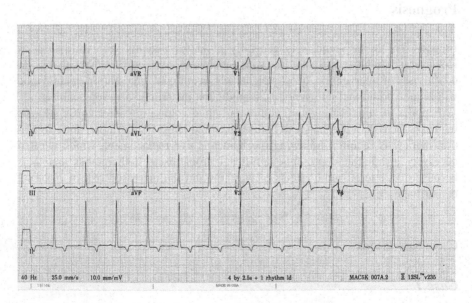

Fig. 11.4 Twelve-lead ECG: evidence of increased leftward forces with LV strain pattern as evidence by tall R waves and inverted T waves in left chest leads (V4-6)

Differential diagnosis. The combination of syncope with physical examination findings of an ejection murmur and ECG abnormalities point to a significant left ventricular outflow obstruction. While this obstruction could be secondary to a number of lesions, including hypertrophic cardiomyopathy, coarctation of the aorta, or sub- or supravalvular aortic stenosis, the click is diagnostic of aortic stenosis.

Assessment. Based on symptoms and physical exam findings in the setting of a history of rheumatic heart disease, this patient is likely to have valvular aortic stenosis. Echocardiography is indicated for confirmation of the diagnosis and evaluation of the pressure gradient across the aortic valve.

   Echocardiogram demonstrates a thickened and calcified aortic valve with severe restriction of ~50 mmHg between the left ventricle and the aorta. There is concentric hypertrophy of the left ventricle without evidence of regional wall motion abnormalities. There is a mild amount of aortic and mitral regurgitation. The aorta is normal in size and caliber with no evidence of aortic coarctation.

   Given that the valve itself is markedly abnormal and there is already aortic regurgitation, balloon dilation is not likely to be effective. Surgical options must be considered. The surgeons must consider the patient's size and interest in continued sports participation in their surgical planning. If this patient wants to continue sports participation, a valve that does not require life-long anticoagulation (Ross procedure or porcine valve) should be chosen.

Case 2

History. A 2-week-old infant is brought into the pediatrician's office for a routine checkup. His birth history was unremarkable: the patient was born by normal, spontaneous vaginal delivery at 3.5 kg. He breastfed with ease and was discharged at 48 h of life. The patient's mother reports that he was feeding well until 2 days ago, when he began to tire more quickly and fall asleep during feeds.

Physical examination. On physical examination, the patient appears happy but tachypneic infant with mild subcostal retractions. Heart rate is 160, respiratory rate 50, and oxygen saturation in the right hand is 97%. Mucous membranes are moist and acyanotic. Lungs are clear to auscultation bilaterally. On cardiac exam, the precordium is hyperdynamic. There is a 2–3/6 systolic ejection murmur heard over the entire precordium with a gallop is present. There is mild hepatomegaly with the liver tip palpated at 4 cm below the costophrenic angle. Pulses are present but not bounding and capillary refill is ~3 s.

Investigative studies. Chest radiographs and ECG may be helpful in assessing for cardiomegaly, pulmonary venous congestion, and specific chamber hypertrophy.

- ECG: sinus tachycardia with biventricular hypertrophy.
- CXR: cardiomegaly with pulmonary edema.

Differential diagnosis. This infant is demonstrating signs and symptoms of heart failure, with decreased feeding, tachycardia, tachypnea, and a physical exam notable for a gallop, liver congestion, and a mild decrease in capillary refill time. The differential diagnosis for progressive heart failure in the early newborn period would include causes of intrinsic myocardial dysfunction, such as viral myocarditis, congenital heart lesions associated with left-to-right shunts if very severe, such as ventricular septal defect or endocardial cushion defects, or congenital heart lesions that lead to obstruction of ventricular outflow, such as aortic stenosis, pulmonic stenosis, or coarctation of the aorta. This patient's murmur is suggestive of aortic stenosis.

Assessment. The patient is emergently transferred to a pediatric facility with the capacity to start prostaglandins, intubate to reduce myocardial demand, and obtain central vascular access to start vasopressors if necessary. An echocardiogram demonstrates a bicuspid aortic valve. The mean gradient is 40 mmHg across the aortic valve with poor left ventricular function and systolic blood pressure of 65 mmHg.

In the setting of poor ventricular function, the guidelines for repair based on mean gradient across the aortic valve are set aside, as the left ventricle cannot generate adequate pressure to overcome the obstruction and maintain cardiac output. In this case, this patient was stabilized and taken to the cardiac catheterization lab for balloon dilation of his aortic valve. His parents were counseled about the risks of this procedure, including the likely need for reintervention in the first year of life and the possibility of aortic regurgitation. In the future, the patient will likely require additional aortic valve dilations or valve replacement surgery.

Chapter 12
Coarctation of the Aorta

Sawsan Mokhtar M. Awad and Megan A. McCarville

Key Facts

- Coarctation of the aorta is typically asymptomatic in older children and adults, however, presents with cardiac shock in severe cases in the neonatal period.
- Higher blood pressure in upper extremities when compared to blood pressure in lower extremities is diagnostic of coarctation of the aorta.
- ECG in older children show left ventricular hypertrophy and possible left ventricular strain pattern (ST, T changes in V4–V6), while in neonates right ventricular hypertrophy pattern is noted due to in utero pressure overload of the right ventricle which is the chamber pumping blood to the narrow area of aortic arch through the ductus arteriosus.
- Repair of coarctation of the aorta is surgical in early childhood and through balloon dilation with or without stent placement in older children. Recoarctation of the aorta is almost always managed through balloon dilation in the cardiac catheterization laboratory unless associated with hypoplasia of the aortic arch which would require repeat surgical intervention.

Definition

Coarctation of the aorta is narrowing of the aortic arch such that it causes obstruction to blood flow. This may be the result of discrete narrowing or more diffuse hypoplasia of the aortic arch. Typical coarctation of the aorta is discrete narrowing of the distal aortic arch close to the origin of the ductus arteriosus, this may involve the origin of the left subclavian artery, just proximal or just distal to it. Coarctation of the aorta is a lesion noted in patients with DiGeorge syndrome.

S.M.M. Awad (✉)
Department of Pediatrics, Rush University Medical Center, 1653 W. Congress Parkway, Suite 770 Jones, Chicago, IL 60612, USA
e-mail: sawsan_m_awad@rush.edu

Ra-id Abdulla (ed.), *Heart Diseases in Children: A Pediatrician's Guide*,
DOI 10.1007/978-1-4419-7994-0_12, © Springer Science+Business Media, LLC 2011

Incidence

Congenital heart defects involving stenosis, or hypoplasia of the aortic arch, the descending aorta, or both, are defined as coarctation of the aorta. Coarctation of the aorta represents a relatively common defect, accounting for 5–8% of all congenital heart diseases.

Pathology

Aortic coarctation results from narrowing of the aortic arch of variable length and extension, usually at the insertion of the ductus arteriosus (Fig. 12.1a, b). Severe constriction may lead to interruption of the aortic arch. Coarctation of the aorta may be isolated or associated with other cardiac defects, most commonly bicuspid aortic valve, followed by left-sided obstructive lesions such as aortic valve stenosis. Coarctation may be associated with ventricular septal defect and complex congenital heart disease such as truncus arteriosus and transposition of the great arteries. Several noncardiac defects are associated with coarctation of the aorta. Cerebral aneurysm is found in around 10% of patients with coarctation of the aorta. Coarctation of the aorta is the most common cardiac defect in Turner syndrome, found in 30% of affected patients.

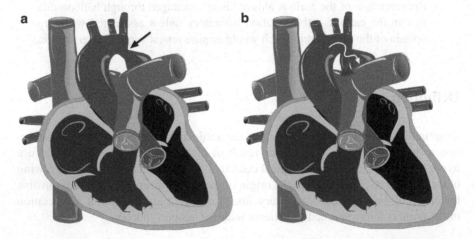

Fig. 12.1 Anatomy of coarctation of aorta. (**a**) The aortic arch is constricted at the distal arch around the region of take off of the left subclavian artery (*black arrow*). (**b**) This is the same region where the ductus arteriosus connects the aortic arch to the pulmonary artery, thus providing widening of the constricted area while the ductus arteriosus is patent (*white arrow*). In many instances, coarctation of the aorta is not uncovered till the ductus arteriosus closes at few days of life

Pathophysiology

In severe coarctation of the aorta, closure of the ductus arteriosus exposes the left ventricle to an acute increase in afterload, leading to hypotension and shock. The area connecting the ductus arteriosus to the aortic arch serves as an area to widen the narrow aortic arch, therefore once the ductus arteriosus starts to close, this connecting area also constricts leading to worsening of obstruction. Furthermore, there are theories suggesting that ductal tissue surrounds the aortic arch in a lasso fashion, therefore causing narrowing of the aortic arch when ductal tissue constricts. In lesions associated with milder obstruction, collateral vessels develop between the aorta proximal to the coarctation and distal to the coarctation. In cases of milder obstruction, the initial presentation may be delayed until childhood or even adulthood. Increased afterload results in left ventricular hypertrophy. Upper extremity blood pressure is higher than that in the lower extremities, opposed to normal situations where the lower extremities blood pressure is 10–15 mmHg higher than the upper extremities blood pressure in ambulating patients.

Clinical Manifestations

Newborn children with coarctation of the aorta are usually asymptomatic at birth. The onset of symptoms is related to closure of the ductus arteriosus within the first 7–10 days of life. The degree of severity of symptoms following ductal closure depends on the severity of the coarctation. With ductal closure, newborn children with severe coarctation may initially have periods of poor color, appearing ashen or dusky, or present with poor feeding and irritability. Children with severe coarctation present with circulatory collapse and shock, with poor or no palpable pulses and usually no audible murmurs. Other congenital heart lesions that may have a similar presentation include other left ventricular outflow tract obstructive lesions such as hypoplastic left heart syndrome, critical aortic stenosis and interrupted aortic arch. Differential cyanosis may be apparent on clinical exam or on pulse oximetry due to less oxygenated blood supplying the lower extremities through the patent ductus arteriosus.

Patients with milder forms of constriction of the aorta may present in a variety of ways. Coarctation of the aorta may present in childhood or adulthood with systemic hypertension, usually resistant to medications. Alternatively, coarctation may be diagnosed after patients are noted to have one of several heart murmurs, including a continuous murmur of the blood flow across the well-developed collaterals, a systolic murmur in the infraclavicular area that corresponds to the segment of coarctation (Fig. 12.2), or an ejection click with a systolic ejection murmur at the right upper sternal border if a bicuspid aortic valve and aortic stenosis coexists with the coarctation. Headaches, chest pain, fatigue, or intracranial hemorrhage may be a less common presentation of coarctation of the aorta.

On examination, severe coarctation may be suggested by the differential cyanosis as mentioned above. In less severe cases, coarctation may be detected through the identification of a delay in the femoral pulse relative to the brachial pulse

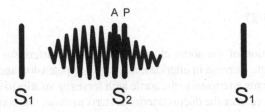

Fig. 12.2 Heart sounds and murmur in coarctation of aorta. *S1* first heart sound, *S2* second heart sound, *A* aortic valve closure, *P* pulmonary valve closure. Constriction of the aorta causes the pressure in the ascending aorta to be higher than the poststenotic region of the aorta causing the blood flow to be turbulent producing a murmur. The murmur is mostly systolic, however, may spill over into diastole

(brachiofemoral delay). Upper and lower extremity blood pressure evaluation is critical in the evaluation of as suspected coarctation. In normal individuals, the systolic blood pressure in the thigh or calf should be higher than or at least equal to that in the arm; thus the finding of a systolic pressure that is lower in the leg than in the arm may suggest the presence of a coarctation.

Chest X-Ray

In severe cases, chest radiographs may demonstrate cardiomegaly, pulmonary edema, and signs of congestive heart failure. In cases diagnosed later in life, chest radiographs may show cardiomegaly, a prominent aortic knob and rib notching secondary to the development of collateral vessels (Fig. 2.10).

Electrocardiography

Electrocardiography (ECG) in patients with coarctation of the aorta may be normal. Severe coarctation in newborn and children and young infants may show evidence of right ventricular hypertrophy due to pressure overload of the right ventricle which pumps blood in utero to the descending aorta through the patent ductus arteriosus (Fig. 12.3a).

Increased left ventricular voltage may be seen in older children and adults with coarctation of the aorta secondary to left ventricular hypertrophy (Fig. 12.3b).

Echocardiography

Transthoracic echocardiography is the gold standard diagnostic tool for coarctation of the aorta. Detailed anatomy of the aortic arch, the coarctation segment, and the ductus arteriosus patency is identified by two-dimensional echocardiography

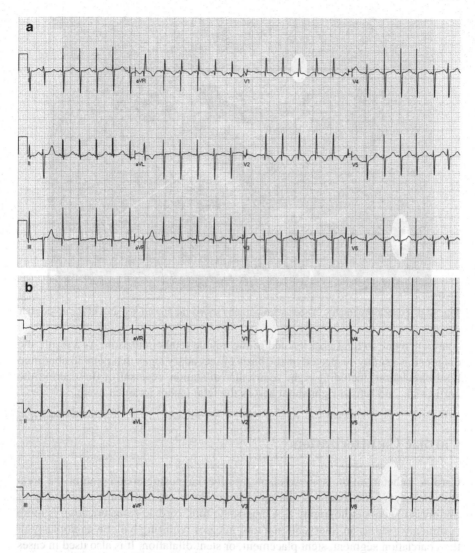

Fig. 12.3 ECG in coarctation of aorta. (**a**) In neonates, severe coarctation of the aorta is manifested on ECG as right ventricular hypertrophy since the right ventricle is the ventricular chamber which pumps blood into the descending aorta in utero. qR wave pattern of the QRS complex in V1 is noted in this infant with coarctation of the aorta. (**b**) Elevated systemic pressure in the proximal aorta will cause pressure overload of the left ventricle, resulting in left ventricular hypertrophy. Tall R in V6 and deep S in V1 is noted in this, half standard, ECG of a patient with coarctation of the aorta

(Fig. 12.4), along with any associated cardiac defects. Color Doppler is used to assess the pressure gradient across the narrow segment, although usually no significant gradient is detected if the ductus arteriosus is patent, and the direction of blood flow across the ductus arteriosus. Prenatal diagnosis can be made by fetal echocardiography, although it is technically difficult to evaluate the fetal aortic arch for

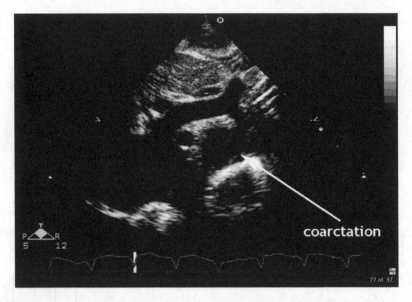

Fig. 12.4 Echocardiography. 2D echocardiography shows the constricted area of the aortic arch

coarctation due to fetal position and/or the unique fetal circulation. As a result, the diagnosis is usually suspected on the basis of secondary signs that point to abnormal fetal circulation, including right ventricular dilatation, reversal of flow across the aortic arch, and left-to-right shunt across the fetal patent foramen ovale.

Cardiac Catheterization

Cardiac catheterization is an excellent tool for diagnosing coarctation of the aorta and identifying the extent of the narrowing. However, due to the availability of noninvasive echocardiography as a diagnostic tool, cardiac catheterization is more commonly used as an interventional tool in cases requiring balloon angioplasty of the coarctation segment, stent placement, or stent dilatation. It is also used in cases that require cardiac catheterization for further characterization of or intervention for other associated cardiac lesions.

Treatment

Treatment of coarctation of the aorta depends on the degree of narrowing and the severity of its presentation. Cases of coarctation that present in the newborn period typically require more invasive interventions than those that present later.

Newborn children who present with shock, poor or absent pulses, or differential cyanosis should be started on prostaglandin E2 until ductal-dependent lesions are excluded. Upon confirmation of the diagnosis, prostaglandin should be continued until the time for definitive intervention, along with continued medical management of metabolic acidosis and shock. Neonatal coarctation of the aorta is almost always treated by surgical approach. The most common technique is resection of the coarctation segment and end-to-end anastomosis via a left lateral thoracotomy incision. An alternative technique is the subclavian flap, which involves using the left subclavian artery to augment the narrow aortic segment and replace resected tissue. Over time, the left upper extremity will be supplied by collateral arteries that develop in lieu of the resected subclavian artery. As a result, the left upper extremity may be smaller than the right upper extremity.

Following repair of coarctation, patients may develop varying degrees of recoarctation and will require life-long cardiology follow-up. If significant recoarctation develops, patients are usually treated by balloon angioplasty with possible stent placement in the coarctation segment.

Patients who present later in life with coarctation of the aorta are usually treated by balloon angioplasty with stent placement of the coarctation segment. Stent use is avoided in younger children since the stent may not be possible to dilate to adult aortic arch diameter dimensions.

Case Scenarios

Case 1

History. A 10-year-old male patient presents to his pediatrician's office for a regular checkup. His past medical history is remarkable for occasional headaches, but the patient otherwise has no complaints.

Physical examination. Initial vital signs are notable for elevated blood pressure (154/78 mmHg) in the right upper extremity. In general, the patient is well developed and well appearing, in no acute distress. Cardiac examination is notable for weak femoral pulses bilaterally. On auscultation, the patient is noted to have a 3/6 systolic murmur in the left infraclavicular area. On recheck of the patient's triage vital signs, the patient is noted to have a blood pressure of 159/79 mmHg in the upper extremity and 110/60 mmHg in the lower extremity.

Investigative studies. Chest radiographs and ECG will help evaluate for chamber hypertrophy and cardiomegaly given the presence of hypertension.

• Chest X-ray: mildly enlarged cardiac silhouette and prominent aortic knob.
• ECG: deep S wave in V1 and tall R in V6 indicative of left ventricular hypertrophy.

Differential diagnosis. This patient is presenting with hypertension and headaches. The differential diagnosis for hypertension includes essential hypertension, endocrine disorders, renovascular disease, or cardiac causes, such as coarctation of the aorta or conditions associated with a large stroke volume; the differential blood pressure between upper and lower extremities strongly suggests coarctation of the aorta.

Assessment. Echocardiography confirms the diagnosis of coarctation of the aorta. Associated cardiac defects, including bicuspid aortic valve and ventricular septal defect, are not found. The patient undergoes percutaneous balloon angioplasty with stent placement given in his older age at presentation and the ability to dilate implanted stent in the future to adult dimensions.

Case 2

History. A 10-day-old newborn presents to the emergency room with increased irritability and poor feeding in the last 2–3 days. He was born full term via normal vaginal delivery with no history of complications during pregnancy. He did well in the first week of life, but started to have episodes of intermittent irritability and decreased oral intake in the last 3 days with noticeable ashen discoloration. Mother denies fever, vomiting, diarrhea, or history of illnesses with other family members.

Physical examination. On examination, the patient is awake but has decreased activity with stimulation. Heart rate is 180, respiratory rate 40, and oxygen saturation 95% on room air. On cardiac examination, no murmurs were detected. However, pulses were markedly diminished in all four extremities with reduced capillary refill (4 s).

Investigative studies. Chest radiographs and ECG may be helpful in assessing for cardiomegaly, pulmonary venous congestion, and specific chamber hypertrophy.

- Chest X-ray: normal heart size and moderately increased pulmonary vascular markings.
- ECG: right axis deviation and right ventricular hypertrophy.

Differential diagnosis. This infant is demonstrating signs of acute circulatory shock, without respiratory distress. His clinical picture is suggestive of a left heart obstructive lesion, including subaortic obstruction secondary to hypertrophic cardiomyopathy and septal hypertrophy, critical aortic stenosis, coarctation of the aorta, interrupted aortic arch, or hypoplastic left heart syndrome. Other causes of cardiogenic shock such as sepsis should also be considered.

Assessment. The patient is emergently started on prostaglandin to maintain patency of the ductus arteriosus resulting in the improvement of systemic perfusion. Echocardiography confirms the diagnosis of coarctation of the aorta. Given the early onset of symptom in this child, surgery with resection of the coarctation segment and end-to-end anastomosis of the aortic segments is planned once the child is stabilized from metabolic acidosis secondary to shock. His parents are counseled that he will need life-long cardiology follow-up to assess for recurrence of the coarctation and possible future need for balloon dilation of recoarctation of the aorta.

Chapter 13
Tetralogy of Fallot

Douglas M. Luxenberg and Laura Torchen

Key Facts

- TOF is seen in patients with DiGeorge syndrome and may be present in combination with AVC defect in children with trisomy 21.
- Harsh systolic ejection murmur is detected in the first week of life.
- Hypercyanotic spells are life threatening and typically not seen in the first few months of life. This may be induced by dehydration.
- Surgical repair is planned at about 4–6 months of age.
- Severe restriction to pulmonary blood flow due to pulmonary stenosis or atresia may initially require a systemic to pulmonary arterial shunt.
- Free (severe) pulmonary regurgitation resulting from surgical enlargement of pulmonary valve annulus eventually causes right ventricular dilation and fibrosis which ultimately may result in ventricular arrhythmias.
- Severe pulmonary regurgitation after TOF repair should be corrected by surgery or interventional cardiac catheterization (currently experimental). Homograft valves (and other biological material) are used for this type of repair.

Definition

Tetralogy of Fallot is the most common cyanotic congenital heart disease. It results from anterior displacement of the outflow ventricular septum resulting in a ventricular septal defect and overriding of the aorta over the VSD. In addition the anterior displacement of the outflow septum will result in narrowing of the right ventricular outflow tract and pulmonary stenosis. Right ventricular hypertrophy results from obstruction of flow at the right ventricular outflow tract and pulmonary valve.

D.M. Luxenberg (✉)
Pediatric Cardiology of Long Island, 100 Port Washington Boulevard, Suite 108,
Roslyn, NY 11576, USA
e-mail: pdcardio@mac.com

Ra-id Abdulla (ed.), *Heart Diseases in Children: A Pediatrician's Guide*,
DOI 10.1007/978-1-4419-7994-0_13, © Springer Science+Business Media, LLC 2011

Incidence

Tetralogy of Fallot (TOF) is one of the most common cyanotic congenital heart defects. In all of its forms, it occurs in approximately 0.3 per 1,000 live births and accounts for about 6% of all congenital heart disease. There does not appear to be any significant bias toward gender or race. There is, however, a tendency toward genetic or chromosomal abnormalities such as DiGeorge and Down syndromes.

Pathology

As the name implies, there are four basic components that make up TOF (Fig. 13.1):

1. A large ventricular septal defect (VSD)
2. Pulmonary stenosis (PS)
3. An overriding aorta
4. Right ventricular hypertrophy (RVH)

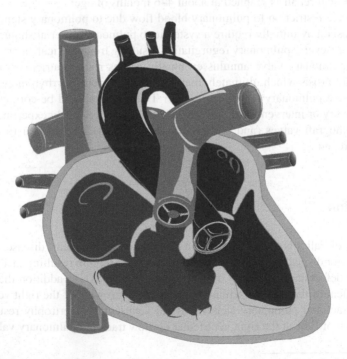

Fig. 13.1 Anatomy of tetralogy of Fallot. The outflow tract septum is anteriorly deviated causing a defect in the ventricular septum with overriding aorta and narrowing of the right ventricular outflow tract (RVOT). Reduced blood flow across the RVOT will eventually cause the pulmonary valve and arteries to be small

Like most congenital heart defects, TOF is not uniform in all patients. There are other, more rare forms which generally vary based on the severity of the pulmonary stenosis. In the most extreme form known as TOF/pulmonary atresia, the pulmonary valve is replaced with a membrane which prevents any blood from flowing into the lungs. In the rarest form, TOF with absent pulmonary valve, there is no pulmonary valve at the base of the pulmonary artery. Blood can flow back and forth across this area without restriction which often results in very large, dilated pulmonary arteries. The main focus in this chapter will be on the more common lesion with the four classic components.

Pathophysiology

The VSD in this defect is generally very large, allowing the pressure on the right and left sides of the heart to equalize. The aorta "overrides" the VSD allowing easy access of blood flow into the aorta from the left and right ventricle. Pulmonary stenosis causes increased resistance to blood flow into the pulmonary circulation and encourages blood flow from the right ventricle into the overriding aorta. Therefore, blood that would normally flow into the pulmonary artery shunts right to left to the systemic circulation causing reduced pulmonary blood flow and cyanosis. Cyanosis is a product of the right to left shunting at the ventricular level as well as the reduced volume of pulmonary blood flow resulting in less oxygenated blood return to the left atrium.

The pressure overload of the right ventricle due to pulmonary stenosis and large VSD results in RVH.

Clinical Manifestations

TOF is well tolerated in utero. Once born, newborn children are frequently asymptomatic and often do not exhibit cyanosis. The first heart sound is normal while the second heart sound is often single, loud, and accentuated. This is due to the lack of pulmonary valve component of the second heart sound due to its deformity. A harsh crescendo–decrescendo systolic ejection murmur is appreciated at the upper left sternal border due to flow of blood across the narrowed pulmonary valve (Fig. 13.2). The VSD is large and not restrictive to flow and therefore is generally silent. Oxygen saturation is often in the high 80s/low 90s.

Once the diagnosis is made, newborn children with adequate oxygen saturations are often followed in the hospital for at least a few days. Occasionally, children with what appears to be severe right ventricular outflow tract (RVOT) and pulmonary valve stenosis do not show significant cyanosis; this may be the result of augmented pulmonary blood flow through a patent ductus arteriosus. In these cases, it is wise to monitor clinical status closely until the ductus arteriosus closes. If oxygen

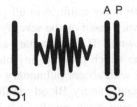

S_1 S_2 S_1

Fig. 13.2 Heart sounds and murmur in tetralogy of Fallot. *S1* first heart sound, *S2* second heart sound, *A* aortic valve closure, *P* pulmonary valve closure. Narrowing of the RVOT and pulmonary stenosis cause a systolic ejection murmur heard best over the left mid to left upper sternal border. The pressures in the right and left ventricles are equal due to RVOT obstruction and large ventricular septal defect (VSD); therefore, blood flow across the VSD is not turbulent and as such does not produce a murmur

saturation remains within an acceptable range (higher than 75%), the patient can be discharged with close follow up. On the other hand, if oxygen saturation drops significantly with closure of the ductus arteriosus, it becomes necessary to keep the ductus arteriosus patent with a prostaglandin infusion. This is followed by surgical interposition of a systemic to pulmonary arterial shunt to secure adequate pulmonary blood flow until complete surgical repair can be performed.

Many patients with TOF do well during the first few months of life and as long as adequate weight gain is observed, no intervention is necessary. Complete surgical repair is planned when the child is about 6 months of age.

Infants and children with unrepaired TOF are at risk for episodes of severe cyanosis known as hypercyanotic spells, commonly referred to as "tet spells." These episodes rarely occur in children less than 9–12 months of age. During a tet spell, the degree of pulmonary stenosis increases due to hypertrophied muscle bundles causing narrowing of the RVOT. The surge in catecholamines brought on by stress or anxiety can further constrict this narrowing. The net result is a severe drop in pulmonary blood flow. Patients will be noticeably cyanotic and hyperpneic. On auscultation, the murmur is diminished or eliminated due to significant reduction in pulmonary blood flow. Hypercyanotic spells are true emergencies and are often cause for patients to undergo palliative or complete repair soon after the episode. Older children often instinctively assume a squatting position in an effort to relieve cyanosis. This is effective because squatting increases the systemic vascular resistance above that of the pulmonary vascular resistance via kinking of the femoral vessels with resultant increase in pulmonary blood flow. In infants and younger children, bringing their knees up to their chests can break a tet spell.

In the hospital setting, treatment of hypercyanotic spells should start with attempts to reduce any cause of anxiety to the child. Allow the child's mother to hold him or her in a knee-to-chest position to increase systemic vascular resistance, preferably in a dark quiet room to assist in calming the child. Observation from a distance with minimal intervention is best if the child appears to be responding to this measure. If this intervention is not effective, sedation can be assisted by morphine, which in addition to sedation provides negative inotropic effect, assisting in relaxation of RVOT muscle bundles, thus allowing increase in pulmonary blood flow.

In the event these measures are not fruitful, the child will require hospitalization with placement of an intravenous line and the use of an intravenous beta blocking agent such as esmolol which reduces muscle contractility through its negative inotropic effect. On occasion, vasopressive drugs such as phenylephrine are used to increase systemic vascular resistance, thus forcing blood to flow through the pulmonary valve.

If all medical measures fail, emergency surgical procedure is indicated. In unstable children, it is best to avoid complete repair and therefore, augmentation of pulmonary blood flow through systemic to pulmonary arterial shunt can be placed. On the other hand, complete surgical repair can be considered if children can be somewhat stabilized prior to surgical repair.

Unrepaired children are at significant risk for developing brain embolization and possible brain abscess due to right to left shunting although these complications do not typically occur in the first year of life.

Children do well after surgical repair of TOF; however, most are left with an incompetent pulmonary valve following surgical enlargement of the pulmonary valve annulus. Over time, the resulting pulmonary regurgitation causes the right ventricle to dilate and become fibrotic and the child becomes prone to ventricular arrhythmias. There has been a tendency lately to be aggressive in managing this potentially damaging pulmonary regurgitation through implantation of competent pulmonary valves before adulthood. Homograft or bovine valves are used for this purpose. Although these valves are currently implanted surgically, implantation via interventional cardiac catheterization (currently an experimental approach) has been successful and may become the method of choice in the near future.

Chest X-Ray

In general, the cardiac silhouette is normal in size and the mediastinum is narrow due to the small pulmonary arteries. The apex can seem to be upturned due to RVH resulting in the classically described "coeur en sabot" or boot-shaped heart. The lung fields are often dark due to the lack of pulmonary blood flow (Chap. 2, Fig. 2.11).

Electrocardiography

The main finding on ECG is RVH. This is often noted by tall R-waves in lead V1 and deep S-waves in lead V6. An upright T-wave in lead V1 is sometimes seen as well and is a hallmark of RVH (but not at all isolated to patients with TOF) (Fig. 13.3). Postoperatively, as a result of patch closure of the VSD, most patients

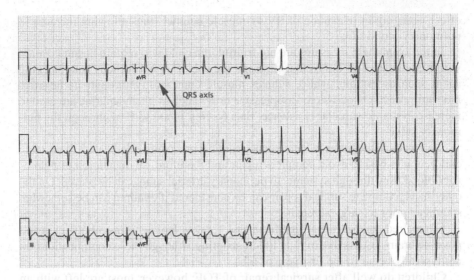

Fig. 13.3 ECG in tetralogy of Fallot. Right ventricular hypertrophy is the dominant feature of ECG in patients with tetralogy of Fallot. RVH may manifest itself in different ways such as tall R in V1 and deep S in V6, rsR′, pure R-wave or qR pattern of QRS complex in right chest leads. In this ECG, RVH is manifested as a pure R in V1, deep S in V6, and right axis deviation

develop right bundle branch block due to interference with the right bundle of His. Electrical conduction abnormalities as well as right ventricular fibrosis due to chronic pulmonary regurgitation may cause ventricular arrhythmias such as premature ventricular contractions and ventricular tachycardia.

Echocardiography

Echocardiography is the mainstay of diagnosis in the modern era of pediatric cardiology. A combination of subcostal, apical, and parasternal 2D imaging help demonstrate the classic anatomy of VSD, RVH, and aortic override. Color Doppler delineates the degree of pulmonary stenosis. The ductus arteriosus is also seen early on in neonates and patients are frequently followed in the hospital until the ductus is closed to ensure that there is adequate pulmonary blood flow across the narrowed pulmonary valve (Fig. 13.4).

Cardiac Catheterization

While no longer necessary for diagnosis in most cases, there remains a role for cardiac catheterization. Anomalous origin of the left anterior descending (LAD) artery from the right coronary artery is seen in about 5% of TOF patients. Such

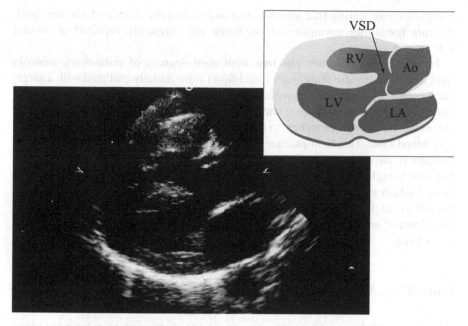

Fig. 13.4 Echocardiography. Parasternal long axis view of an infant with unrepaired tetralogy of Fallot. The left ventricle is seen in its long axis (apex to the left of the screen). *Black arrow* points to VSD underneath the overriding aorta

coronary artery anomalies may not be readily visualized by echocardiography. Because congenital heart surgeons often have to surgically incise the anterior wall of the RVOT and pulmonary valve annulus during the repair, in cases where this coronary artery anomaly exists, there is a risk of accidentally transecting the coronary artery. Therefore, patients with TOF may be studied in the cardiac catheterization laboratory prior to complete surgical repair to assess the origin and course of the coronary arteries.

Treatment

In the modern era of congenital heart surgery, with patients being successfully operated on at smaller weights and younger ages with excellent results, it is now often possible for patients to undergo complete anatomic repair as their initial operation. Palliative procedures are now often reserved for extreme cases. Complete repair of TOF can be safely performed at 4–6 months of age.

In general, unrepaired patients are watched closely at home. Parents are instructed to look for signs of inadequate pulmonary blood flow such as hyperpnea, cyanosis, or general failure to thrive. If any are seen, children are referred for surgery at an earlier age for repair. In addition, patients with hypercyanotic spells are admitted for treatment of the episode and invariably scheduled for complete repair during that admission so as to avoid the chance of another spell. Patients remaining asymptomatic at home are surgically repaired at around 4–6 months of age.

In years past, newborn children with high degrees of pulmonary stenosis (and hence inadequate pulmonary blood flow) were initially palliated with a surgically created systemic to pulmonary arterial shunt (Blalock–Taussig shunt or BT shunt). A systemic to pulmonary arterial shunt is a synthetic vascular tube connecting the aorta, or one of its branches, to the pulmonary arteries thus augmenting pulmonary blood flow. This is in essence an artificially created patent ductus arteriosus. Patients requiring a systemic to pulmonary arterial shunt are followed closely and are brought back to the operating room for complete repair. The VSD is closed which allows the formerly overriding aorta to receive blood solely from the left ventricle. The RVOT is enlarged and pulmonary stenosis is relieved with take down of any previously placed BT shunt. This is performed often in the first year of life.

Long-Term Management

During the initial repair, it is important to relieve obstruction to pulmonary blood flow. Depending on the degree of pulmonary stenosis and the location of the obstruction (subvalvar, valvar, or supravalvar), surgeons may find it necessary to cut across the pulmonary valve to enlarge the outflow tract (transannular patch) rendering the valve ineffective, resulting in significant pulmonary regurgitation. This is typically well tolerated initially, however, after many years of free pulmonary insufficiency; the right ventricle becomes dilated and less compliant, eventually becoming a possible source of potentially lethal ventricular arrhythmias. Sudden death in older children with repaired TOF is felt to be secondary to ventricular arrhythmias. These patients with poorly functioning pulmonary valves are followed on a yearly basis with electrocardiography and echocardiography. Holter monitoring and exercise stress tests are done periodically and if significant changes are found, prompt referral for electrophysiology testing is made. In addition, such patients often undergo pulmonary valve replacement as outlined above.

Case Scenarios

Case 1

A 2-day-old newborn boy is noted to have a loud murmur in the newborn nursery. The patient is otherwise well, feeding without any difficulty and breathing comfortably. On physical examination, the heart rate is normal at 100 bpm. Respiratory rate is 40 breaths/min and blood pressure is normal in the upper and lower extremities.

Pulse oximetry measures 88% in the right upper extremity and is not significantly different in the legs. Pulses are equal in the upper and lower extremities, and the lungs are clear to auscultation. There is a hyperactive precordium. On cardiac auscultation there is normal S1 and a mildly increased S2. A loud, harsh III/VI systolic ejection murmur is heard best at the upper left sternal border. Diastole is clear.

Chest X-ray is significant for generally decreased pulmonary vascularity. Cardiac silhouette is normal in size. There is a concavity along the left heart border due to diminished pulmonary artery segment and the apex is slightly upturned.

Electrocardiogram shows evidence of RVH (pure R-wave in V1, 2).

Echocardiography confirms the diagnosis of TOF by demonstrating a large VSD, overriding aorta, RVH, and moderate pulmonary stenosis. There is also a small patent ductus arteriosus with a left to right shunt.

This patient is followed in the neonatal ICU for few days. The ductus arteriosus is noted to be closed by echocardiography prior to discharge with no significant drop in oxygen saturation, indicating adequate pulmonary blood flow through the RVOT. The patient is seen every few weeks in cardiology clinic with no significant change noted. At 5 months of age he undergoes complete repair. Discussion:

This is the classic "pink tet." The patient has classic anatomy of TOF without hemodynamically significant pulmonary stenosis. Because there is adequate pulmonary blood flow, the patient remains "pink" and has normal development both before and after surgery.

Case 2

A 3-month-old girl was diagnosed with TOF by her pediatrician. She has been doing well since discharge from the hospital after birth with excellent growth and development. Her baseline oxygen saturation has been in the mid to high 80s.

Her parents report that she has not been eating well for the past 2 days and that her diapers are not as wet as usual for her. She has had some diarrhea as well and they are concerned because she is not at all "herself."

Upon exam you notice that she is somewhat withdrawn (she is usually a very interactive child) and her skin appears much darker than you had previously appreciated. She is grunting and noticeably uncomfortable. Her blood pressure is normal and her pulses are strong, yet on auscultation the usually very loud murmur is no longer appreciated. Discussion:

This patient is having a hypercyanotic spell (tet spell) likely brought on by dehydration from gastrointestinal illness. Worsening right ventricular outflow obstruction is causing blood in the right ventricle to favor flow through the VSD and into the aorta, thus exacerbating cyanosis. Because there is little pulmonary blood flow, the loud murmur which is due to pulmonary stenosis is no longer audible.

The child must be referred immediately to a tertiary care center for management of a hypercyanotic spell using the emergency medical transport system. In the meantime, turn out the lights in the exam room (calming effect) and ask the mother to hold the baby while bringing her knees to her chest to increase the systemic resistance by kinking the femoral blood vessels. This may resolve the problem. At the tertiary care center, this patient will be given IV fluids to restore her hydration status and a few days later will undergo complete repair of her TOF.

Hypercyanotic spells are medical emergencies. They are frequently brought on by dehydration which is why it is vital to closely watch all TOF patients especially when they become ill. Once a hypercyanotic spell has occurred, it is generally accepted that the best course of action is to undergo complete surgical repair to avoid occurrence of future similar spells.

Chapter 14
Double Outlet Right Ventricle

Douglas M. Luxenberg and Jacquelyn Busse

Key Facts

- DORV is a Conotruncal lesion associated with DiGeorge syndrome.
- The aorta and pulmonary artery emerge predominantly from the right ventricle.
- The great vessels may be normally related to each other or transposed.
- Clinical presentation can mimic lesions such as VSD, TOF, or TGA and is mainly determined by the presence and extent of pulmonary stenosis and the relation of the great arteries to one another.
- Timing of surgical repair is determined by the extent of pulmonary blood flow.

Definition

Double outlet right ventricle (DORV) is a cyanotic congenital heart disease where both great arteries (pulmonary artery and aorta) emerge completely or predominantly from the right ventricle. The output of the left ventricle is through a ventricular septal defect which allows escape of LV output into the great vessels. This lesion is known to be associated with DiGeorge syndrome.

Incidence

Double outlet right ventricle (DORV) is one of the less common congenital heart lesions occurring in just under 0.1 per 1,000 births and accounting for just over 1% of all congenital heart disease. The prevalence appears to be similar in males and

D.M. Luxenberg (✉)
Pediatric Cardiology of Long Island, 100 Port Washington Boulevard,
Suite 108, Roslyn, NY 11576, USA
e-mail: pdcardio@mac.com

Ra-id Abdulla (ed.), *Heart Diseases in Children: A Pediatrician's Guide*,
DOI 10.1007/978-1-4419-7994-0_14, © Springer Science+Business Media, LLC 2011

females and across various ethnic groups. DORV is a conotruncal lesion associated with DiGeorge syndrome. Other conotruncal lesions include truncus arteriosus, tetralogy of Fallot (TOF), and transposition of the great arteries (TGA).

Pathology

DORV encompasses a large variety of congenital heart lesions, the details of which are beyond the scope of this text. One largely accepted definition is to classify as DORV, all heart lesions in which both great arteries (aorta and pulmonary artery) arise predominantly from the right ventricle. Because the word "predominantly" is somewhat vague, it is generally accepted that if >50% of a great artery is supplied by the right ventricle, it is to be considered to have arisen from that ventricle. It is this lesion that will be the main focus of this chapter (Fig. 14.1).

There is almost always a ventricular septal defect (VSD) in this lesion and there are frequently (in at least 70%) varying degrees of pulmonary stenosis (PS) as well. Coronary artery anomalies are also somewhat common.

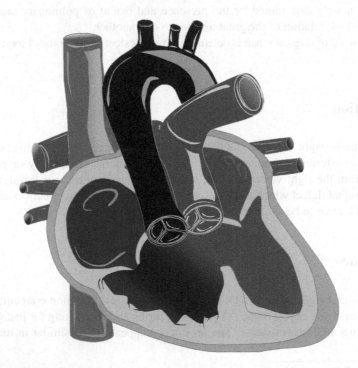

Fig. 14.1 Anatomy of DORV. Both the aorta and pulmonary artery emerge mainly from the right ventricle. The only outlet of blood from the left ventricle to the right ventricle is through the VSD. While the relationship of the great vessels to each other varies, in this diagram the great vessels are transposed with no appreciable pulmonary stenosis

Pathophysiology

The hemodynamics in DORV depends on the relationship of the great arteries to one another, the location of the VSD, and the degree of pulmonary stenosis present (Fig. 14.2a–c).

As always, blood follows the path of least resistance. In the presence of a large VSD and normal pulmonary vascular resistance (typically the case in a newborn after the first few days/weeks of life), blood will flow in a left to right fashion toward the pulmonary circuit. If there is pulmonary stenosis (PS), there will be resistance forcing blood to the aorta (right-to-left shunting). The balance or imbalance between these two shunts is what makes each form of DORV unique.

Clinical Manifestations

How a patient does prior to any repair or palliation varies based in large part on the underlying anatomy and generally falls into one of three categories:

1. Subaortic VSD and pulmonary stenosis: These patients generally do quite well in the newborn period and their presentation is similar to those with TOF. Because of the large VSD, there is a tendency for increased pulmonary blood flow but the PS in these patients can often effectively balance out the lesion,

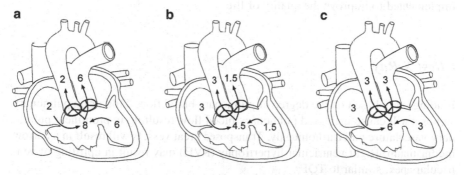

Fig. 14.2 Left-to-right shunting. Numbers represent volume of blood flow in liters per minute per square meter (l/min/m^2). (**a**) In this scenario, there is no pulmonary stenosis, resulting in excessive pulmonary blood flow and reduced systemic blood flow. The former will cause congestive heart failure and the latter will cause poor cardiac output. (**b**) In this scenario, there is severe pulmonary stenosis restricting blood flow to the lungs. A patient with this type of pathophysiology will not have congestive heart failure and the cardiac output will be adequate. However, the limited volume of pulmonary blood flow will result in significant cyanosis. This patient will typically have oxygen saturation below 70%. (**c**) In this scenario, there is moderate pulmonary stenosis resulting in balanced pulmonary and systemic circulations with reasonable oxygen saturation (80's). There is a tolerable increase in pulmonary blood flow and adequate cardiac output

resulting in a stable hemodynamic state. On physical examination the classic systolic ejection murmur of PS is noted and a hyperactive precordium is often seen. Of course if there is too much PS, it can result in pulmonary undercirculation (much like that seen during a "tet-spell") resulting in cyanosis.
2. Subaortic VSD and no pulmonary stenosis: These patients have no obstruction to pulmonary flow. There is a large left-to-right shunt across the VSD and into the pulmonary artery resulting in significant pulmonary overcirculation. Tachypnea, diaphoresis, and failure to thrive are common symptoms. Congestive heart failure develops early on, often at just a few weeks of age, requiring anti-CHF medicines such as digoxin and lasix.
3. Subpulmonary VSD: This is also referred to as the "Taussig-Bing Anomaly." Presentation is similar to TGA with a VSD with patients quickly becoming cyanotic and exhibiting signs of congestive heart failure from pulmonary over-circulation. If left untreated, they exhibit extreme failure to thrive and eventually succumb due to complications such as respiratory infections. On examination, these patients are quite cyanotic and sickly appearing with the degree of cyanosis worsening in proportion to the amount of pulmonary stenosis. If pulmonary stenosis is absent, there may be no murmur on examination.

If left untreated, DORV patients will eventually develop irreversible lung changes known as pulmonary vascular obstructive disease. The lung beds are no longer reactive to changes in circulation or oxygen level thus rendering them ineffective. Pulmonary resistance is high resulting in less pulmonary blood flow. Eventually, such patients develop a net right-to-left shunt across the VSD resulting in systemic cyanosis often referred to as Eisenmenger's syndrome. Once having reached this point, heart-lung transplantation may be considered; or palliative measures can be implemented to improve the quality of life.

Chest X-Ray

Findings vary based on the degree of pulmonary blood flow. Mild or no pulmonary stenosis will cause increased pulmonary blood flow resulting in prominent pulmonary vasculature and cardiomegaly. Transposed great vessels will result in a narrow mediastinum. Right ventricular hypertrophy (RVH) may result in uplifting of ventricular apex, similar to TOF.

Electrocardiography

As would be expected, DORV patients invariably have EKG evidence of RVH as evidenced by a tall R in V1 and V2 and a deep S in V5 and V6 (Fig. 14.3). Other forms of RVH patterns may also be noted as well.

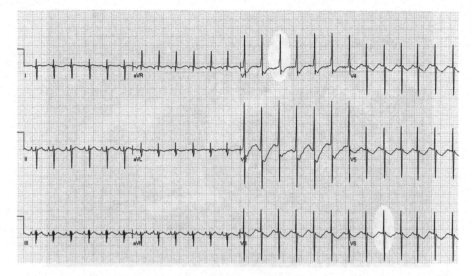

Fig. 14.3 ECG in DORV. Right ventricular hypertrophy (RVH) is the dominant feature in the ECG of patients with DORV due to volume and pressure overload of the right ventricle. In the ECG shown here RVH is manifested through tall and pure R in V1 and deep S in V6. This ECG also shows right axis deviation

Echocardiography

A combination of subcostal, apical, parasternal, and suprasternal 2D imaging allow the cardiologist to definitively make the diagnosis of DORV (Fig. 14.4). The great arteries are well visualized in these views and one can make the determination of whether or not there is >50% "commitment" of the aorta to the right ventricle.

In addition, pulsed and continuous wave Doppler allow interrogation of the pulmonary valve and right ventricular outflow tract so as to assess any pulmonary stenosis that may be present.

Cardiac Catheterization

Cardiac catheterization is generally not indicated for diagnosis, although in complicated cases it can certainly aid in delineating the anatomy. Interventions are usually not needed.

Treatment

As with most congenital heart defects, the goal is to undergo a complete repair resulting in a physiologically normal heart. The way to effectively do this varies

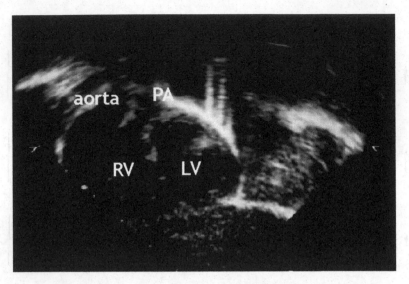

Fig. 14.4 Echocardiography in DORV. Both the aorta and pulmonary artery emerge from the right ventricle in the subcostal view of a patient with double outlet right ventricle

based on the specific form of DORV but generally involves closing the VSD "to the aorta." A patch, usually made of Dacron or Gore-Tex, is sewn into place so the left ventricular blood flow is directed out to the aorta. Care must be taken to assure there is no obstruction to blood flow. The right ventricular outflow is then addressed. If there is considerable PS, significant reconstruction may be needed to assure proper pulmonary blood flow. This may include interpositioning of an RV to PA conduit in extreme forms of the disease but most often requires only relieving obstructive muscle bundles and tissue from the region.

In some complex forms of DORV, an arterial switch operation (ASO), such as that used in TGA, is needed to put the aorta in the proper position above the left ventricle.

Patients generally do quite well in the long term following a complete repair. Depending on what was done to the pulmonary outflow tract, further operations may be necessary. If an RV to PA conduit was used, it will likely need to be upsized later in life to allow for growth, or a pulmonary valve may need to be implanted if a significant amount of pulmonary insufficiency resulted from the repair.

Case Scenarios

Case 1

A newborn male is noted to have a loud murmur while in the nursery. He is otherwise doing well. On physical examination, he is comfortable, pink, and in no acute distress. His heart rate is 155 beats/min and his blood pressure measures 86/54 in all four extremities. Pulse oximetry is 99% on room air.

EKG demonstrates RVH and right axis deviation (normal for a newborn).

His chest X-ray is generally unremarkable with normal cardiac silhouette and lung markings.

Echocardiogram demonstrates the anatomy of DORV with a large VSD and moderate pulmonary stenosis. There is bidirectional shunting across the VSD.

Discussion

This patient has a very well balanced form of DORV. The moderate PS is, in effect, balancing out the left-to-right shunt across the VSD, keeping the patient both out of heart failure (from too much pulmonary blood flow) and from becoming cyanotic (from too little systemic blood flow).

Management

This patient can be followed closely at home and observed for any sign that the lesion is becoming unbalanced (tachypnea, diaphoresis, failure to thrive in the case of not enough PS, or cyanosis in the case of too much PS) at which time a complete surgical repair will be needed.

Case 2

A newborn is discharged home after an unremarkable stay in the newborn nursery. Now 3 months old, he is noted to be falling off of the growth chart. His parents relate that he starts out well with a bottle but then "loses steam" and often falls asleep before finishing.

On physical examination you note that while initially thought to be comfortable, he is in fact quite tachypneic with a respiratory rate >60 breaths/min. His blood pressures are normal in all extremities and he is somewhat tachycardic at 155 beats/min. His liver is palpable 3 cm below the right costal margin and his pulses are strong throughout.

On auscultation he has a very active precordium with a III/VI holosystolic murmur noted at the left sternal border. In addition, an S3 gallop is appreciated as is a diastolic rumble at the apex.

Chest X-ray demonstrates a large cardiac silhouette with a significant amount of pulmonary overcirculation.

Echocardiogram demonstrates the anatomy of DORV with no associated pulmonary stenosis.

Discussion

This lesion behaves much like a large, nonrestrictive VSD with excessive pulmonary blood flow resulting in congestive heart failure.

Management

These patients are often started on anitcongestive medications such as digoxin and lasix, if failure to thrive persists despite aggressive medical therapy, they will need to be referred for complete repair. Because of the large VSD, the murmur is often not as loud as one would expect, especially in the first days of life, the diagnosis can easily be missed only to present a few weeks later as heart failure.

Chapter 15
Transposition of the Great Arteries

Douglas M. Luxenberg and Megan A. McCarville

Key Facts

- d-TGA typically presents early after birth with severe cyanosis.
- Children with large VSD and d-TGA may present later without VSD, since mixing at the ventricular level in children with VSD allow better oxygenation.
- Second heart sound is single due to posteriorly positioned pulmonary valve rendering its closure inaudible.
- Children with d-TGA and intact ventricular septum will require prostaglandin infusion to maintain patency of ductus arteriosus.
- Balloon atrial septostomy (Rashkind procedure) is often needed in children with a small atrial communication to improve atrial level mixing of blood and therefore better oxygenation.
- Arterial switch procedure is performed during first 1–2 weeks of life.
- Atrial switch operation is no longer the procedure of choice.
- Lifelong followup is recommended for all patients after surgical repair. During follow up, branch pulmonary arterial stenosis is frequently encountered.

Definition

Transposition of the great arteries is a cyanotic congenital heart diseases where the great arteries (pulmonary artery and aorta) are connected to the wrong ventricle. This leads to an abnormal circulatory pattern where poorly oxygenated blood from the systemic veins is ejected back to the body and well oxygenated pulmonary venous blood is ejected back to the lungs. The separation of the 2 circulations in this fashion

D.M. Luxenberg (✉)
Pediatric Cardiology of Long Island, 100 Port Washington Boulevard,
Suite 108, Roslyn, NY 11576, USA
e-mail: pdcardio@mac.com

Ra-id Abdulla (ed.), *Heart Diseases in Children: A Pediatrician's Guide*,
DOI 10.1007/978-1-4419-7994-0_15, © Springer Science+Business Media, LLC 2011

leads to profound cyanosis and hypoxia. Patients typically have on or 2 levels of blood mixing (atrial septal defect and patent ductus arteriosus) allowing some improvement in systemic oxygenation. Patients with this lesion and a ventricular septal defect present with less cyanosis as it provides an additional level of blood mixing.

Incidence

Transposition of the great arteries (TGA) occurs in approximately 2–3 per 10,000 live births with a strong (65%) predilection towards male gender. It had previously been thought that infants of diabetic mothers had a higher incidence of TGA, but this has not been proven to be true.

Pathology

Although there are technically many different variations of TGA, the main focus of this chapter will be on dextro-transposition of the great arteries (d-TGA). In this lesion, the visceroatrial and atrioventricular connections are normal. That is, the inferior and superior vena cavae return deoxygenated blood to the right atrium. Deoxygenated blood then passes through the tricuspid valve and enters the right ventricle. Oxygenated blood returns to the left atrium via the pulmonary arteries and then passes through the mitral valve and enters the left ventricle. It is at this point that the problem arises. In d-TGA, the right ventricle is connected to the aorta and the left ventricle is connected to the pulmonary artery, leading to ventricular-arterial discordance. While the pulmonary artery and the aorta normally crisscross each other, with the aorta arising posterior and to the right of the pulmonary artery and then traveling leftward and anterior to cross the pulmonary artery, in d-TGA, the pulmonary artery and the aorta arise from the heart parallel to each other with the aorta arising from the right ventricle and the pulmonary artery arising from the left ventricle (Fig. 15.1).

In about half of cases, d-TGA occurs only in association with a patent foramen ovale (PFO) or a small PDA. In the remainder of cases, associated anomalies are present, most commonly ventricular septal defect which is present in 30–40% of cases. Significant left ventricular outflow tract obstruction can also be seen.

A different lesion, discussed briefly here is levo-transposition of the great arteries (l-TGA), also known as congenitally corrected TGA. In l-TGA, the right and left atria connect to the wrong ventricles and the ventricles then connect to the wrong arteries. In this case, two wrongs actually do make a right with deoxygenated blood draining from the right atrium to the left ventricle to the pulmonary artery and oxygenated blood draining from the left atrium to the right ventricle to the aorta. This leads to normal pattern of blood flow and there is no cyanosis present. Unfortunately, the fact that the right ventricle becomes the pumping chamber to the body (systemic circulation) rather than to the lungs can eventually lead to heart failure. L-TGA is also associated with other congenital anomalies, such as Ebstein malformation of the tricuspid valve and complete heart block.

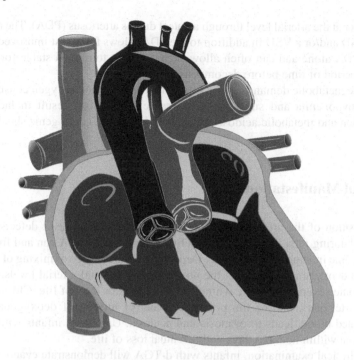

Fig. 15.1 Anatomy of d-TGA. The great vessels are switched; the aorta emerges from the right ventricle while the pulmonary artery emerges from the left ventricle. In d-TGA, the great vessels assume a parallel course, rather than the normal crisscross relationship. The parallel course of great vessels gives the narrow mediastinal appearance on chest X-ray

Pathophysiology

In the normal heart, the pulmonary and systemic circulations are in series with one another. Deoxygenated blood from the body returns to the right side of the heart and then travels via the pulmonary artery to the lungs where it becomes oxygenated. Oxygenated blood returns to the left side of the heart via the pulmonary veins and is pumped out of the aorta where is it delivered to the body, becomes deoxygenated once more, and returns to the right side of the heart.

In d-TGA, the pulmonary and systemic circulations are in parallel with one another. The deoxygenated blood that enters the right side of the heart is pumped into the aorta which is abnormally connected to the right ventricle, and therefore deoxygenated blood returns to the body without the benefit of improving its oxygenation. In the parallel circulation, oxygenated blood returning to the left heart goes back to the lungs through the abnormally connected pulmonary artery, therefore, depriving the body from receiving oxygenated blood.

Mixing of oxygenated and deoxygenated blood at one or more of three levels is required for survival. Mixing can occur at the atrial level via an atrial septal defect (ASD) or a PFO, at the ventricular level if a ventricular septal defect (VSD) is present, or at the arterial level through a patent ductus arteriosus (PDA). The presence of an ASD and/or a VSD in addition to the PDA allows for a vast improved mixing over a PDA alone and can often allow such a patient to remain stable for a much greater period of time before decompensation occurs.

As the metabolic demands of the infant increases, so does oxygen consumption. Severe hypoxemia and subsequent anaerobic metabolism result in lactic acid production and metabolic acidosis, eventually leading to cardiogenic shock.

Clinical Manifestations

Transposition of the great arteries, as with most congenital heart defects, is well tolerated during fetal life. Following delivery, however, d-TGA can and frequently does become incompatible with life. Depending on the degree of mixing of oxygenated and deoxygenated blood at the atrial, ventricular, and arterial levels, patients can become severely cyanotic within the first hours or days of life. Closure of the ductus arteriosus, one of the potential levels of mixing of deoxygenated and oxygenated blood, leads to cyanosis and acidosis. Untreated, infants with d-TGA deteriorate within hours to days with eventual loss of life.

On physical examination, infants with d-TGA will demonstrate cyanosis, worsening as time passes. After a few days of life, infants often become more tachypneic, but this can be subtle and easily missed. One of the hallmarks of d-TGA is "reverse differential cyanosis"; that is, preductal oxygen saturations (measured by a pulse oximeter on the right arm) will be lower than postductal oxygen saturations (taken by a pulse oximeter on one of the feet). The differential finding is due to mixing of oxygenated blood from the pulmonary artery with deoxygenated blood in the aorta through the PDA (right to left shunt). The vast majority of congenital heart lesions have the opposite finding making reverse differential cyanosis virtually pathognomonic for the diagnosis of d-TGA. The heart sounds are generally normal and murmurs are often absent. The second heart sound is single as the pulmonary valve closure becomes inaudible due to its posterior position far away from the chest wall (Fig. 15.2). Occasionally, a continuous murmur caused by flow across the patent ductus arteriosus may be heard.

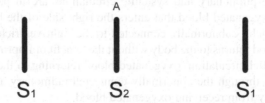

Fig. 15.2 Heart sounds in d-TGA. *S1*, first heart sound; *S2*, second heart sound; *A*, aortic valve closure. The second heart sound is single due to the posterior displacement of the pulmonary valve away from the chest wall. Murmurs may be absent in d-TGA unless there are additional defects

Chest X-Ray

Chest radiographs of patients with d-TGA are classically described as having an "egg on a string" appearance, which results from the oval/egg-shaped cardiac silhouette combined with the front-to-back orientation of the aorta and pulmonary artery leading to a narrowed mediastinum. Although the classic appearance occurs in some cases, in most instances, the chest radiograph of newborn children afflicted with d-TGA is often quite normal. Over time, chest X-ray may demonstrate an enlarged cardiac silhouette with a marked increase in pulmonary vasculature (Fig. 15.3).

Electrocardiography

Initially, the electrocardiogram (ECG) in cases of d-TGA commonly appears normal. As time progresses, right ventricular hypertrophy may become apparent, demonstrated by tall R in V1 and deep S in V6. Other forms of right ventricular

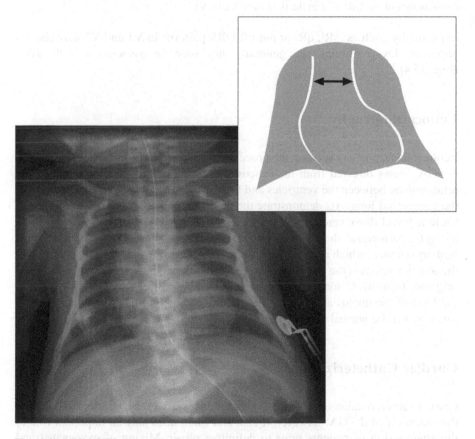

Fig. 15.3 d-TGA CXR. The mediastinum is narrow due to the parallel arrangement of the transposed great vessels

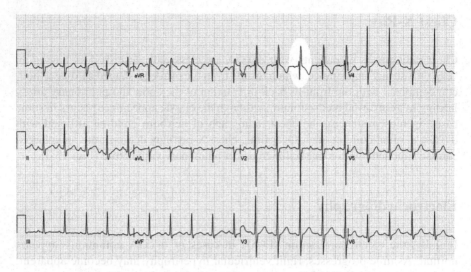

Fig. 15.4 ECG in d-TGA. Right ventricular hypertrophy is noted in this ECG manifested as rsR′ configuration of the QRS axis in the right chest leads (V1)

hypertrophy such as rsR′, qR, or pure R QRS patterns in V1 and V2 may also be apparent. Dysrhythmias are generally not seen in association with TGA (Fig. 15.4).

Echocardiography

Echocardiography has become the procedure of choice in making the diagnosis of d-TGA. Views directed from the subcostal region allow the determination of the relationships between the ventricles and their respective great arteries. Views along the parasternal long axis demonstrate the great artery that arises from the left ventricle to travel downward and bifurcate, thus making it a pulmonary artery. Views along the parasternal short axis demonstrate both semilunar valves (aortic and pulmonary) *en face*, which is not typical in a normal heart. Further imaging reveals that the anterior vessel is the aorta (achieved by demonstrating that the coronary arteries originate from it). Color Doppler flow studies demonstrate a right to left shunt at the level of the ductus arteriosus. In general, the right and left ventricular systolic function will be normal (Fig. 15.5).

Cardiac Catheterization

Cardiac catheterization is generally no longer necessary in most centers to establish the diagnosis of d-TGA; however, it can, and often does play an important role in the stabilization of patients prior to definitive repair. Mixing of oxygenated and

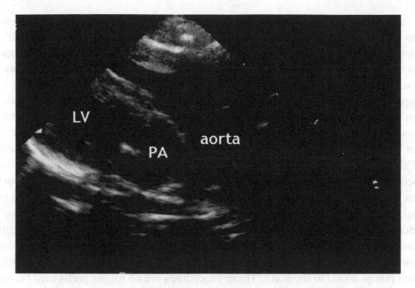

Fig. 15.5 Echocardiography in d-TGA. *LV*, left ventricle; *PA*, pulmonary artery. Parasternal long axis. The aorta and pulmonary arteries are transposed and parallel to each other, the aorta is anterior, emerging from the right ventricle, while the pulmonary artery is posterior, emerging from the left ventricle

deoxygenated blood at one or more levels is necessary for survival in d-TGA. The foramen ovale is a relatively small communication that does not permit a significant amount of flow across it. In an effort to stabilize the patient prior to surgical repair, a larger defect at the atrial level can be created by balloon atrial septostomy (BAS). A balloon tipped catheter is fed, most often from the right groin, into the right atrium and passed across the foramen ovale into the left atrium. At this point, the balloon is inflated and then rather harshly pulled back into the right atrium, creating a tear in the atrial septum that allows more adequate mixing of blood and thus increasing oxygen saturation, at least temporarily. Some centers perform BAS in the intensive care unit under echocardiogram guidance rather than in a cardiac catheterization lab.

Treatment

The initial approach to an infant with d-TGA is aimed at stabilization. Once the ductus arteriosus spontaneously closes, patients develop a severe metabolic acidosis and often rapidly deteriorate. This is especially apparent in those infants without a secondary source of mixing such as an ASD or a VSD. It is therefore vital to obtain IV access and begin an infusion of prostaglandin which will often reopen and then maintain the ductus arteriosus. Once this has been achieved (often confirmed by echocardiogram), the patient can undergo the BAS procedure to further improve mixing of oxygenated and deoxygenated blood.

The current standard treatment for d-TGA is an anatomic surgical repair referred to as the arterial switch operation (ASO), sometimes called the "Jatene Switch" in honor of the surgeon who first successfully performed it in 1975. This surgical intervention involves transecting each great artery above the valves, which stay in place. The arteries are then "switched" back to their normal locations resulting in a complete anatomic correction for this lesion. The coronary arteries are also removed from the native aortic root with a "button of tissue" from the native aorta surrounding the orifice and are reimplanted in the "new" aortic root. Once repaired, the relocated great vessels are frequently referred to as the "neo-aorta" and "neo-pulmonary artery."

Prior to the development of the currently used anatomic repair, an "atrial switch" procedure was the treatment of choice for d-TGA (there were actually two variations on this operation known as the Mustard and Senning procedures). The two atrial switch procedures differed in technical aspects, but shared the objective of switching the atrial flow of blood via crisscrossing baffles across the atria. Ultimately, deoxygenated blood is directed to the left ventricle, which pumps blood to the pulmonary artery and the oxygenated blood is directed to the right ventricle which pumps blood to the aorta. These procedures are no longer performed because they leave the right ventricle in the systemic position which can fail over time. In addition, the atrial baffles create excessive scarring within the atria resulting in significant atrial arrhythmias.

Lifelong followup is indicated in all patients with d-TGA often with yearly ECG and echocardiograms. Following the modern ASO, patients often develop some degree of supravalvar neo-pulmonary stenosis. The etiology is frequently multifactorial consisting most commonly of a combination of excessive tension on the branch pulmonary arteries following the switch procedure as well as a discreet narrowing along the suture lines of the repair. In addition, neo-aortic insufficiency is common due to the fact that the neo-aortic valve is actually the native pulmonary valve and is not normally exposed to systemic pressures.

Because the coronary arteries are manipulated during the repair, their ECG is monitored for changes that would indicate coronary compromise. Regular stress testing is performed every few years for this indication as well.

Case Scenarios

Case 1

History. A newborn infant is evaluated by the on call pediatrician because the nurse notes that the child appears "dusky." The baby was born at full term via normal spontaneous vaginal delivery. The pregnancy and delivery were uncomplicated and the patient had previously been doing fine in the nursery, breastfeeding without difficulty.

Physical examination. On initial examination, the child appears to be in no distress. On closer examination, he is quite tachypneic with a respiratory rate greater than 60.

His skin color appears darker than usual. A pulse oximeter placed on the right arm measures 55%; on the left leg, it reads 75%. The oxygen saturations remain unchanged after the patient is placed on 100% oxygen by nasal cannula for several minutes. The remainder of his exam, including cardiac auscultation, is unremarkable.

Investigative studies. Chest radiographs and ECG will help in assessing pulmonary vascularity, cardiac size, and chamber hypertrophy.

- Chest X-ray: The lung fields are clear and the mediastinum appears somewhat narrowed.
- ECG: Normal with no evidence of chamber hypertrophy.

Differential diagnosis. This infant is presenting with cyanosis and tachypnea in the newborn period. On initial assessment, this presentation could point to a range of anomalies, including respiratory or neurologic disease, along with systemic infection; however, the presence of tachypnea without associated retractions, decreased breath sounds, or grunting, and the failure of his oxygen saturations to improve even marginally with supplemental oxygen point towards a cyanotic congenital heart lesion with right-to-left shunting. Most likely potential causes of severe cyanosis include transposition of the great arteries, tricuspid atresia, pulmonary atresia, and total anomalous pulmonary venous return. The reverse differential cyanosis noted in this child strongly suggests transposition of the great arteries.

Assessment. Given the likelihood of a ductal-dependent cyanotic heart lesion, the patient is started on prostaglandin with improvement in both pre- and post-ductal oxygen saturations. An echocardiogram confirms the diagnosis of d-transposition of the great arteries, and the patient is transferred to the NICU for further care. The following morning, he undergoes a BAS, following which the oxygen saturations in the arm increase from 60 to 75%. At 1 week of age the child undergoes an arterial switch procedure.

Case 2

History. A 16-year-old young woman presents to her pediatrician for a routine physical exam. She is a very active young woman who participates in multiple varsity sports in her high school. She has no particular complaints, but is noted to have a low resting heart rate of 45 beats per minute on initial vital signs. Following exercise for 30s, her heart rate increases to 75 beats per minute. Although her pediatrician feels that her low heart rate is reflective of her status as an athlete, she is referred to a cardiologist for further evaluation.

Physical examination. Resting heart rate is 45 beats per minute. Oxygen saturation is 100% on room air. The remainder of the physical exam, including cardiac auscultation, is unremarkable except for single second heart sound.

Investigative studies. ECG may be useful in assessing for conduction abnormalities. Chest radiography is unlikely to be helpful in this situation.

• ECG: Leftward axis with mildly widened QRS in a left bundle branch block pattern.

Assessment. Because of her abnormal findings on ECG, an echocardiogram is performed which demonstrates the anatomy of congenitally corrected transposition of the great arteries (l-TGA). Her left sided ventricle is morphologically consistent with that of a right ventricle and her right sided ventricle appears to be a morphologically left ventricle. There is little to no tricuspid or mitral valve regurgitation and her biventricular systolic function is normal. An exercise stress test is scheduled for the next day and she performs remarkably well, exercising well into stage V (over 15 min) on a standard Bruce protocol. She has no evidence of dysrhythmia during the stress test and her heart rate and blood pressure appropriately increase with peak exercise.

The patient has l-TGA. At this time she is completely healthy and able to participate fully in competitive athletics. No medication or intervention is warranted at this time and she is followed on yearly basis for signs of ventricular failure such as exercise intolerance. She and family are aware that in the future, the systemic right ventricle may "tire out" necessitating medical and possibly surgical therapy.

Chapter 16
Pulmonary Atresia with Intact Ventricular Septum

Zahra J. Naheed, Ra-id Abdulla, and Daniel E. Felten

Key Facts

- The pathology of pulmonary atresia with intact ventricular septum ranges between two extremes. One extreme is that of a hypoplastic right ventricle (RV) with no significant regurgitation of tricuspid valve with RV to coronary arterial sinusoids. The other extreme is that of a dilated right ventricle with tricuspid regurgitation and typically no RV to coronary sinusoids.
- Holosystolic murmur in patients with pulmonary atresia suggests severe tricuspid regurgitation. The right ventricle in such cases is typically dilated.
- Patients with hypoplastic right ventricle and competent tricuspid valves do not exhibit holosystolic murmur.
- Abnormal coronary arteries with supply from the right ventricular cavity and stenosis constitute high risk patients with possibilities of sudden death due to myocardial ischemia and ventricular arrhythmias.
- Ductus arteriosus patency is needed preoperatively as it provides the only source of pulmonary blood flow. After surgical or interventional cardiac catheterization repair, patency of ductus arteriosus is still needed till forward flow across the right heart and pulmonary valve is established; this may require several days or weeks to achieve.

Definition

Pulmonary atresia with intact ventricular septum PA-IVS is a cyanotic congenital heart disease. The pulmonary valve/arteries are atretic, thus preventing blood from the right heart to reach the pulmonary circulation. The pulmonary circulation is

Z.J. Naheed (✉)
Department of Pediatrics, John H. Stroger, Jr. Hospital of Cook County,
5742 N. Chrishana Ave. 15, Chicago, IL 60659, USA
e-mail: amekha2000@yahoo.com

Ra-id Abdulla (ed.), *Heart Diseases in Children: A Pediatrician's Guide*,
DOI 10.1007/978-1-4419-7994-0_16, © Springer Science+Business Media, LLC 2011

fed by blood through the patent ductus arteriosus. In PA-IVS there is no ventricular septal defect, therefore blood in-utero will have the tendency to cross the patent foramen ovale or atrial septal defect to the left heart and small volume of blood will enter the right ventricle. Over time, this will lead to hypoplasia of the right ventricle. In a variation of this lesion, there may be incompetence of the tricuspid valve, leading to severe tricuspid regurgitation with dilation of the right ventricle due to back and forth flow of blood through the incompetent tricuspid valve.

Incidence

Pulmonary atresia with intact ventricular septum (PAIVS) is rare disorder that accounts for 2.5–3% of the total cases presenting as sick infants with congenital heart disease. Its prevalence has been described as 4.5–8.1 per 100,000 live births. There is no known genetic predilection of this disease.

Pathology

The primary defect in this lesion is complete obstruction of the right ventricular outflow tract due to an imperforate pulmonary valve; the ventricular septum in this subset of lesion is intact. The pulmonary valve may be well formed, consisting of three fused cusps, or the valve may be atretic. This lesion does not allow for normal blood flow through the right side of the heart to the lungs, and it is accompanied by a spectrum of right ventricular and tricuspid valve abnormalities. The right ventricle can range in size from severely dilated to extremely small, and the tricuspid valve ranges from enlarged but severely regurgitant to extremely stenotic. Rarely the lesion presents with Ebstein-like malformation of the tricuspid valve (apically displaced and regurgitant). The size of the ventricle and tricuspid valve generally are directly related to one another, that is if the ventricle is normal in size, the valve is usually large and regurgitant. If the ventricle is small, the valve is usually stenotic. In the case of a small ventricle, the endocardium is usually quite thickened (Fig. 16.1).

In some cases, the right ventricle will form communications with the coronary arteries called ventriculo-coronary connections (sinusoids), particularly in cases with high right ventricular pressures. These may represent the predominant source of blood flow to the myocardium. The coronary arteries supplied by these connections may be stenotic to a variable degree. Abnormalities at the myocardial level include ischemia, fibrosis, infarction, spongy myocardium, and endocardial fibroelastosis. The number of sinusoids is inversely related to the severity of endocardial fibroelastosis.

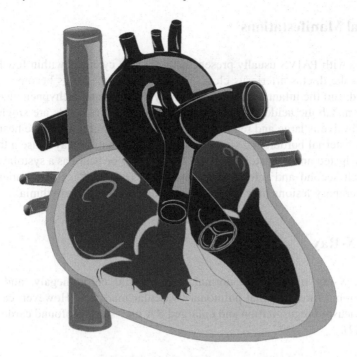

Fig. 16.1 Anatomy of pulmonary atresia – intact ventricular septum. The pulmonary valve is atretic with no forward flow across it. Blood in the right ventricle regurgitates into the right atrium. The only exit for systemic venous return is across an atrial septal defect and into the left heart. Blood supply to the lungs is achieved through a patent ductus arteriosus (as depicted in this diagram) or through systemic to pulmonary arterial collaterals. The right ventricular size may be small (hypoplastic) as shown in this diagram, or dilated due to severe tricuspid regurgitation

Pathophysiology

Due to the complete obstruction of the right outflow tract, blood entering the right atrium can either flow in and out of the right ventricle through a large and regurgitant tricuspid valve or it will bypass the right ventricle entirely if the tricuspid valve is atretic. Regardless, the only way for the blood to move forward is via a patent foramen ovale or an atrial septal defect. There is mixing of deoxygenated and oxygenated blood in the left atrium, which is then supplied to the body through a normally formed left ventricle and aorta. Therefore, newborn children with this lesion are cyanotic from birth.

Since venous blood does not return through the right side of the heart to the lungs, pulmonary blood flow is dependent on retrograde flow through the ductus arteriosus. As the ductus closes in the first hours to days of life, the newborn child with this lesion will become progressively more tachypneic, cyanotic, and develop metabolic acidosis. Outcome is fatal unless the ductus arteriosus is maintained patent to allow for pulmonary blood flow.

Clinical Manifestations

Neonates with PAIVS usually present with obvious cyanosis within few hours of birth. As the ductus arteriosus closes, blood flow to the lungs becomes severely restricted, and the infant becomes profoundly cyanotic and tachypneic due to progressive metabolic acidosis. The first and second heart sounds are single. If the tricuspid valve is large and regurgitant, a pansystolic murmur may be heard in the left lower sternal border, and severe tricuspid regurgitation may cause a thrill that can be palpated and a diastolic rumble. A PDA may be heard as a systolic murmur in the left second and third intercostals space (Fig. 16.2). Some patients with severe coronary lesions may be prone to sudden death and arrhythmia.

Chest X-Ray

A chest X-ray might show normal size to mild cardiomegaly, and usually decreased but rarely normal pulmonary vascular markings. However, cases with severe tricuspid regurgitation and enlarged RA may show profound cardiomegaly (Fig. 2.12).

Electrocardiography

Infants with PAIVS lack the pattern of right axis deviation due to right ventricular predominance inherent to normal newborns. Instead, ECG in these patients usually shows an axis 30–90° manifested by a dominant R wave in lead I. Left ventricular dominance can be noted by absence of dominant R waves in VI and their presence in leads V5 and V6. Cases with dilated right atrium may show prominent P waves in VI and lead II. ST–T wave abnormalities should alert the viewer for a strong possibility of presence of ventriculo-coronary artery connections or coronary artery stenosis suggesting subendocardial ischemia (Fig. 16.3).

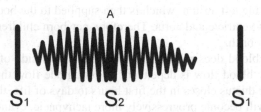

Fig. 16.2 Heart sounds and murmur in PAIVS. *S1*, first heart sound; *S2*, second heart sound; *A*, aortic valve closure; *P*, pulmonary valve closure. Continuous murmur caused by blood flow across the PDA or systemic to pulmonary arterial collaterals may be heard

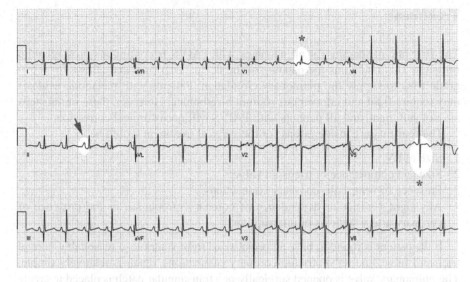

Fig. 16.3 ECG in PAIVS. Right ventricle may be dilated and hypertrophied (qR in V1 and deep S in V5). Tricuspid regurgitation leads to right atrial enlargement (tall P wave)

Echocardiography

A definitive diagnosis can be made with the two dimensional echocardiography, which will reveal pulmonary atresia and an intact ventricular septum. It can also evaluate the size of the right atrium, tricuspid valve, right ventricle, and pulmonary branches as well as the patency of the ductus arteriosus. Color Doppler is helpful in further delineating right to left shunt across the atrial septum, regurgitation through the tricuspid valve, and the presence of ventriculo-coronary connections. However, although echocardiography is excellent for making the initial diagnosis, it is limited in identifying coronary artery stenosis and right ventricular dependent coronary circulation.

Cardiac Catheterization

Cardiac catheterization is done as an important supplemental test that resolves the two questions that echocardiography cannot reliably answer. First, the presence of ventriculo-coronary connections and right ventricular dependent coronary circulation can be shown by a right ventricular angiogram. Second, a balloon occlusion aortograph can highlight the proximal coronary arteries and presence, if any, of stenosis or interruption. In rare cases of very restrictive atrial shunt, a balloon atrial septostomy might be needed to make the obligatory R to L shunt widely open.

Treatment

The first line of therapy for all neonates with PAIVS is continuous prostaglandin infusion. This maintains the patency of the ductus arteriosus and allows for retrograde flow to supply the pulmonary circulation. Patients with metabolic acidosis may require fluid and intravenous sodium bicarbonate. However, these initial steps are not sufficient, and all patients with PAIVS will need surgical correction.

The four major considerations for the surgical treatment would be:

1. Size of RV.
2. Size and competence of tricuspid valve.
3. Presence of ventriculo-coronary connections.
4. Any right ventricular dependence of coronary circulation or the presence of coronary artery stenosis or interruption.

If the patient is found to have a normal sized right ventricle, a reasonably normal tricuspid valve, and no ventriculo-coronary connections, repair is relatively simple. The pulmonary valve is opened surgically or a transannular patch is placed to create an open pulmonary artery. Alternatively this may be performed in the cardiac catheterization laboratory using interventional measures to perforate the atretic pulmonary valve followed by balloon dilation. If adequate flow is not initially established, a BT shunt may be placed while the RV and PA grow. Alternatively, continuous use of prostaglandin or stent placement in the ductus arteriosus can achieve similar results to placement of systemic to pulmonary arterial shunt. If these structures grow adequately, eventually, the systemic to pulmonary arterial shunt is taken down (or prostaglandin is withheld versus device occlusion of previously stented PDA). This would achieve a 2-ventricle repair, in which case the right and left ventricles pump blood to the pulmonary and systemic circulation normally.

If the right ventricle is hypoplastic and the tricuspid valve is dysfunctional, repair depends on the presence or absence of ventriculo-coronary connections. If there are no connections, a surgical valvotomy may be done to allow flow through the right ventricle, but a systemic to pulmonary arterial shunt must be placed to provide adequate pulmonary blood flow. The patient is allowed to grow with the systemic to pulmonary arterial shunt until big enough to tolerate Fontan repair. If there are ventriculo-coronary connections, but no evidence of stenosis or interruptions, which would suggest right ventricle dependent coronary circulation, surgical valvotomy would be done and transannular patch placed in addition to systemic to pulmonary arterial shunt placement. Fontan procedure would be done at a later date as above. However, if there are stenotic or interrupted coronaries, valvotomy should not be done, as flow through these coronaries is dependent on elevated right ventricular pressure. A systemic to pulmonary arterial shunt is placed and Fontan is done at a later date or, in severe cases of right ventricle dependent coronary circulation, heart transplant may be required.

CPR training should be provided to the caretakers close to discharge because of risk of sudden death.

Case Scenarios

Case 1

A full-term newborn boy was born via normal spontaneous vaginal delivery. Obstetrical ultrasound at 20 weeks of gestation revealed abnormal heart structures. This was followed by a fetal echocardiogram which demonstrated a hypoplastic right ventricle and no foreword flow across the pulmonary valve and reverse flow of blood across a small tortuous patent ductus arteriosus from the aorta to small pulmonary arteries. Parents were counseled prenatally that there appeared to be pulmonary atresia and that the anatomy of the coronary arteries were not well demonstrated by fetal echocardiography. The child developed cyanosis soon after birth with oxygen saturation of 75% while breathing room air. Physical examination was significant for mild tachypnea and cyanosis. First heart sound was normal, second heart sound was single; no significant murmurs were audible soon after birth. Prostaglandins were initiated.

In many similar cases, the concept of differential diagnosis is no longer applicable as diagnosis is already made through in utero investigative studies. It is important to repeat echocardiographic assessment of cardiac structures soon after birth to confirm diagnosis and obtain further details. At few hours of life, the oxygen saturation increased to 88% while on prostaglandin infusion and breathing room air. The child was breathing spontaneously; however, he was intubated and mechanically ventilated soon thereafter due to a period of apnea felt to be secondary to prostaglandin infusion.

Postnatal echocardiography confirmed diagnosis and right ventricle to coronary sinusoids were noted. The right ventricle was small with well developed inlet and outlet regions and hypoplastic apical region, pulmonary atresia were small, but not hypoplastic. The ductus arteriosus was patent and moderate in size.

In view of the coronary artery anomalies, cardiac catheterization was performed at 5 days of life. This demonstrated right ventricle to coronary sinusoid which appeared to be small with no evidence of stenosis or interruption of coronary arteries. The right ventricle was felt to be adequate to support biventricular circulation, therefore, the pulmonary valve was perforated and dilated with balloon catheters and the ductus arteriosus patency was maintained with stent placement. The prostaglandin infusion was discontinued and oxygen saturation remained around 85%.

Parents were counseled that if antegrade flow through the right ventricle and now patent pulmonary valve continues, future interventional cardiac catheterization will be performed to occlude the stented PDA to examine if antegrade flow across the right ventricle and pulmonary valve is adequate. If the flow is deemed adequate, then device closure of the PDA can be performed, otherwise, surgical intervention to convert to univentricular repair may be considered. This repair would initially include enlarging atrial communication and Glenn shunt placement, followed at about 18 months of age with a Fontan procedure (IVC to pulmonary artery connection).

Case 2

A 1-day-old girl was noted to be tachypneic and mildly cyanotic while in the newborn nursery. Physical examination revealed mild depression of oxygen saturation (90%) while breathing room air. Respiratory rate was slightly increased. Peripheral pulses and perfusion were within normal limits. No hepatomegaly was detected. Auscultation was significant for a harsh holosystolic murmur and a mid-diastolic murmur.

Differential diagnosis with this type of presentation includes tricuspid regurgitation associated with elevated right ventricular pressure such as what is noted with pulmonary hypertension secondary to persistent fetal circulation. Mitral regurgitation and ventricular septal defects result in holosystolic murmur; however, there should be no drop in oxygen saturation with the later two pathologies.

Chest X-ray revealed severe cardiomegaly with reduced pulmonary vascular markings indicating reduced pulmonary blood flow. Electrocardiography showed right atrial enlargement and right ventricular hypertrophy (qR pattern of QRS complex in V1 and V2).

Cardiology consult was requested and echocardiogram revealed severely dilated right atrium and right ventricle with severe tricuspid regurgitation and pulmonary valve atresia. The ductus arteriosus was patent and shunting was left to right providing the only supply of blood to the pulmonary circulation.

Prostaglandin was initiated to maintain patency of the ductus arteriosus. At 1 week of life, the child was taken to the operating room where surgical valvotomy was performed. The ductus arteriosus was left patent. Postoperative course demonstrated progressive reduction of tricuspid regurgitation and no residual pulmonary stenosis. Prostaglandin infusion was discontinued 3 days after surgical repair and forward flow across the pulmonary valve was adequate. Child was discharged home 10 days after surgical repair.

In this child, the right ventricle was of adequate size to maintain biventricular repair. Coronary artery abnormalities are typically not noted in children with severe tricuspid valve regurgitation and dilated right ventricle. Alternatively, the pulmonary valve could have been opened through interventional cardiac catheterization measures without the need for surgical intervention. Flow through a patent ductus arteriosus allows for adequate pulmonary blood flow until tricuspid regurgitation lessens as the pulmonary vascular resistance drops favoring forward flow through the pulmonary valve.

Chapter 17
Pulmonary Atresia with Ventricular Septal Defect

Karim A. Diab and Thea Yosowitz

Key Facts

- There is no forward flow across the pulmonary valve in pulmonary atresia with ventricular septal defect (PA-VSD); right ventricular output is thorough a VSD to the LV.
- Pulmonary atresia may affect the pulmonary valve alone with normal size pulmonary arteries, or at the other extreme the pulmonary arteries may be severely atretic with pulmonary blood flow (PBF) carried into the distal pulmonary vasculature through numerous systemic to pulmonary arterial (SP) collaterals.
- Patients with PA-VSD present with either cyanosis due to low PBF or congestive heart failure due to excessive PBF through large collaterals.
- The murmur heard in PA-VSD is continuous due to blood flow through PDA or SP collaterals.
- Planning of surgical repair is determined by magnitude of SP collaterals.
- Surgical outcome is better when the pulmonary arteries are well developed and less favorable with severe pulmonary arterial hypoplasia and higher dependence on SP collaterals.
- Balloon and stent dilation of abnormal pulmonary arterial branches and collaterals may be required repeatedly in severe cases to secure unobstructed PBF.

Definition

Pulmonary atresia with ventricular septal defect (PA-VSD) is a cyanotic congenital heart disease characterized by the absence of direct communication between the right

K.A. Diab (✉)
Department of Pediatrics, St. Joseph Hospital and Medical Center, 500 W. Thomas Rd. Suite 500, Phoenix, AZ 85013, USA
e-mail: kdiab@email.arizona.edu

Ra-id Abdulla (ed.), *Heart Diseases in Children: A Pediatrician's Guide*,
DOI 10.1007/978-1-4419-7994-0_17, © Springer Science+Business Media, LLC 2011

ventricle and the pulmonary artery (i.e. atresia of the pulmonary valve), a large ventricular septal defect and overriding aorta. It could be considered as a severe form of tetralogy of Fallot; however, the pulmonary anatomy is usually more complex in PA-VSD than that noted in patients with tetralogy of Fallot.

Incidence

PA-VSD is a rare type of cyanotic congenital heart disease occurring in about 0.07 per 1,000 live births and representing about 1–2% of all forms of congenital heart malformations. It is slightly more prevalent in males than in females. Although a clear genetic etiology has not been elucidated, there is a clear association with certain risk factors during pregnancy as well as with certain genetic syndromes. There is a higher risk for development of this lesion in fetuses of diabetic mothers and in those exposed to certain teratogens such as retinoic acid. A clear association with DiGeorge syndrome/velocardiofacial syndrome (VCFS) and with Alagille syndrome has also been described. DiGeorge/VCFS syndrome involves a chromosome 22q11 deletion and is characterized by distinct facial features, palatal anomalies, immunodeficiency, hypocalcemia, renal anomalies, and congenital heart disease. Certain studies have shown that patients with PA-VSD who have the 22q11 deletion have more complex pulmonary artery anatomy.

Pathology

PA-VSD is characterized by a spectrum of variable extension of the severity of the atresia of the pulmonary arteries. At one end of the spectrum, the atresia is limited to the pulmonary valve resulting in an imperforate pulmonary valve (i.e. membranous atresia). In this case, the main pulmonary artery and branch pulmonary arteries are usually normal in size. The other end of the spectrum includes atresia of the pulmonary valve and arteries with systemic to pulmonary arterial collaterals providing blood flow to the lung parenchyma. More commonly, the pulmonary valve and proximal pulmonary artery are affected, with small branch and distal pulmonary arteries supplied with blood through a patent ductus arteriosus and systemic to pulmonary arterial collaterals (Fig. 17.1).

A hallmark of PA-VSD is the presence of aortopulmonary collaterals that provide at least part of the pulmonary blood supply. These are vessels that arise from the aorta (usually the abdominal aorta) and connect to the pulmonary arteries at various levels. These collaterals can be minimal (in case of isolated membranous pulmonary valve atresia) or more typically multiple and very tortuous in the more

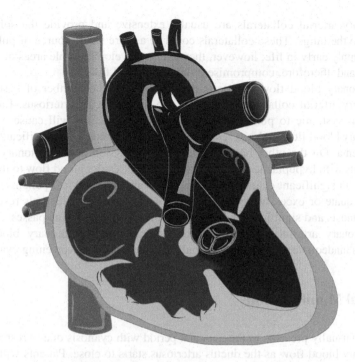

Fig. 17.1 Anatomy of PA-VSD. The pulmonary valve is atretic with no forward flow. Blood in the right ventricle exits through a VSD and into the left ventricle. Pulmonary blood flow is secured through a patent ductus arteriosus (shown in this diagram) or systemic to pulmonary arterial collaterals

complex forms of PA-VSD. This is in contrast to tetralogy of Fallot, where systemic to pulmonary arterial collaterals are extremely unusual.

In addition to the complex pulmonary arterial tree anatomy, PA-VSD, like TOF, is characterized by an overriding aorta and a large malalignment type perimembranous ventricular septal defect. There is also moderate to severe right ventricular hypertrophy.

Pathophysiology

In PA-VSD, there is no communication between the right ventricle and the pulmonary arterial tree. Hence, all blood supply to the pulmonary circulation has to be derived from the systemic circulation. This is provided by two main sources: the patent ductus arteriosus and systemic to pulmonary arterial collaterals.

When a PDA is present, the pulmonary arteries are usually continuous or confluent in most cases. On the other hand, when the PDA is absent, the systemic to pulmonary arterial collaterals are usually extensive and provide the sole blood supply to the lungs. These collaterals could be a more stable source of pulmonary blood supply early in life; however, they tend to develop multiple areas of stenosis later on and, therefore, compromise pulmonary blood flow.

Pulmonary blood flow is determined by the size and number of systemic to pulmonary arterial collaterals as well as the patent ductus arteriosus. Large and numerous systemic to pulmonary arterial collateral vessels will cause excessive pulmonary blood flow and as a result no significant cyanosis but significant pulmonary edema. On the other hand, limited or small systemic to pulmonary arterial collaterals with hypoplastic pulmonary arteries will restrict blood flow to the lungs, resulting in significant cyanosis and no pulmonary edema. Most patients are born with adequate or excessive systemic to pulmonary arterial collaterals resulting in mild cyanosis and significant pulmonary edema, however, as time passes, systemic to pulmonary arterial collaterals become stenotic and pulmonary blood flow becomes inadequate resulting in less pulmonary edema and worsening cyanosis.

Clinical Manifestations

PA-VSD usually presents in the neonatal period with cyanosis due to restriction of pulmonary blood flow as the ductus arteriosus starts to close. Patients with ductus arteriosus which remains patent, or those with multiple and/or large systemic to pulmonary arterial collaterals providing adequate or excessive pulmonary blood flow, will have near normal oxygen saturation. The latter subset of patients can even present in heart failure with tachypnea and minimal cyanosis due to the excessive pulmonary blood flow. However, within weeks or months these patients will outgrow their source of pulmonary blood flow as the collaterals develop stenosis resulting in progressive hypoxemia.

On physical examination, the degree of cyanosis is inversely related to the extent of pulmonary blood flow. Children with numerous and/or large systemic to pulmonary arterial collaterals or PDA will have excessive pulmonary blood flow which will lessen cyanosis, however, at the expense of developing pulmonary edema and congestive heart failure. Therefore, these patients will present with shortness of breath and easy fatigability. There may be mild cyanosis with oxygen saturation in high 80s to low 90s. Capillary refill may be prolonged with diminished peripheral pulses. Hepatomegaly may be present. The precordium in these patients is hyperactive with prominent right ventricular impulse. Auscultation will reveal a single second heart sound due to pulmonary atresia and a continuous murmur reflecting flow across systemic to pulmonary arterial collaterals and PDA (Fig. 17.2).

Patients with small systemic to pulmonary arterial collaterals will present predominantly with cyanosis. There may be tachypnea due to low oxygen saturation; however, there are no significant symptoms of pulmonary edema or congestive heart failure. Single second heart sound and continuous murmur are again heard in

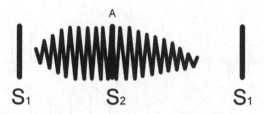

Fig. 17.2 Heart sounds and murmur in PA-VSD. *S1*, first heart sound; *S2*, second heart sound; *A*, aortic valve closure. Second heart sound is single due to atresia of the pulmonary valve. Continuous murmur due to flow through PDA or collaterals is present

these patients. The continuous murmur reflects systemic to pulmonary arterial collaterals that are present, but restrictive.

Although a VSD is an integral part of this congenital heart disease, like tetralogy of Fallot the VSD does not produce the typical holosystolic murmur associated with VSD due to the elevated right ventricular pressure and the right to left shunting across the VSD which occurs in a laminar fashion, consequently not producing any murmur.

Chest X-Ray

Typical radiologic features are similar to those seen in classic tetralogy of Fallot. A boot-shaped heart is seen due to elevation of the apex of the heart because of right ventricular hypertrophy and concavity in the area of the main pulmonary artery because of hypoplasia or atresia of this artery. The heart size is usually normal or slightly enlarged. Pulmonary vascular markings are usually decreased. A right aortic arch is more commonly seen than in classic TOF, particularly in those patients with DiGeorge syndrome. An absent thymus shadow can also sometimes be appreciated in these latter patients.

Electrocardiography

Findings on electrocardiography are also similar to those seen in TOF: right axis deviation and right ventricular hypertrophy (Fig. 17.3). In those patients with excessive pulmonary blood flow secondary to extensive systemic to pulmonary arterial collaterals, there might be left atrial enlargement and biventricular hypertrophy due to the increase in blood return from the pulmonary veins.

ECG can be helpful in differentiating PA-VSD from PA with intact ventricular septum. The latter shows diminutive anterior QRS forces because of the small right ventricle. In addition, ECG is different than that seen in tricuspid atresia where there is left superior axis deviation and small anterior QRS forces.

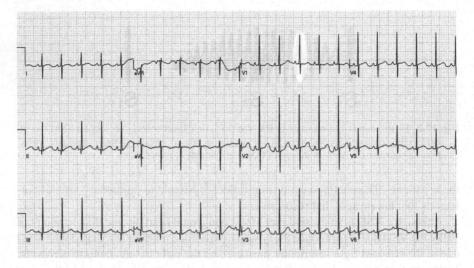

Fig. 17.3 ECG in PA-VSD. Right ventricular hypertrophy (RVH) is seen in this ECG. RVH is manifested as tall R in V1

Echocardiography

PA-VSD can be readily diagnosed by echocardiography. The features are similar to those in TOF except that in PA-VSD there is no communication between the right ventricle and the main pulmonary artery. Echocardiography can also be helpful to evaluate the size of the pulmonary arteries and determine whether they are confluent or discontinuous. It can also help detect the presence of systemic to pulmonary arterial collaterals, although it is not a sufficient test to completely define these tortuous vessels. Additional information such as patency of the ductus arteriosus, presence of a right aortic arch and additional lesions can also be clearly assessed.

Cardiac Catheterization

Although echocardiography can establish the diagnosis of PA-VSD, it provides limited details about the anatomy of the pulmonary arteries and systemic to pulmonary arterial collaterals. Therefore, cardiac catheterization continues to be a helpful procedure to delineate the distribution of the true pulmonary arteries and of the collaterals. In addition, cardiac catheterization can provide helpful therapeutic interventions in PA-VSD. This could be applied initially during the newborn period in those patients with a membranous type of pulmonary atresia in whom the atretic valve area can be perforated and then balloon-dilated to establish continuity between the RV and the main pulmonary artery. In those patients with more extensive atresia of the outflow tract and more complex systemic to pulmonary arterial collaterals, cardiac catheterization is important in the long-term follow up of these patients to relieve stenotic areas in these vessels.

MRI and CT

Cardiac MRI or CT scan can also delineate the source of pulmonary blood flow by determining the anatomy of the pulmonary arteries and systemic to pulmonary arterial collaterals. This is often obtained prior to surgical repair in newly diagnosed newborn children unless those patients will undergo an interventional catheterization, in which case cardiac catheterization will provide the information needed.

Management

Management of PA-VSD depends on the source of pulmonary blood flow which dictates the clinical presentation. Infants relying on the patent ductus arteriosus for adequate pulmonary blood flow, require immediate institution of prostaglandin infusion after birth. Those who have significant pulmonary blood flow through multiple systemic to pulmonary arterial collaterals can maintain adequate oxygen saturations even after the PDA closes and, thus, do not require prostaglandin infusion. Rare cases where pulmonary blood flow is excessive, secondary to extensive collaterals might require anticongestive heart failure therapy with diuretics.

The main goal of therapy is to establish a reliable source of pulmonary blood flow by creating a communication between the right ventricle and the pulmonary arteries. If the pulmonary arteries are confluent, a PDA typically feeds the confluent pulmonary arteries. These patients benefit from opening the atretic pulmonary valve in cases of membranous pulmonary valve atresia and patent main pulmonary artery with or without placement of a systemic to pulmonary arterial shunt. On the other hand, if pulmonary atresia is more extensive, affecting the pulmonary valve and main pulmonary artery, then a systemic to pulmonary arterial shunt is necessary to maintain a reliable source of pulmonary blood flow till the child is about 4–6 months of age when a right ventricle to pulmonary arterial conduit can be placed with closure of the ventricular septal defect.

Children with multiple systemic to pulmonary arterial collaterals typically have poorly developed pulmonary arteries and numerous collateral vessels feeding different segments of the two lungs. Management in such cases is challenging and requires multiple staging of operative repair. Repair starts by good understanding of the pulmonary arterial and collateral anatomy. The initial surgical step brings together as many collaterals and the pulmonary artery on one side of the chest to a single source of blood supply (systemic to pulmonary arterial or BT shunt). This procedure is known as unifocalization since it connects all blood vessels supplying the lung to a single source of blood supply. Unifocalization is performed through a lateral thoracotomy. After few weeks, the same surgical procedure is performed for the other side of the chest. A third surgical procedure is then performed to bring the two "unifocalized" sides together and connect to the right ventricle through a conduit (homograft). In some instances, the pulmonary arteries are poorly developed and therefore pulmonary arterial pressure is elevated requiring the VSD to be left open to prevent right heart failure, this may be closed at a later date.

Overall, patients with PA-VSD in whom the true pulmonary arteries are well developed fare well and their prognosis is comparable to those with TOF. Those patients with abnormal pulmonary artery anatomy and extensive systemic to pulmonary arterial collaterals have poorer prognosis with less certain long-term results.

Case Scenarios

Case 1

A female newborn was noted to be severely cyanotic shortly after birth. She was born at term by Cesarean section because of non-reassuring fetal status. There were no complications during pregnancy. Birth weight was 3.8 kg. Apgars were 7 and 8 at 1 and 5 min, respectively. She was noted to have cyanosis and labored breathing since birth. The child was transferred to the neonatal intensive care unit for further evaluation.

Physical Exam

On physical examination, the patient was cyanotic, but did not otherwise appear sick. Heart rate was 148 bpm, respiratory rate 50, blood pressure was 62/38 mmHg, oxygen saturation 74% while breathing room air. On auscultation, the first heart sound was normal and the second heart sound was single. A systolic ejection murmur was heard over the left upper sternal border. Lungs were clear and the liver was not enlarged. Mucosa had bluish discoloration. Pulses were adequate.

Chest X-ray: The heart size is normal. "Boot-shaped" heart is seen secondary to right ventricular hypertrophy and hypoplasia of the main pulmonary artery. The pulmonary vascular markings are decreased, suggesting decreased pulmonary blood flow.

ECG: Evidence of right axis deviation and right ventricular hypertrophy are noted.

Differential Diagnosis

This patient presented with cyanosis and increased work of breathing at birth. The differential at this juncture should include pulmonary pathology, cardiac pathology, as well as sepsis. A systolic murmur in the upper sternal border in a cyanotic newborn is suggestive of a congenital cyanotic heart defect. The boot shaped heart on CXR is due to right ventricular hypertrophy, which is seen in many right sided obstructive lesions such as tetralogy of Fallot and PA-VSD. The lack of pulmonary vascular markings also can help in forming the differential diagnosis in favor of a lesion associated with reduced pulmonary blood flow such as tetralogy of Fallot and PA-VSD with limited collateral circulation. The ECG is helpful in distinguishing this case of PA-VSD from two other common causes of severe cyanosis in the newborn: PA with intact ventricular septum where the anterior forces are small due to the hypoplastic RV; and tricuspid atresia where there is left superior axis deviation.

An echocardiogram revealed PA-VSD in this case; as well as small pulmonary arteries, moderate RVH with normal systolic function. There was a dilated aorta overriding a large VSD. There was no communication between the RV and the main pulmonary artery, which was found to be normal in size with normal size confluent branch pulmonary arteries. A moderate size PDA was present. Small systemic to pulmonary arterial collateral arteries were seen.

Assessment

This patient has cyanosis at birth with decreased pulmonary blood flow and findings by echocardiography diagnostic of PA-VSD. *In this case, pulmonary blood flow depends on a patent ductus rather than numerous systemic to pulmonary arterial collaterals.*

Management

The patient should be immediately initiated on prostaglandin infusion to keep the ductus arteriosus patent and maintain an adequate source of pulmonary blood flow. In this particular case, the patient might benefit from catheter perforation and dilatation of the pulmonary valve area to create a connection between the RV and the pulmonary artery. This can be done in the cardiac catheterization laboratory; however, if not possible, surgical reconstruction of the right ventricular outflow tract can then be performed.

Case 2

A 16-month-old boy presented to the emergency department because of increased work of breathing and "progressively turning blue" during the prior recent months. The patient was born at term and was discharged home after few days. The child received limited medical care during his life. He had occasional upper respiratory tract infections in the past. In his first months of life, he was tachypneic and struggled with weight gain, but then improved until a few months ago when cyanosis developed.

Physical Exam

On physical examination, the patient was cyanotic and in respiratory distress. Heart rate was 145 bpm, RR 40, BP was 90/65, weight was 8 kg, and oxygen saturation was 82% on room air. The patient had micrognathia, hypertelorism, and short palpebral fissures. Lungs were clear. Cardiac auscultation revealed a single second heart sound and a blowing continuous murmur was heard over the precordium as well as over the back. Liver was 2 cm below the costal margin. Pulses were mildly decreased but symmetric.

CXR: Showed a normal to mildly-enlarged heart with an upwardly displaced apex. Pulmonary vascular markings were decreased.

ECG: Showed evidence of RVH and right axis deviation.

Differential Diagnosis

Cyanosis, tachypnea, and a history of respiratory infections can occur in pulmonary disease such as BPD, Cystic Fibrosis, pulmonary hypertension, a-v malformations to name a few. In the acute setting, pneumonia can present with tachypnea and hypoxia. Heart disease becomes more apparent once you examine this child and hear the continuous murmur over the precordium and back. The upward displaced apex of the heart on CXR is consistent with RVH, also seen on the EKG. The dysmorphic facial features along with cyanotic heart disease can help the practitioner with the differential diagnosis.

An echocardiogram was done and revealed PA-VSD with multiple systemic to pulmonary arterial collaterals with areas of stenoses. There was a small PDA. The branch pulmonary arteries were discontinuous.

Assessment

This patient has significant cyanosis. He also has dysmorphic features common to DiGeorge/Velocardiofacial syndrome and this should prompt the suspicion for possible associated congenital heart disease commonly involving the conotruncal lesions such as tetralogy of Fallot and pulmonary atresia. As noted by the mother, this patient was not significantly cyanotic at birth, but actually had increased pulmonary blood flow causing his failure to thrive and increased work of breathing initially. The presence of major systemic to pulmonary arterial collaterals as well a persistent PDA provided excessive pulmonary blood flow to the point of causing symptoms of congestive heart failure. As the patient grew older, he outgrew this source of pulmonary blood flow and started getting more cyanotic. In addition, the development of areas of stenoses in the systemic to pulmonary arterial collaterals caused a decrease in pulmonary blood flow. Typical of patients with DiGeorge syndrome (chromosome 22q11 deletion), the pulmonary arteries are commonly abnormal or discontinuous as in this case.

Management

This patient needs surgical intervention to improve his pulmonary blood flow. This is done through multiple surgical and interventional procedures that aim at unifocalizing the pulmonary arteries and systemic to pulmonary arterial collaterals and ultimately closing the VSD and achieving a full repair. In order to plan these steps, cardiac MRI or CT scan as well as cardiac catheterization will be helpful in detailing the anatomy of these collaterals. This patient should also be evaluated for findings associated with 22q11 deletion. Calcium and phosphorus and immune function studies should be done. Finally, the family should be counseled regarding importance of proper pediatric followup since this is an unusual late presentation.

Chapter 18
Tricuspid Atresia

Karim A. Diab and Daniel E. Felten

Key Facts

- Clinical presentation of TA varies depending upon the extent of pulmonary blood flow. Children with ventricular septal defect tend to have increased pulmonary blood flow, while those with intact ventricular septal defect rely on the patency of ductus arteriosus to supply pulmonary blood flow. As the ductus arteriosus constricts, pulmonary blood flow is severely limited resulting in cyanosis.
- Second heart sound is single when the ventricular septum is intact due to associated pulmonary atresia.
- ECG shows a QRS axis of 0 to −90° (leftward and superior axis).
- Early intervention includes initiating prostaglandin infusion when pulmonary blood flow is ductal dependent and cardiac catheterization atrial septostomy if the atrial communication is restrictive.

Definition

Tricuspid atresia (TA) is defined as complete absence of a tricuspid valve orifice resulting in no direct communication between the right atrium and the right ventricle. This leads to a significantly hypoplastic right ventricle.

K.A. Diab(✉)
Department of Pediatrics, St. Joseph Hospital and Medical Center,
500 W. Thomas Rd. Suite 500, Phoenix, AZ 85013, USA
e-mail: kdiab@email.arizona.edu

Ra-id Abdulla (ed.), *Heart Diseases in Children: A Pediatrician's Guide*,
DOI 10.1007/978-1-4419-7994-0_18, © Springer Science+Business Media, LLC 2011

Incidence

TA is a rare congenital heart disease with a frequency of about 0.057 per 1,000 live births. It has been reported to occur in about 2.6–3.7% of patients with congenital heart malformations. This makes it the third most common form of cyanotic congenital heart disease after tetralogy of Fallot and transposition of the great arteries. There is no sex predilection.

Anatomy/Pathology

The absence of a tricuspid valve orifice causes blood from the right atrium to flow into the left atrium through a foramen ovale or atrial septal defect. The development of the right ventricle relies largely on blood flow during fetal life, so it is invariably hypoplastic. Blood may flow into the right ventricle through a ventricular septal defect (VSD), which is usually of the perimembranous type. If a VSD is present, the degree of right ventricular hypoplasia is determined by its size. If there is no VSD, the right ventricle tends to be severely hypoplastic and there is associated pulmonary atresia (Fig. 18.1).

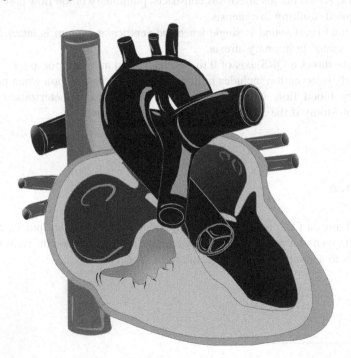

Fig. 18.1 Anatomy of tricuspid atresia. Atresia of the tricuspid valve prevents antegrade flow into the right ventricle, thus causing hypoplasia of the right ventricle. Pulmonary blood flow is supplied to the pulmonary arteries through patent ductus arteriosus

TA is classified into three groups depending on the relationship of the great arteries:

1. Type I: when the great arteries are normally related (approximately 70% of cases).
2. Type II: when there is d-transposition of the great arteries; this can be associated with subaortic stenosis and coarctation of the aorta (approximately 25% of cases).
3. Type III: when there are other associated complex lesions such as l-transposition of the great arteries; this is a very rare form of TA (less than 5% of cases).

Each of these types is further subclassified depending on the presence or absence of a VSD. Type I is the typical example of TA; whereas Types II and III are mixed lesions that present more variably and require more complicated management approaches. This chapter will focus predominantly on type I.

Pathophysiology

Venous blood enters the right atrium and is forced by the atretic tricuspid valve to shunt to the left atrium across an atrial communication (PFO or ASD). Systemic and pulmonary venous blood then mixes in the left atrium and passes through the mitral valve to the left ventricle. Blood flow from the left ventricle depends on the type of TA and presence or absence of a VSD.

In TA with normally related great arteries (type I) and intact ventricular septum, pulmonary blood flow is supplied through a PDA. Blood flows from the left ventricle to the aorta which then supplies the systemic circulation as well as the pulmonary arteries through the PDA. These patients become more cyanotic over the first hours of life as the ductus arteriosus constricts resulting in drop in pulmonary blood flow.

In patients with normally related great arteries and a VSD, blood flows from the left ventricle both to the aorta and through the hypoplastic right ventricle to the pulmonary artery. Pulmonary blood flow depends on the size of the VSD and the presence of a patent ductus arteriosus (PDA). A larger VSD will allow for improved flow to the pulmonary artery and make a PDA less necessary. Over time, the VSD tends to decrease in size, which results in decreasing pulmonary blood flow and increasing cyanosis.

In those patients with d-transposed great arteries (type II), the ascending aorta arises from the right ventricle and the pulmonary artery from the left ventricle. If a VSD is present, blood can flow from the left ventricle through the hypoplastic right ventricle to the aorta and systemic circulation. A large VSD will allow for unobstructed blood flow to the systemic circulation. However, as systemic vascular resistance increases and pulmonary vascular resistance decreases over the first few days of life, blood will preferentially flow into the pulmonary artery causing excessive pulmonary blood flow and congestive heart failure. As the VSD gets smaller over time, there will be increasing restriction of the systemic flow leading to hypotension and shock. Alternatively, if the VSD is small or absent systemic circulation relies on the presence of a PDA. In this case, blood flows from the left ventricle to the pulmonary artery and through the PDA to the aorta, similar to blood flow pattern in children with hypoplastic left heart syndrome. As the PDA closes, flow to the systemic circulation is restricted, and the patient will develop hypotension and shock.

In patients with the rare type of TA and l-TGA, the morphologic left (systemic) ventricle is hypoplastic because it is located on the right side of the heart and does not receive blood flow from the right atrium. This situation mimics mitral atresia because although the ventricle on the left side of the heart develops normally, but it is morphologically the right ventricle, which is intended to handle pulmonary pressures and not systemic pressures.

Clinical Manifestations

The clinical presentation of patients with TA varies depending on the type of great artery relationship as well as on the presence or absence of a VSD. However, due to the complete mixing of blood in the left atrium, all these patients have some degree of cyanosis that is usually noticeable before the first week of life. The clinical manifestation is divided into the two major groups of patients as follows:

Patients with Normally Related Great Arteries

Patients with no VSD have a severely hypoplastic right ventricle and pulmonary atresia, and they manifest cyanosis soon after birth as they rely on the PDA for pulmonary blood flow. On physical examination, these newborn infants have a single second heart sound and might have a PDA murmur, which is a long systolic or continuous murmur heard best over the left upper sternal border and left subclavicular region.

On the other hand, those patients with TA-VSD will have varying degrees of cyanosis depending on the size of the defect and the degree of pulmonary stenosis. Those with a small restrictive VSD or with significant pulmonary valve stenosis will present similarly to those without a VSD, that is, with significant cyanosis in the newborn period. On physical examination, they might have a palpable thrill from a small VSD or pulmonary valve stenosis. The second heart sound is single if there is severe pulmonary valve stenosis; otherwise it splits in a normal fashion. A holosystolic murmur may be heard because of flow across the VSD, whereas a systolic ejection murmur may be a reflection of pulmonary stenosis (Fig. 18.2).

Patients with a large VSD and no pulmonary stenosis have excessive pulmonary blood flow, particularly after the pulmonary vascular resistance drops in the first weeks after birth. Therefore, these patients will present with symptoms of congestive

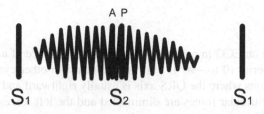

Fig. 18.2 Heart sounds and murmur in tricuspid atresia. *S1*, first heart sound; *S2*, second heart sound; *A*, aortic valve closure; *P*, pulmonary valve closure. Continuous murmur of blood flow through the PDA is audible. The second heart sound may be single due to pulmonary atresia secondary to tricuspid atresia and hypoplastic right ventricle. Pulmonary valve may be normal if patient has a ventricular septal defect allowing for blood flow from the left ventricle and into the right ventricle and pulmonary valve

heart failure. On physical examination, they are tachypneic and only mildly cyanotic. Auscultation reveals a single second heart sound and a systolic ejection murmur due to increased flow across the pulmonary valve. A third heart sound may be heard as well. The liver is usually enlarged. It is important to note that the VSD in these patients tends to get smaller with time, which will limit pulmonary blood flow and improve symptoms of CHF. However, limiting pulmonary blood flow will also result in increasing cyanosis.

Patients with Transposed Great Arteries

Patients with d-TGA and a large VSD usually present with symptoms of congestive heart failure, as described above, and mild cyanosis. Those who have a small VSD or those in whom the VSD gets smaller with time will have symptoms of decreased systemic perfusion and increased pulmonary blood flow. On examination, these patients are tachypneic, mildly cyanotic, and likely hypotensive depending on the degree of restriction of systemic flow. On auscultation, they have a single and loud S2, as the aortic valve is anterior when the great arteries are transposed.

Diagnostic Testing

Chest X-Ray

Two things to notice on CXR: heart size and pulmonary vascular markings. The degree of cardiomegaly is proportional to the degree of pulmonary blood flow, i.e. increased blood flow to the lungs will increase the volume load on the heart and result in cardiomegaly. Most patients with TA will, therefore, have a normal heart size on CXR with decreased pulmonary vascular markings. The exception is those patients with a large VSD and no pulmonary stenosis.

ECG

A typical finding on ECG in patients with TA is the presence of a QRS axis that is leftward and superior (0 to −90°). This is in contrast to other cyanotic congenital heart disease lesions where the QRS axis is usually rightward and inferior. In addition, the right ventricular forces are diminished and the left forces are dominant in TA. Left axis deviation is less common in those patients with transposed great arteries. There might also be right or sometimes bilateral atrial enlargement as evidenced by tall or wide P waves, respectively (Fig. 18.3).

Echocardiography

Echocardiography readily establishes the diagnosis and is the diagnostic procedure of choice. The basic anatomic features can be easily assessed including the absence of a tricuspid valve, the size of the atrial and ventricular defects, the small right ventricle, the relationship of the great arteries, presence of pulmonary or subaortic stenosis, the size of the PDA and the presence of coarctation in those with transposed vessels and a small VSD (Fig. 18.4).

Echocardiography is also essential to evaluate these patients following surgical palliative procedures to monitor for valve regurgitation, ventricular dysfunction, pulmonary flow obstruction and development of clots.

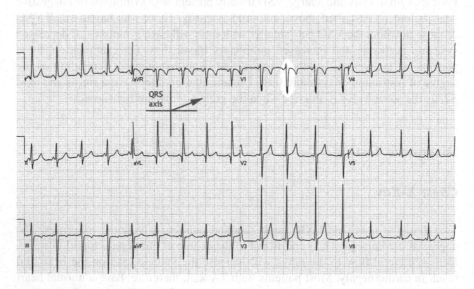

Fig. 18.3 ECG in tricuspid atresia. Hypoplastic right ventricle is demonstrated through small "r" wave in the right chest leads and left axis deviation (newborn QRS axis tends to be rightwards)

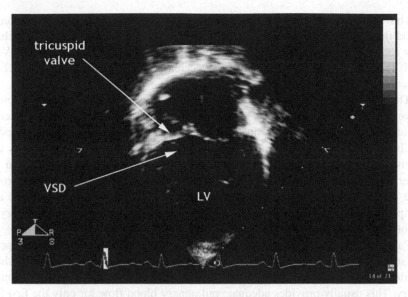

Fig. 18.4 Echocardiography. *LV* left ventricle, *VSD* ventricular septal defect 2D echocardiography demonstrates anatomy of tricuspid valve. The right ventricle is hypoplastic. A ventricular septal defect is noted in this patient

Cardiac Catheterization

Cardiac catheterization is no longer necessary during the newborn period as echocardiography provides a reliable non-invasive means to diagnose this entity. In the rare case where the ASD is restrictive, a balloon atrial septostomy might be needed to relieve obstruction to the egress of blood from the right atrium.

On the other hand, cardiac catheterization is essential in the older patient who has undergone previous palliative surgical interventions. This mainly helps determine pulmonary vascular resistance, pulmonary pressures and size of the pulmonary arteries, all of which would help plan future surgical management.

Management

Initial management of patients with TA depends on the adequacy of pulmonary blood flow. Newborn children with decreased pulmonary blood flow, who represent the majority of cases, will present with severe cyanosis and will require prompt prostaglandin infusion in order to maintain patency of the ductus arteriosus and improve pulmonary blood supply.

Those infants with increased pulmonary blood flow, such as those with normally related or transposed great arteries with a large VSD and no pulmonary stenosis, will have minimal cyanosis and are not dependent on a PDA for adequate pulmonary blood flow. Since these patients present with symptoms of congestive heart failure, they can benefit from diuretic therapy. It is important to note again that the VSD tends to get smaller with time resulting in decreased pulmonary blood flow in these patients.

The ultimate goal of management is to separate systemic and pulmonary flow to prevent mixing and to utilize the single functional ventricle to supply the systemic circulation. Thus, the single ventricle heart will provide fully oxygenated blood to the body (systemic circulation), the pulmonary circulation in these cases can receive passive blood flow, without the benefit of a pumping chamber, from the superior and inferior vena cava. This is performed initially through a Glenn procedure (superior vena cava to pulmonary artery) at about 6–9 months of age and completion of the Fontan procedure (inferior vena cava to pulmonary artery at about 12–18 months of age).

Patients with decreased pulmonary blood flow are initially managed with prostaglandin to keep the PDA open until a systemic-to-pulmonary arterial shunt (Blalock–Taussig) is placed between the innominate artery and the right pulmonary artery. This usually provides adequate pulmonary blood flow for only the first few months of age since the shunt does not grow with the patient. At around 6 months of age, when the pulmonary vascular resistance is low, a bidirectional Glenn procedure is performed. This involves connecting the superior vena cava to the right pulmonary artery. At around 2 years of age, a Fontan operation is then performed to direct the rest of the systemic venous blood (from the inferior vena cave) to the right pulmonary artery. This is done through the use of a tunnel conduit and provides the last step in separating the pulmonary and systemic circulations.

Patients with increased pulmonary blood flow might require a band to be placed across the main pulmonary artery to limit the amount of pulmonary blood flow if anti-congestive heart failure treatment is inadequate. Limiting pulmonary blood flow is critical to avoid damage to the pulmonary vasculature and allow for a Glenn and then a Fontan operation to be feasible later on.

Course and Prognosis

Without treatment, TA is fatal in infancy in the majority of cases. The introduction of the Fontan procedure in 1971, and its later modifications, drastically changed the outcome of this disease. These patients are currently expected to live into adulthood and lead a nearly normal life. It is important to note that the Fontan surgery is not the last procedure that is needed as the Fontan conduit might need to be changed after several years. In addition, these patients require follow-up with a cardiologist throughout their lives, as they can develop other complications such as cardiac dysfunction, arrhythmias and effusions. These patients will usually be able to participate in physical activities but most likely not the competitive types.

Case Scenarios

Case 1

History. A 2-day-old male newborn was noticed to be cyanotic in the newborn nursery and to have poor oral intake. The patient is a product of full term gestation with no complications during pregnancy; Apgars were 8 at 1 min and 9 at 5 min.

Physical examination. Heart rate was 148 bpm, respiratory rate 48, blood pressure was 62/40 mmHg, oxygen saturation was 80% while breathing room air, and weight was 3.5 kg. Cardiac auscultation revealed single S1 and S2, a 2/6 systolic ejection murmur heard best at the left upper sternal border. Lungs were clear to auscultation. There was bluish discoloration of the mucosa; femoral pulses were equal.

Investigational studies

– CXR: showed normal heart size and decreased pulmonary vascular markings.
– ECG: showed a left and superior axis with dominant left forces.

Differential diagnosis. This newborn is clearly cyanotic and has decreased pulmonary blood flow as evidenced by decreased pulmonary blood flow on CXR. These findings suggest shunting from right to left either due to increased pulmonary pressures or due to decreased flow to the pulmonary vasculature. The only primary pulmonary issue to consider is pulmonary hypertension given decreased pulmonary blood flow. Cardiac anomalies include TA, Ebstein anomaly, tetralogy of Fallot, pulmonary atresia, and severe pulmonary stenosis. However, normal heart size and contour make pulmonary hypertension and TA most likely.

Assessment. Since the patient developed cyanosis early in the newborn period, a ductal dependent lesion is likely – in this case TA without VSD. The finding of a single second heart sound and lack of findings of congestive heart failure are consistent with TA without VSD. The right ventricle is severely hypoplastic, therefore there is no second heart sound from the pulmonary valve, and flow to the systemic circulation is unobstructed, so there is no backup into the pulmonary or venous system. CXR also supports the diagnosis as pulmonary vascular markings are diminished and the heart size is normal, both indicating that blood flow is being shunted away from the pulmonary circulation and is not backing up in the venous system. However, severe pulmonary stenosis or atresia with VSD could present with most of the same findings above, so the ECG further narrows the diagnosis in this case. Unlike other cases of cyanotic congenital heart disease where there is some degree of RV hypertrophy and right axis deviation, this ECG shows left superior axis as seen in TA due to the normal LV and hypoplastic RV. Echocardiogram would be indicated to establish the diagnosis and determine the type of TA, and in this case would confirm TA with no VSD.

Management. After stabilization of the patient with institution of prostaglandin infusion to maintain the patency of the ductus arteriosus and provide a source of pulmonary blood flow, this patient should undergo surgical palliation by placement of a BT shunt to connect the innominate artery to the right pulmonary artery. Further palliation is done through a Glenn procedure at about 6 months then Fontan procedure at 2 years of age to completely separate the pulmonary from the systemic circulation.

Case 2

History. A 15-day-old female infant was admitted to the hospital because of cyanotic episodes while feeding. The patient was born full term with unremarkable pregnancy. Her birth weight was 4.8 kg. She was discharged home in 2 days. However, the mother noted that her lips would turn blue with crying or feeding.

Physical examination. The patient looked well developed, in no distress. Vital signs were normal except for mild tachypnea and an oxygen saturation of 92–93% on room air that dropped to 80s with crying. Cyanosis was noticed especially when the patient was irritable. Lungs were clear. Cardiac auscultation revealed a single second heart sound and a grade 3/6 systolic ejection murmur was heard best over the left upper sternal border. The liver was palpable 2 cm below the costal margin. Pulses were normal.
Investigational studies

– CXR: showed mild cardiomegaly and increase in pulmonary vascular markings.
– ECG: showed left axis deviation.

Differential diagnosis. Unlike the previous case, this patient was not cyanotic shortly after birth, so is unlikely to have a ductal dependent lesion. Instead, with increasing difficulty over the first few weeks of life, this patient is more likely to have a lesion that causes progressive heart failure as pulmonary vascular resistance decreases. Such lesions include large VSD, TA with VSD, truncus arteriosus, Tetralogy of Fallot with large VSD and minimal pulmonary stenosis, anomalous pulmonary venous drainage, and transposition of the great arteries with large VSD. These lesions can lead to increased pulmonary flow and CHF over the first weeks of life.

Assessment. This child likely has TA with large VSD. As mentioned above, the progressive cyanosis over the first weeks of life make a ductal dependent lesion unlikely. Physical findings of mild tachypnea and hypoxia at rest with an enlarged liver suggest congestive heart failure, which can be seen with most of the above lesions due to increase in pulmonary blood flow, but the single second heart sound suggests either TA or truncus arteriosus. The systolic ejection murmur is a reflection of the increased blood flow across the pulmonary area. The CXR shows increased pulmonary vascular markings and mild cardiomegaly, which is also consistent with many of the above lesions; however, the left axis deviation on ECG is not consistent with right ventricular hypertrophy that is seen with the other lesions except for TA. An echocardiogram would confirm the diagnosis of TA with normally related great arteries, large VSD and no pulmonary stenosis. The large VSD without pulmonary stenosis allowed for unobstructed blood flow to the pulmonary vasculature causing excessive pulmonary blood flow and symptoms of congestive heart failure.

Management. This patient will benefit from anti-congestive heart failure medications and ultimately will need palliative surgical intervention to aim at separating her pulmonary and systemic circulations through a staged Fontan surgery.

Chapter 19
Total Anomalous Pulmonary Venous Return

Karim A. Diab and Daniel E. Felten

Key Facts

- TAPVR typically presents in early infancy due to excessive pulmonary blood flow and mild cyanosis. Presentation is earlier when there is obstruction to pulmonary venous flow where neonates present with severe cyanosis and cardiogenic shock, surgical repair must be planned immediately.
- Mixing of well oxygenated blood through the anomalous connection of pulmonary veins with the systemic blood in the right atrium results in similar oxygen saturation in all cardiac chambers and arteries, therefore pre and post ductal oxygen saturations are equal.
- Increased blood flow across the right heart causes delay in closure of the pulmonary valve, presenting as fixed splitting of second heart sound as well as systolic flow murmur over the pulmonic region.
- Supra-cardiac drainage of anomalous pulmonary veins to the superior vena cava result in figure-eight or snow man appearance of the cardiac silhouette on CXR.

Definition

Total anomalous pulmonary venous return (TAPVR) is a cyanotic congenital heart disease where blood from all four pulmonary veins returns anomalously to the right atrium instead of the left atrium. The pulmonary veins may either connect directly to the right atrium, or they may connect to a systemic vein that drains into the right atrium.

K.A. Diab (✉)
Department of Pediatrics, St. Joseph Hospital and Medical Center, 500 W. Thomas Rd.
Suite 500, Phoenix, AZ 85013, USA
e-mail: kdiab@email.arizona.edu

Ra-id Abdulla (ed.), *Heart Diseases in Children: A Pediatrician's Guide*,
DOI 10.1007/978-1-4419-7994-0_19, © Springer Science+Business Media, LLC 2011

The oxygenated blood from the lungs mixes with poorly oxygenated systemic venous blood in the right atrium and is supplied to the left atrium through an atrial communication (patent foramen ovale or atrial septal defect). Thus, partially deoxygenated blood is sent into systemic circulation causing cyanosis.

Incidence

TAPVR occurs in about 0.06 per 1,000 live births or in about 1.5% of all patients with congenital heart malformations. There is no clear sex predilection; however, some studies have shown some male preponderance in the infracardiac type of TAPVR. TAPVR is usually an isolated lesion but can be associated with other defects as part of a syndrome such as heterotaxy syndrome or cat-eye syndrome.

Anatomy/Pathology

During normal embryologic cardiac development, the pulmonary veins migrate posterior to the developing heart and join to form a common pulmonary vein. The common pulmonary vein then fuses with the posterior wall of the left atrium allowing drainage of pulmonary venous blood into the left atrium. Failure of this vein to unite with the left atrium forces blood returning from the lungs to find an alternative pathway resulting in TAPVR. Unlike partial anomalous pulmonary venous return where some of the pulmonary veins drain into the systemic circulation, in TAPVR all pulmonary veins drain in an abnormal fashion (Fig. 19.1).

TAPVR can be classified into one of the following four groups depending on the site of pulmonary venous drainage:

1. Supracardiac or supradiaphragmatic type: This is the most common type occurring in more than 50% of cases. In this case, all pulmonary veins drain into a common pulmonary confluence behind the left atrium, which then drains into a left vertical or ascending vein returning blood to the innominate vein which connects to the superior vena cava, thus draining pulmonary venous blood to the right atrium.
2. Cardiac type: Occurs in about 25% of cases. In this type, all pulmonary veins drain into the common pulmonary vein which then drains into the right atrium either directly or, more commonly, through the coronary sinus.
3. Infracardiac or infradiaphragmatic type: Occurs in about 20% of cases. The four pulmonary veins connect to a common pulmonary vein that travels down through a long venous vessel and connects to the intra-abdominal veins (such as the portal or hepatic vein).

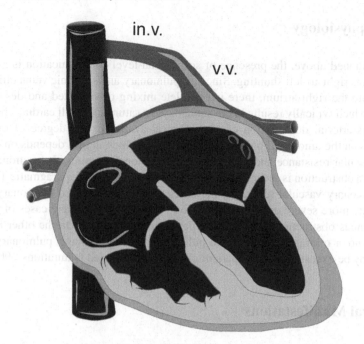

in.v.

v.v.

Fig. 19.1 Anatomy of TAPVR. *IV* innominate vein, *VV* vertical vein. All pulmonary veins drain into a vertical vein which carries all pulmonary venous return to the innominate vein and finally into the superior vena cava. Blood reaches the left atrium through an atrial septal defect

4. Mixed type: (about 5% of cases). In this type, the right and left pulmonary veins drain to different sites. An example would be the right pulmonary veins draining directly into the right atrium and the left pulmonary veins into a vertical vein and then into the superior vena cava.

A few findings are common to all these types and are worth mentioning:

– All types have some atrial communication (patent foramen ovale or atrial septal defect) which is essential for survival since such a communication constitutes the only source of blood flow into the left atrium.
– A common pulmonary vein (usually located behind the left atrium) is common to all types, other than the mixed type. Surgical repair in these cases is easier as it only requires connecting this common collecting vein to the back of the left atrium.
– The right atrium and ventricle are usually dilated while the left atrium is small as it receives less blood.
– Pulmonary venous obstruction may be present in any type of TAPVR, and it may be anything from mild to severe. Obstruction may occur in any type but is most common in the infradiaphragmatic type (obstruction occurring at the level of the diaphragm) and is less common with the cardiac type.

Pathophysiology

As mentioned above, the presence of some atrial level communication is essential to provide right-to-left shunting. Since all pulmonary and systemic veins ultimately drain into the right atrium, there is complete mixing of saturated and desaturated blood, which typically results in the same oxygen saturation in all cardiac chambers and thus arterial desaturation causing clinical cyanosis. The degree of cyanosis depends on the amount of pulmonary blood flow, which in turn depends on pulmonary vascular resistance and the presence of pulmonary venous obstruction.

When obstruction is severe, such as in some cases of infradiaphragmatic TAPVR, the pulmonary vascular resistance increases resulting in reduced pulmonary blood flow with more severe cyanosis (saturation below 80%). In severe cases of pulmonary venous obstruction pulmonary hypertension will result. On the other hand, if there is no or minimal obstruction to pulmonary venous drainage, pulmonary blood flow may be excessive and the patient can be well saturated (saturations >90%).

Clinical Manifestations

Clinical presentation of patients with TAPVR depends on the degree of pulmonary venous obstruction, with severe obstruction at one end of the spectrum and absence of obstruction at the other.

Patients with Severe Pulmonary Obstruction

This is typical of the infradiaphragmatic type of TAPVR, which is invariably obstructed, but it also occurs in about 50% of the supradiaphragmatic type. The pulmonary venous obstruction causes significant pulmonary hypertension and pulmonary edema. As a result, infants are usually acutely ill within the first few hours after birth with severe cyanosis, tachypnea and respiratory distress. Untreated, these infants will deteriorate quickly and die within a short period of time. Findings on physical examination include severe cyanosis, tachypnea and tachycardia. On cardiac auscultation, the first and second heart sound is louder than normal and a soft systolic murmur may be heard in the pulmonary area, although a murmur is often absent. Findings of pulmonary congestion are found on lung auscultation. Hepatomegaly is invariably present.

Patients Without Pulmonary Venous Obstruction

Infants with TAPVR but no pulmonary venous obstruction are usually not ill-looking and have only mild cyanosis that could go undetected in the early newborn period. These patients present with symptoms similar to a very large atrial septal defect shunt.

Poor feeding, tachypnea, failure to thrive and recurrent pulmonary infections occur within the first few months of life. More commonly, these patients are diagnosed as newborns due to the detection of a murmur or mild cyanosis. On physical examination, these infants are thin, tachypneic and might be slightly cyanotic. On cardiac auscultation, the first and second heart sounds are increased. The second heart sound is widely split. There often is a gallop rhythm from a prominent filling third heart sound. The increased flow across the tricuspid valve results in a tricuspid stenosis-like murmur producing a diastolic rumble murmur at the left lower sternal border. In addition, a systolic ejection murmur at the left upper sternal border can be heard due to increased flow across the pulmonary valve. A continuous murmur can be heard in cases of supracardiac TAPVR to a left vertical vein. The liver is usually enlarged.

Chest X-Ray

In patients with obstructed TAPVR, CXR shows a normal size heart and marked pulmonary edema with diffuse reticular pattern. On the other hand, in patients with non-obstructed TAPVR, CXR shows significant cardiomegaly and increased pulmonary vascular markings. A classic CXR appearance in the older child with non-obstructed supracardiac TAPVR reveals a figure-eight, or what is known as a snowman appearance (Fig. 2.14).

ECG

The findings on ECG include peaked P waves indicating right atrial enlargement and evidence of right ventricular hypertrophy with right axis deviation and qR pattern in V1.

Echocardiography

Echocardiography is essential in making the diagnosis of TAPVR. It reveals dilated right sided cardiac chambers and smaller left sided chambers. It can determine the type of pulmonary venous drainage and presence or absence of obstruction to pulmonary venous return.

Cardiac Catheterization

With the availability of advanced non-invasive imaging techniques such echocardiography and MRI, cardiac catheterization is not usually indicated in this lesion. If performed, it would reveal similar oxygen saturation measurements in all cardiac chambers.

MRI or CT

In infants, echocardiography usually provides adequate and detailed information on the precise anatomic type of TAPVR. In older patients, poor echocardiographic windows or more complicated cases where venous drainage is not well defined by echocardiography, MRI provides a noninvasive technique to determine precise anatomic details. Cardiac CT with angiography can also be obtained; however, it would involve more radiation exposure.

Management

Since the advent of prostaglandin infusion, obstructed TAPVR remains the only surgical emergency for newly diagnosed congenital heart disease lesions. All other congenital heart diseases can be stabilized with prostaglandin infusions and/or balloon atrial septostomy (Rashkind procedure). Children with no obstruction to total anomalous pulmonary venous drainage are stable and actually tend to present at 1–2 months of age. On the other hand patients with obstructed TAPVR become critically ill soon after birth due to severe elevation of pulmonary vascular resistance causing significant reduction in pulmonary blood flow and severe cyanosis. Interventions that could help while awaiting surgery in sick patients include intubation and mechanical ventilation while using 100% oxygen as well as correction of metabolic acidosis. The use of prostaglandins is controversial as it might help increase cardiac output by allowing right-to-left shunting across the ductus arteriosus but at the expense of further decrease in pulmonary blood flow.

Surgical repair is performed immediately once the diagnosis of obstructed TAPVR is made (e.g., in most cases of infradiaphragmatic TAPVR), but it can be postponed and performed at a more convenient time in early infancy in cases of non-obstructed TAPVR. The repair involves creation of an anastomosis between the common pulmonary vein and the wall of the left atrium. The vertical vein is ligated.

Although mortality remains high for obstructed TAPVR, mortality associated with non-obstructed TAPVR is low. The results of surgical repair are excellent with mortality of about 5%. Long-term potential complications include pulmonary venous obstruction at the site of anastomosis and arrhythmias.

Case Scenarios

Case 1

History. A 3-month-old male infant was noted to have poor weight gain. He also had history of recurrent upper respiratory infections and the mother reports that he breathes rapidly during feedings. She occasionally notices his lips to turn blue. He was born by normal vaginal delivery at term and was discharged from the hospital at 2 days of life. Birth weight was 4.5 kg. There were no complications during pregnancy.

Physical exam. Weight was 5.2 kg, heart rate was 145 bpm, RR 48, BP was 76/48, and oxygen saturation was 88% on room air. The precordium was hyperdynamic with increased RV impulse, S1 was loud, S2 was widely split. A 2/6 systolic ejection murmur was heard over the left upper sternal border and a 2/6 diastolic rumble murmur was heard over the left lower sternal border. Lungs were clear with some scattered rhonchi. Liver was palpable 3 cm below the costal margin. Pulses were normal.

Investigative studies

- CXR: Revealed cardiomegaly and increased pulmonary vascular markings.
- ECG: Tall P waves indicating right atrial enlargement and right axis deviation with qR pattern in V1 indicating RV enlargement.

Differential diagnosis. This infant presents in heart failure at 3 months of life, which suggests a lesion with significant left to right shunting (large ASD or VSD, large PDA, tetralogy of Fallot with only mild pulmonary stenosis), cardiomyopathy, or TAPVR. Findings of auscultation reflect increased flow across the pulmonary valve producing a systolic ejection murmur and increased flow across the tricuspid valve resulting in diastolic rumble, which would be unlikely in cardiomyopathy. Moreover, left to right shunt lesions and cardiomyopathy should not present with this degree of cyanosis unless the patient were in severe heart failure due to significant pulmonary edema. The combination of heart failure with cyanosis should suggest TAPVR. Since this patient presents outside of the newborn period, it is likely to be a case where the anomalous pulmonary venous return is not obstructed, therefore likely to be of the supracardiac, cardiac, or mixed types.

Diagnosis and management. Echocardiography can accurately establish the diagnosis of TAPVR. Surgical repair is scheduled soon after the diagnosis is made to avoid the development of pulmonary and cardiac changes secondary to long standing cyanosis and volume overload.

Case 2

History. A female newborn was found to be cyanotic soon after birth. She was born at term by normal vaginal delivery with no complications during pregnancy. Her birth weight was 4.2 kg. She was promptly admitted to the neonatal intensive care unit.

Physical exam. The patient looked ill with poor perfusion. Pre- and postductal saturations were 70 and 73% on room air, respectively. She was tachypneic, her HR was 160 bpm, and BP 42/28. On auscultation, the second heart sound was loud and no murmurs were appreciated. The liver was 3 cm below the costal margin. Lung auscultation revealed rales at the bases. The patient was intubated and placed on 100% oxygen and started on inotropic support.

Investigative studies

– ECG: shows peaked P waves indicative of right atrial enlargement; right axis deviation.
– CXR: shows mild cardiomegaly and marked pulmonary edema.

Differential diagnosis. This newborn is severely ill with significant cyanosis and respiratory distress. The findings on CXR are similar to those seen with hyaline membrane disease in premature newborns. Early presentation secondary to a congenital heart disease is unique to very few lesions, these are:

• d-transposition of the great arteries: in this lesion the right ventricle pumps deoxygenated blood to the aorta resulting in severe cyanosis, lower extremity oxygen saturation is slightly higher as shunting across the ductus arteriosus delivers some oxygenated blood to the descending aorta.
• Hypoplastic left heart syndrome (HLH) with intact atrial septum: patients with HLH who have atrial level communication (patent foramen ovale or ASD) may not be diagnosed until a few days of life when the ductus arteriosus starts to constrict causing the reduction of the only blood supply to the body. On the other hand, patients with the rare variety of hypoplastic left heart syndrome associated with intact atrial septum are immediately and gravely ill at birth due to inability of pulmonary venous blood to drain out of the left atrium due to combination of mitral atresia and intact atrial septum, thus preventing delivery of oxygenated pulmonary venous blood.
• TAPVR with obstruction to pulmonary venous drainage: in this lesion, drainage of pulmonary venous blood is prevented due to stenosis of pulmonary veins resulting in severe pulmonary hypertension and interference with pulmonary blood flow, thus presenting as severe cyanosis soon after birth. Pre- and postductal saturations in this case are the same since oxygenated and deoxygenated blood mixes in the right atrium resulting in identical oxygen saturations in all cardiac chambers.

Diagnosis and management. Although diagnosis may be difficult at times, echocardiography should establish the diagnosis and determine the type of TAPVR and the site of obstruction. Classically this would be infracardiac TAPVR with obstruction occurring at the portal-hepatic system. If a PDA is present, it will be shunting right to left because of pulmonary hypertension. If the exact drainage site of the anomalous pulmonary vein is not well delineated by echocardiography, MRI could be done. The patient can be kept on 100% oxygen, started on pressors and possibly on prostaglandins to try to increase the cardiac output, although prostaglandins can further decrease the pulmonary blood flow and can be less helpful in this lesion. Meanwhile, emergent surgical repair is planned to reconnect the anomalous pulmonary venous drainage to the left atrium, which will bypass the obstructed region within the anomalous pulmonary venous connection.

Chapter 20
Truncus Arteriosus

Shannon M. Buckvold, Thea Yosowitz, and Joan F. Hoffman

Key Facts

- Patients with truncus arteriosus have a significant probability of having DiGeorge syndrome.
- Auscultation findings include single second heart sound and systolic murmur due to excessive blood flow through the pulmonary arteries, this may present as continuous murmur.
- Presentation of truncus arteriosus may be at 1–2 months of age due to mild cyanosis and prominent respiratory symptoms.
- Children with truncus arteriosus should be assessed for genetic, parathyroid and immune defects.
- Surgical repair requires placement of a right ventricle to pulmonary artery homograft which will require replacement 2–3 times during childhood due to development of stenosis and regurgitation.

Definition

Truncus arteriosus is a cyanotic congenital heart disease. In this lesion, there is only one (truncus) artery receiving blood ejected from both ventricles. The truncus then continue as the aortic arch and providing pulmonary arteries. The pulmonary arteries emerge form the truncus as a main pulmonary artery which bifurcates into a right and left pulmonary arteries, or the 2 pulmonary arteries emerge separately from the truncus. Truncus arteriosus is known to be associated with DiGeorge syndrome.

J.F. Hoffman (✉)
Department of Pediatrics, Rush University Medical Center, 1653 W. Congress Parkway, Suite 770 Jones, Chicago, IL, 60612, USA
e-mail: joan_hoffman@rush.edu

Ra-id Abdulla (ed.), *Heart Diseases in Children: A Pediatrician's Guide*,
DOI 10.1007/978-1-4419-7994-0_20, © Springer Science+Business Media, LLC 2011

Incidence

Truncus arteriosus is rare, with a prevalence of 1–2% of all congenital heart defects. It is commonly found in association with the microdeletion 22q11 syndromes also known as DiGeorge, Velocardiofacial, or CATCH-22 syndromes.

Pathology

In truncus arteriosus, the heart has a single outlet through a single semilunar (truncal) valve and into a common arterial trunk. *The valve may be incompetent.* The defining feature of this common arterial trunk is that the ascending portion gives rise to all circulations: systemic, pulmonary, and coronary. The common arterial trunk usually overrides the crest of the ventricular septum, such that it has biventricular origin. Both ventricles are well-developed and in communication by a large ventricular septal defect, which is always present and roofed by the common arterial trunk (Fig. 20.1).

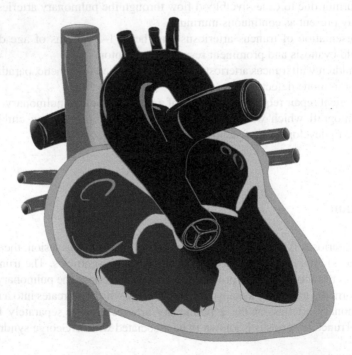

Fig. 20.1 Anatomy of truncus arteriosus. A single valve and great vessel overrides a ventricular septal defect, thus emerging from both ventricles. The pulmonary arteries originate directly from the truncus. The pulmonary arteries may emerge as a single main pulmonary artery, then bifurcating into left and right branches (type I) as depicted in this image, or emerge as two separate pulmonary arteries, either close together (type II) or apart from either sides of the truncus (type III)

Two classification systems (Collett and Edwards 1949; Van Praagh 1965) have been devised, both based on the description of the anatomic origin of the pulmonary arteries from the common arterial trunk. The pulmonary arteries arise from the ascending portion of the common arterial trunk in two main ways:

- From a single orifice, with a main pulmonary artery segment of variable length, which then branches and gives rise to left and right pulmonary artery.
- From separate orifices at about the same level on the common arterial trunk, and these orifices can either be side-by-side or on opposite sides of the common arterial trunk.

The classifications based on the anatomic position of the pulmonary arteries are as follows:

Type 1: There is a main pulmonary artery arising from the ascending portion of the truncus. The left and right pulmonary arteries arise from the MPA.

Type 2: Both pulmonary arteries arise side by side in the posterior aspect of the truncus.

Type 3: The pulmonary arteries arise opposite each other on the lateral aspects of the ascending truncus.

Type 4: Also known as pseudotruncus is not a true type of truncus arteriosus since it represents pulmonary atresia with ventricular septal defect. The pulmonary arteries in this lesion arise opposite each other on the lateral aspects of the descending aorta, these vessels are in reality collateral vessels feeding pulmonary segments and not real pulmonary arteries. It is best to avoid classifying this lesion as a truncus arteriosus.

Stenosis at one or both branches of the pulmonary artery has been described, but is generally rare.

Associated Anomalies

In contrast to the normal aortic valve, the truncal valve may have from one to six leaflets. Most common is three leaflets (~60%), followed by four (~25%), and two (~10%), with one, five and six leaflets being quite rare. Furthermore, the valve leaflets may be thickened, dysplastic, fused, and of unequal size, and the truncal sinuses which support the valve leaflets are often poorly developed.

A right aortic arch with mirror-image brachiocephalic branching is present in up to 35% of patients. A right aortic arch courses over the right mainstem bronchus and passes to the right of the trachea, in contrast to a left aortic arch, which courses over the left mainstem bronchus and passes to the left of the trachea.

An interrupted aortic arch may be present (~15%), such that the common arterial trunk gives rise to the coronary circulation, to the ascending aorta which supplies the head and neck, and to a large ductus arteriosus which gives rise to the pulmonary arteries and continues on to supply the descending aorta. This type of truncus arteriosus is important to mention because in this type, the systemic blood flow that supplies the lower body is ductal dependent. It is also frequently associated with DiGeorge syndrome.

A branch pulmonary artery may be absent in up to 10% of patients, usually on the left if the aortic arch is left-sided, or on the right if the aortic arch is right-sided.

Coronary artery anomalies are common in truncus arteriosus, and vary from unusual origin and course to stenosis of the coronary ostium.

Pathophysiology

In truncus arteriosus, outflow from both ventricles is directed into a dilated common arterial trunk. Consequently, a mixture of oxygenated and deoxygenated blood enters systemic, pulmonary, and coronary circulations. The actual oxygen saturation in the common arterial trunk will depend on the ratio of pulmonary blood flow to systemic blood flow, with greater systemic oxygenation reflecting a greater magnitude of pulmonary blood flow. The magnitudes of pulmonary and systemic blood flow are determined by the relative resistances of the pulmonary and systemic vasculature. In the newborn period, when pulmonary vascular resistance is high, pulmonary blood flow may be only twice as much as the systemic blood flow. As pulmonary vascular resistance declines in infancy, the magnitude of pulmonary blood flow relative to systemic blood flow increases and can be enormous, as flow into the lower resistance pulmonary vasculature occurs throughout systole and diastole. The torrential pulmonary blood flow returns to the left heart and imposes a significant volume overload with attendant increased myocardial work load, which eventually leads to congestive heart failure.

There is both systolic and diastolic blood flow into the pulmonary arteries due to their origin from the truncus. With persistent diastolic flow into the pulmonary vasculature, the common arterial diastolic pressure is low, reducing coronary artery perfusion. Combined with subnormal systemic oxygenation, the myocardium becomes ischemic, which potentiates the progression to heart failure.

The abnormal truncal valve can be significantly regurgitant, which imposes further volume load and oxygen demand on the heart. Left heart dilation may already be present at birth as a result of truncal regurgitation during fetal life. In this case, the substantial decrease in common arterial diastolic pressure associated with truncal regurgitation subjects the fetal heart to reduced coronary perfusion with resultant ischemia, and significantly increases the risk of mortality in the newborn period. Coronary artery anomalies pose additional risks of cardiac ischemia.

The pulmonary arteries exhibit systemic pressure as a result of their origin from common arterial trunk. Chronic exposure to systemic pressure and high flow causes progressive pulmonary vascular disease. If the defect is not corrected, pulmonary vascular resistance progressively increases with remodeling of the vasculature. Once severe pulmonary vascular disease is present, deterioration is rapid and death ensues.

Clinical Manifestations

Truncus arteriosus lesions that are not identified by fetal ultrasound will commonly present in the newborn period. The clinical presentation of truncus arteriosus is determined by the magnitude of pulmonary blood flow, the presence and severity of truncal valve regurgitation, and the presence of ductal-dependent systemic blood flow.

The degree of cyanosis is determined by the amount of pulmonary blood flow. Mild-moderate cyanosis is often present at birth. Severe cyanosis suggests severely reduced pulmonary blood flow, which for this lesion, would occur in the rare instance of branch pulmonary artery stenosis in combination with significant truncal regurgitation that limits diastolic flow into the pulmonary arteries. Stridor may be noted, particularly with left aortic arch and aberrant right subclavian artery creating a vascular ring. It may also be present due to associated airway anomalies such as laryngomalacia.

Cardiac examination in this lesion varies, but may be significant for a hyperdynamic precordium, tachycardia, a normal S1 with a loud and single S2 and an ejection click that corresponds to maximal truncal valve opening. An S3 gallop is appreciated when significant volume overload is present, whether from truncal regurgitation or pulmonary overcirculation. A grade 2 to 4/6 systolic murmur is often audible at the left sternal border due to increase flow across the truncal valve and pulmonary arteries (Fig. 20.2). If truncal valve regurgitation is present, a high-pitched diastolic decrescendo murmur is audible at the mid left sternal border. As the pulmonary vascular resistance declines and pulmonary blood flow increases, a low-pitched apical diastolic mitral flow murmur may become audible. Diastolic runoff into the pulmonary vasculature and truncal valve regurgitation lead to bounding arterial pulses, except in the rare case of associated interrupted aortic arch and ductal constriction, when pulses may be diminished and the infant appears very ill.

Infants may exhibit symptoms of congestive heart failure, characterized by tachypnea, poor feeding, dyspnea, diaphoresis, irritability, and restlessness. Wheezing, grunting, and increased work of breathing will be demonstrated on physical examination. Liver distention is present. Symptoms may be present at birth or progress over initial weeks after birth as the pulmonary vascular resistance declines and pulmonary blood flow increases. Growth failure is often significant.

The occasional patient who presents beyond infancy exhibits cyanosis, exercise intolerance, digital clubbing, facial swelling, and liver enlargement.

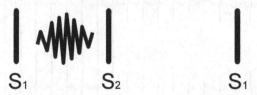

Fig. 20.2 Heart sounds and murmur in truncus arteriosus. *S1* first heart sound, *S2* second heart sound. Second heart sound may be single reflecting a single semilunar valve (truncal valve) or multiple sounds are heard due to abnormal truncal valve cusps. A systolic flow murmur is common due to the increase in blood flow across the truncal valve

Chest X-Ray

Cardiomegaly with increased pulmonary vascular markings is often evident on radiography of the chest, unless pulmonary ostial stenosis is present, which produces dark lung fields. In the unusual case of an absent pulmonary artery, usually on the left, differential pulmonary blood flow may be demonstrated, with increased pulmonary vascular markings on the right and decreased pulmonary vascular markings on the left. Truncal enlargement and absence of the pulmonary trunk segment may be identifiable, as might a right aortic arch, which appears as a slight indent of the right tracheal border. A thymus may be distinctly absent, suggesting 22q11 microdeletion (Chap. 2, Fig. 2.13).

Electrocardiography

The ECG in truncus arteriosus can be normal in a newborn, though often there will be borderline right ventricular hypertrophy, with mild right axis deviation (QRS axis of 120–140) or significant R voltage in V1 and V3R. After a week, evidence of biventricular hypertrophy is often present, with right ventricular hypertrophy suggested by qR and increased R voltage in V1 and V3R, and upright T waves in V1, and left ventricular hypertrophy suggested by significant R voltage in V5 and V6, sometimes accompanied by T wave abnormalities. Left forces (V4–V6) become increasingly prominent as pulmonary blood flow increases (Fig. 20.3).

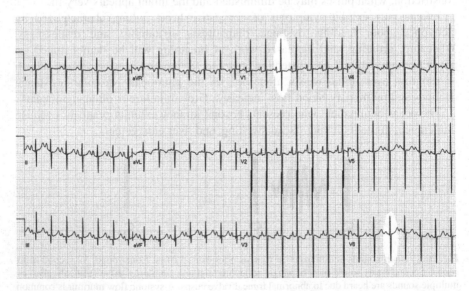

Fig. 20.3 ECG in truncus arteriosus. Right ventricular hypertrophy due to the systemic pressure in the right ventricle is present. R wave is tall in V1 and S wave is deep in V6

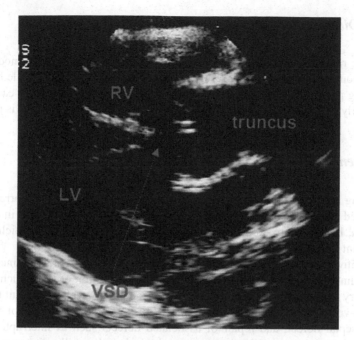

Fig. 20.4 Echocardiography. *LV* left ventricle, *RV* right ventricle, *VSD* ventricular septal defect. The truncus arises from both ventricles, overriding the ventricular septal defect

Echocardiography

Two dimensional, Doppler, and color Doppler echocardiography studies are diagnostic. The standard long-axis image demonstrates the ventricular septal defect, the single great artery which forms the roof of the ventricular septal defect and overrides the crest of the ventricular septum, the abnormal truncal valve, and the dilated common arterial trunk. Truncal regurgitation is readily demonstrated by color Doppler in this same view. Further echocardiographic imaging is performed to define the truncal valve anatomy and function, pulmonary artery origin and anatomy, coronary artery origin and course, anatomy of the aortic arch, and ventricular function (Fig. 20.4).

Cardiac Catheterization

Diagnostic cardiac catheterization is rarely necessary in the newborn period, except in unusual cases when echocardiography is unable to define aortic arch anatomy, coronary anatomy, or pulmonary anatomy. In infants, cardiac catheterization may be indicated to quantify pulmonary and systemic blood flow and calculate pulmonary vascular resistance. Any patient who presents with truncus arteriosus beyond infancy requires cardiac catheterization for hemodynamic assessment, as the risk for irreversible hypertensive pulmonary vascular disease is significant.

Other Diagnostic Modalities

Magnetic resonance imaging can provide additional anatomic and hemodynamic information, and is particularly useful in defining vascular anatomy, while radionuclide lung perfusion scans can be useful for quantifying blood flow to each lung, particularly if concern for unilateral ostial or branch pulmonary stenosis is present.

Treatment

Following medical stabilization in the intensive care unit, surgical correction is performed in the neonatal period because operative delay results in cardiac ischemia, heart failure, and risk of pulmonary vascular disease, which confer significant surgical risk.

Definitive surgical repair is performed through a median sternotomy incision on cardiopulmonary bypass. The procedure involves separation of the branch pulmonary artery from the common arterial trunk, placement of a valved conduit between the right-ventricle and pulmonary artery (RV-to-PA conduit), closure of the ventricular septal defect, and repair of associated defects such as interrupted aortic arch. Large atrial communications are repaired, though small atrial communications are often created to allow for right atrial decompression, as right ventricular hypertrophy is significant and compliance is poor in the early period following complete repair. If the truncal valve requires repair for regurgitation or stenosis, operative difficulty increases considerably. Long-term survival depends on truncal valve function.

Following surgical repair, many infants require outpatient medical therapy for post-operative left ventricular dysfunction and varying degrees of truncal valve regurgitation. Furosemide is commonly prescribed diuretic and carries with it the risk of hypokalemia, hypocalcemia, osteopenia, and hypercalciuria with calcium oxalate urinary stones. Furosemide-associated hearing loss is more commonly associated with rapid intravenous administration of the medication. Angiotensin-converting enzyme (ACE) inhibitors such as captopril and enalapril are provided to decrease systemic vascular afterload if truncal valve regurgitation is present. Caution should be exercised in prescribing or advising ibuprofen to any infant or child receiving ACE inhibitors, as there is a risk of precipitating acute renal failure.

Patients with truncus arteriosus require lifelong cardiology follow-up to monitor for obstruction or stenosis of the conduit, which can be related to patient outgrowth of the conduit or to calcification. When obstruction leads to significant increases in right ventricular pressure (typically 2/3 systemic or greater), re-sternotomy and replacement are indicated. Additionally, at least yearly follow-up allows for monitoring of truncal valve function, branch pulmonary artery stenosis, biventricular function, arterial trunk dilation, exercise tolerance, and arrhythmia surveillance. Any child with a history of truncus arteriosus repair who experiences chest pain or syncope warrants cardiology consultation.

Infective endocarditis prophylaxis is indicated for these patients, as most have some residual lesion in the setting of prosthetic material. Additionally, many have small atrial level communications which put them at risk for paradoxical emboli if right-to-left flow across the atrial septum occurs. While this is extremely rare in children with normal hearts, the risk is appreciably greater in children with residual or progressive right heart lesions, such as RV-to-PA conduit stenosis, which compromises right ventricular diastolic function and promotes right-to-left flow at the atrial level.

Special Considerations of Truncus Arteriosus in the Infant with 22q11 Microdeletion

As upwards of 35% of newborns with truncus arteriosus will have 22q11 microdeletion, all newborns with this defect should receive genetic testing by fluorescent in situ hybridization (FISH) of 22q11. Mothers of infants with 22q11 should be offered genetic testing on future pregnancies, as the risk of a similarly affected sibling is increased.

Hypocalcemia is common and can be profound, particularly in the post-operative period. Most require supplementation throughout the first year of life, which can often be discontinued in early childhood.

As these infants have T cell deficiency associated with thymic hypoplasia, irradiated blood should be selected when transfusion is planned, which will decrease future risk of graft-versus-host disease. Also related to T cell deficiency, these infants should not receive live viral vaccine, as viremia and viral sepsis can cause critical illness in these infants.

Upper airway anomalies, bronchomalacia, and tracheomalacia arc common, and often require otolaryngology consultation. Many 22q11 patients are challenging to intubate. Some infants require tracheostomy.

Poor feeding and growth failure are common, even when the operative result is good. Some infants require gastrostomy tube feedings for nutritional supplementation.

Case Scenarios

Case 1

A full term infant boy born by spontaneous *vaginal* delivery is limp at delivery. He is warmed, dried, stimulated, and provided CPAP for 2 min. Apgars are 2 and 8 at 1 and 5 min, respectively. He *is* vigorous, but is noted to be tachypneic, with mild subcostal retractions, so is brought to the nursery for further evaluation.

Physical Exam

His weight is 2.91 kg. Heart rate is 157 and regular. SpO$_2$ is 92% in room air. He is not apparently dysmorphic. *He does not appear cyanotic*. On cardiac examination, he has a normoactive precordium. On auscultation, he has mild regular tachycardia, with a normal S1, single S2, and systolic ejection click. A 3/6 systolic ejection quality (crescendo-decrescendo) murmur is present along the left sternal border, and a 2/4 diastolic decrescendo murmur is present at the left lower sternal border. Abdomen is soft, with no hepatomegaly. Brachial and femoral pulses are 3+ and somewhat bounding. Extremities are slightly cool.

CXR. The cardiac silhouette is borderline *enlarged*. A thymus *shadow* is absent, suggesting the diagnosis of a 22q11 deletion syndrome. A right aortic arch is suggested. Pulmonary notch is absent. Increased pulmonary vascularity is demonstrated.
ECG. The ECG demonstrates right ventricular hypertrophy, with a pure, tall R and upright T waves in V1.

Differential Diagnosis

This child is presenting with tachypnea, subcostal retractions, and mild hypoxemia. Respiratory pathology should be considered initially in the differential diagnosis and includes RDS, Transient tachypnea of the newborn, pneumonia, and sepsis. The cardiac findings on physical exam, along with the hypoxemia and the CXR findings of borderline cardiomegaly and increased pulmonary vascular markings are more indicative of a cyanotic congenital heart defect. The absent thymic shadow and the right aortic arch should alarm the practitioner to a possible 22q11 deletion syndrome. Heart defects associated with this include tetralogy of Fallot, VSD, interrupted aortic arch and truncus arteriosus. The single S2 is seen in both TOF and truncus arteriosus.

ECHO. Echocardiography demonstrates truncus arteriosus with a single great vessel giving rise to a right aortic arch, the coronary arteries, and the pulmonary arteries. The pulmonary artery branches arise from separate, side-by-side origins. A large ventricular septal defect is present with malalignment of the ventricular septum. Mild truncal valve stenosis and moderate truncal valve insufficiency is demonstrated.

Assessment

This infant has truncus arteriosus. An echocardiogram must be performed quickly to determine whether the arch is interrupted. The infant is only mildly desaturated since pulmonary blood flow occurs throughout systole and diastole, even though pulmonary vascular resistance is likely to remain high so shortly after birth. The tachypnea and mild respiratory distress in this infant may be secondary to mild metabolic acidosis from decreased systemic perfusion secondary to diastolic flow reversal through both the regurgitant truncal valve and the branch pulmonary arteries originating from the ascending arterial trunk.

Management

Medical management initially should include diuretics and digitalis to prevent progression to congestive heart failure as the pulmonary vascular resistance decreases. Urgent consult to a pediatric cardiologist is imperative. Definitive surgical correction of the defect will be necessary. The practitioner will also need to assess for 22q11 deletion by FISH analysis, monitor calcium levels, and assess for other anomalies. Further evaluation of the presumed DiGeorge syndrome should be done.

Case 2

A full term infant girl born by spontaneous *vaginal* delivery develops stridor and increased work of breathing at several minutes of life and is brought to the nursery for further evaluation.

Physical Exam

Her weight is 3.05 kg. Heart rate is 134 and regular. SpO_2 is 88% in room air. She is provided CPAP with 50% oxygen while the examination continues. She is mildly dysmorphic, with small eyes and a small nose. She has audible stridor. On cardiac examination, she has a normoactive precordium. On auscultation, she has normal rate and rhythm, with a normal S1, single S2, and systolic ejection click. A 1 to 2/6 soft systolic ejection quality murmur is present along the left sternal border, and diastole is silent. Abdomen is soft, with no hepatomegaly. Brachial and femoral pulses are normal intensity, not bounding, and symmetric. Extremities are warm and well-perfused.

Labs

An arterial blood gas is performed, with a pH of 7.21, pCO_2 of 62 mmHg, pO_2 of 48 mmHg.

Note: She required intubation prior to the arrival of the transport team, secondary to worsening stridor and respiratory distress.

CXR. The cardiac silhouette is borderline enlarged. A thymus shadow is absent. Lung fields appear normal. The endotracheal and nasogastric tubes are well-positioned.

Differential Diagnosis

The first notable physical exam finding in this neonate is her work of breathing and stridor, suggestive of an airway abnormality. Airway abnormalities that present in the newborn period include laryngomalacia, vocal cord paralysis, and vascular rings. The physical findings on cardiac exam are subtle, the murmur is non-specific and a single S2 is not always appreciated by the non-discriminating ear. The inappropriately low pO2 during oxygen administration and the CXR with the absent thymus and borderline enlarged heart should guide the practitioner to include congenital cardiac defects in the differential, specifically those common with 22q11 deletion syndrome.

ECHO. The echo is indicated secondary to low pO_2 in the setting of oxygen administration and a chest radiograph that suggests an absent thymus. The echo demonstrates truncus arteriosus with a single great vessel giving rise to a left aortic arch, the coronary arteries, and the pulmonary arteries. The pulmonary artery branches arise from separate, side-by-side origins. An aberrant right subclavian artery is demonstrated. A large ventricular septal defect is present with malalignment of the ventricular septum. The dysplastic three-leaflet truncal valve functions well, with no stenosis and no insufficiency.

Assessment

Though this infant has DiGeorge syndrome and truncus arteriosus, the predominant features of her presentation are consistent with airway anomalies, which are common among DiGeorge patients. The suggestion of cardiac disease in this infant is more subtle, with a single S2 and systolic ejection click on physical examination, a low pO2 despite oxygen administration, and an absent thymus on chest radiograph.

Management

Infants who present with stridor require airway evaluation by an otolaryngologist, preferably before cardiac surgery, to allow for a better prediction of the post-operative course. This infant has significant tracheo- and bronchomalacia which will certainly be expected to complicate her course in infancy. Prompt consult with the cardiologist is necessary. Pulmonary blood flow does not seem to be compromised in this case. As pulmonary vascular resistance drops, pulmonary blood flow will increase and diuretics may be necessary. The work up for DiGeorge Syndrome with 22q11 deletion should also include serum calcium and phosphorus levels, CBC with differential, immunoglobins, T and B cell studies, and renal ultrasound. A genetics consult should be obtained to discuss implications of the syndrome and to counsel parents on genetic testing for future pregnancies.

Chapter 21
Single Ventricle

Sawsan Mokhtar M. Awad and Ra-id Abdulla

Key Facts

- In single ventricle there is one ventricle receiving blood from both atria.
- A small outlet chamber is present in single ventricle, however it does not communicate directly with the atria, instead it receives blood from the single ventricle through a bulboventricular foramen.
- The aorta and pulmonary arteries in single ventricle are either normally arranged or transposed.
- Clinical presentation and management in single ventricle is controlled by extent of pulmonary blood flow:

    - Severe pulmonary stenosis (PS): the pulmonary blood flow (PBF) will be restricted resulting in cyanosis. These patients will require systemic to pulmonary arterial shunt to improve PBF.
    - No PS: PBF will be unrestricted resulting in congestive heart failure (CHF) and only mild cyanosis. These patients will require banding of pulmonary artery to restrict PBF.
    - Moderate PS: PBF will be somewhat restricted and the child will present later with mild cyanosis and CHF. These patients can be observed till Glenn shunt is placed at 4–5 months of age.

Definition

Single ventricle is a cyanotic congenital heart disease where there is one ventricle which receives blood from both atria. The single ventricle ejects to the great vessels (pulmonary artery and aorta) directly and through a rudimentary outflow chamber which connects to the single ventricle through a bulboventricular foramen (VSD like communication).

S.M.M. Awad (✉)
Department of Pediatrics, Rush University Medical Center, 1653 West Congress Parkway, Suite 770 Jones, Chicago, IL 60612, USA
e-mail: sawsan_m_awad@rush.edu

Ra-id Abdulla (ed.), *Heart Diseases in Children: A Pediatrician's Guide*,
DOI 10.1007/978-1-4419-7994-0_21, © Springer Science+Business Media, LLC 2011

Incidence

This lesion is very rare. It is seen in about 1% of infants with congenital heart disease and 5 per 100,000 live births.

Pathology

Single ventricle is an arrest of development of an early embryological stage where the two atria communicate with the primitive ventricle (predecessor to the left ventricle) which communicates with an outlet chamber, called bulbus cordis (predecessor to the right ventricle). In a typical single ventricle, many of the features of this early developmental stages is noted, such as the double inlet or common atrioventricular communication between the two atria and single ventricle, the bulboventricular foramen, and the outlet chamber.

Single ventricle is a lesion where both atria are connected to a single ventricle. This is either through two separate atrioventricular valves (double inlet ventricle) or a common atrioventricular valve. The morphology of the single ventricle can be that of a left ventricle, a right ventricle, or a common ventricle (not typical of either ventricular morphology). Other congenital heart lesions as hypoplastic left heart syndrome and tricuspid atresia are not considered single ventricle lesions although they have the same pathophysiology as single ventricle. Please see chapters 18 and 23 for further details.

The most common type of single ventricle lesions is double inlet left ventricle. In this lesion, the single ventricle is of a left ventricular morphology with a small outlet chamber (Fig. 21.1). The communication between the single ventricle and the outlet chamber is known as the bulboventricular foramen. The single ventricle is posterior while the outlet chamber is anterior and to the left. The pulmonary and aortic vessels could be normally related, i.e. the pulmonary artery is anterior and to the left while the aorta is posterior and to the right. With such an arrangement, the pulmonary artery emerges from the small outlet chamber, while the aorta emerges from the main (single) ventricle. On the other hand, the two great vessels could be transposed where the aorta is anterior and to the left (emerging from the outlet chamber) and the pulmonary artery is posterior and to the left (emerging from the single ventricle).

Patients with heterotaxy may have single ventricle similar to what is described here; however, heterotaxy lesions are more complex as they include other pathologies such as situs abnormalities and systemic and/or pulmonary venous drainage. Please refer to chapter 22 for further details.

Pathophysiology

Presentation, course, management and prognosis are determined by the presence and extent of pulmonary stenosis. Arrangement of great vessels does not significantly impact presentation or course since oxygenated and deoxygenated blood

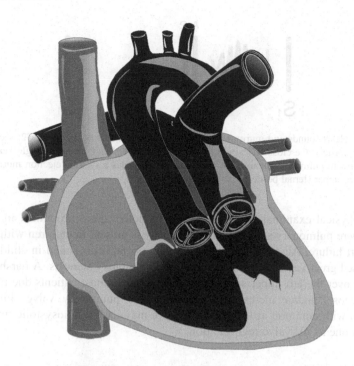

Fig. 21.1 Anatomy of single ventricle. In this type of single ventricle the tricuspid and mitral valves open into the single ventricle of left ventricular morphology, this is connected through an outlet chamber (primitive right ventricle). The pulmonary artery is anterior emerging from the rudimentary outlet chamber while the aorta is posterior emerging from the single ventricle

already mix in the single ventricle and the oxygen saturation in both great vessels tend to be identical. However, the extent of pulmonary stenosis, if present, determines the blood volume to the lungs. The greater the blood volume to the lungs, the milder is cyanosis and the worse is congestive heart failure. Lack of pulmonary stenosis will allow excessive pulmonary blood flow, leading to pulmonary edema and congestive heart failure. However, high pulmonary blood flow brings back more well oxygenated blood into the heart and thus minimizing cyanosis.

Clinical Manifestations

Clinical presentation varies with the extent of pulmonary stenosis. In cases of severe pulmonary stenosis pulmonary blood flow will be restricted and children will present early with cyanosis due to mixing of blood in the single ventricle and restricted pulmonary blood flow. The other extreme of clinical presentation is secondary to little or no pulmonary stenosis resulting in excessive pulmonary blood flow which will cause pulmonary edema and limited or no cyanosis. Patients with excessive pulmonary blood flow will develop respiratory distress, easy fatigability and failure to thrive.

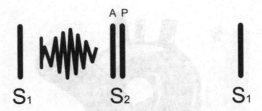

Fig. 21.2 Heart sounds and murmur in single ventricle. S1: first heart sound, S2: second heart sound, A: aortic valve closure, P: pulmonary valve closure. Many cases of single ventricle are associated with pulmonary stenosis. A systolic click precedes a systolic ejection murmur heard over the left upper sternal border

On physical examination cyanosis will be noted, more prominent in children with severe pulmonary stenosis. Hepatomegaly is present in children with congestive heart failure. Auscultation reveals single second heart sound in children with transposed great vessels or those with severe pulmonary stenosis. A harsh systolic murmur over the left upper sternal border is heard in most patients due to pulmonary stenosis and/or increase flow through the pulmonary valve (Fig. 21.2). Children with common atrioventricular valve may have a holosystolic murmur at the apex due to AV valve regurgitation.

Chest Radiography

Findings on chest X-ray are nonspecific. Cardiomegaly and increased pulmonary vascular markings are present in cases of single ventricle with no or little pulmonary stenosis. Normal cardiac silhouette with minimal pulmonary vascular markings (lung oligemia) are present in cases with severe pulmonary stenosis. In patients with mild to moderate pulmonary stenosis the size of the cardiac silhouette can be normal with slight increase in pulmonary vascular markings.

Electrocardiography

Electrocardiography is usually abnormal. Typically there is left ventricular hypertrophy. Later in life, spontaneous complete heart block and junctional rhythm may be present.

Echocardiography

Echocardiography is the gold standard in diagnosing single ventricle. Subcostal and apical views are valuable in determining the anatomical details of the lesion. Identification of the morphology of the dominant chamber (usually left ventricle), the size of bulboventricular foramen, the relation of the great arteries is possible through 2D echocardiography. Doppler flow and color Doppler is used to determine extent of pulmonary stenosis. Atrioventricular valve regurgitation is identified by color Doppler.

Fetal echocardiography is a useful tool in diagnosing such lesions in utero. This allows for preparation for delivery of baby at a tertiary care center with prompt care.

Cardiac Catheterization

Cardiac catheterization is not necessary for making the diagnosis. Cardiac catheterization is reserved for those patients who need interventional procedures or if some of the anatomical details are in doubt. However, cardiac catheterization is typically performed in patients prior to performing Glenn shunt and prior to completion of Fontan procedure to assess pulmonary arterial anatomy and pulmonary vascular resistance.

Treatment

Without surgical treatment, survival of these patients is very poor. Staged surgery is the main stay of treatment. The first stage may include one of the following options depending on the pulmonary blood flow:

- Pulmonary artery banding in patients with no pulmonary stenosis and increased pulmonary blood flow.
- Prostaglandin in patients with pulmonary atresia and ductal dependant pulmonary circulation which will be followed by surgical creation of systemic to pulmonary arterial shunt.
- No intervention and close medical follow up in patients with mild to moderate pulmonary stenosis and just the right amount of pulmonary blood flow.

Second stage includes creation of a cavopulmonary shunt (Glenn shunt). This shunt allows drainage of systemic venous return from the superior vena cava directly to the pulmonary circulation, thus bypassing the heart. During this surgical procedure the systemic to pulmonary arterial shunt is taken down. Glenn shunt is typically performed at about 3–6 months of age. Glenn shunts cannot be performed earlier than 3 months of age due to the relatively elevated pulmonary vascular resistance in early weeks of life leading to failure of passive blood flow from the SVC to the pulmonary circulation. During this procedure the pulmonary artery connection to the heart is disrupted, either through a tight band or resecting the main pulmonary artery, in essence creating pulmonary atresia. In some instances when the aortic valve is stenotic, rather than sacrificing the pulmonary valve, it could be used to deliver blood to the aorta in addition to the stenotic native aortic valve. This is performed through transecting the pulmonary artery a short distance above the pulmonary valve. The distal stump is sutured thus limiting pulmonary blood flow to that coming through the Glenn shunt. The proximal stump of the pulmonary artery is connected to the ascending aorta, thus allowing dual pathways of blood to go from the single ventricle to the aorta, one through the native aortic valve and the other through the native pulmonary valve, now connected to the ascending aorta.

The Fontan procedure is completed at about 18 months of age. The inferior vena cava is connected to the pulmonary circulation either through a baffle within the right atrium or an extracardiac conduit connecting the IVC to the pulmonary arteries. This procedure will allow almost all systemic venous blood to flow passively into the pulmonary circulation without the need for a pumping chamber, thus bypassing the heart. The single ventricle in these cases is dedicated to pumping blood to the systemic circulation through the aorta. The only systemic venous return which continues to drain to the atrium is from the coronary sinus which results in mild drop in oxygen saturation.

Case Scenarios

Case 1

A 3 month old boy was seen by a pediatrician for the first time. The child was brought for a well child care visit; however, the mother did have concerns regarding bluish discoloration of the lips when he cries. On physical examination the heart rate was 110 bpm, regular. Respiratory rate was 35/min. Blood pressure in upper extremity was 90/60 mmHg. Oxygen saturation was 88% in upper and lower extremity. Weight was at 5th percentile and height was at 25th percentile on the growth chart. The child appeared to have mild increase in respiratory effort with noticeable intercostal retractions. The oral mucosa did not show clear cyanosis; however, had a hint of bluish discoloration. Peripheral pulses and perfusion were normal. Mild Hepatomegaly was detected. The precordium was clearly hyperactive with a palpable thrill. On auscultation, first heart sound was normal, S1 and S2 were normal with a harsh 4/6 systolic ejection murmur detected over the left upper sternal border.

The child is not known to the pediatrician; therefore, additional care in assessing this child is required since past medical history is not known. History is significant for bouts of cyanosis with agitation. The mother does not notice cyanosis when the child is quiet; this is perhaps due to milder oxygen desaturation when the child is quiet. The latter supposition is supported by the fact that the child has mild oxygen desaturation (88%) which should not cause obvious cyanosis upon inspection.

Respiratory disease is unlikely in view of lack of significant respiratory symptoms and signs. The harsh systolic ejection murmur over the pulmonic area clearly points to a cardiac abnormality, likely involving the pulmonary valve. Although cyanosis causes increase respiratory effort, the mild oxygen desaturation noted is unlikely the culprit to increase in respiratory effort, which is most probably due to associated increase in pulmonary blood flow and edema.

The child was referred to a pediatric cardiologist. Echocardiographic evaluation revealed single ventricle with moderate pulmonary stenosis (50 mmHg). This is a cyanotic congenital heart disease where blood from both atria mix in the single ventricle. Increase in pulmonary blood flow result in lessening the extent of cyanosis, however, at the expense of pulmonary edema. This child does have pulmonary edema and congestive heart failure, however, mild. The cyanotic congenital heart disease this child has is well balanced. Cyanosis is mild and congestive heart failure has not resulted in significant symptoms.

The child continued follow up with pediatric cardiology after initiating anti-congestive heart failure medications including digoxin and furosemide. The child will be scheduled for cardiac catheterization at about 6 months of age to assess pulmonary vascular resistance prior to undergoing Glenn shunt at 3–6 months of age.

Case 2

A 10 day old newborn previously healthy was noticed to have increase work of breathing and poor feeding. On examination, intercostals and subcostal retractions were noticed. The liver was 3 cm below the costal margin. Saturation was noticed to be in the low 90s. Auscultation revealed normal S1, single S2 and a 2/6 systolic murmur heard over the upper midsternal region with radiation into both axillae.

ECG was abnormal with increased left ventricular forces. Chest radiography showed increased cardiothoracic ratio and prominent pulmonary vascular markings.

The child was admitted for further assessment of potential congenital heart disease. The dominant features in this child are that of increase pulmonary blood flow, pulmonary edema and congestive heart failure. Although cyanosis could be due to pulmonary edema, it is more likely that it is due to cyanotic congenital heart disease since cyanosis secondary to pulmonary disease alone is associated with severe respiratory symptoms. The respiratory symptoms in this child are moderate, rather than severe.

Echocardiography was performed and showed single ventricle with transposed great vessels and no pulmonary stenosis.

The congenital heart disease in this child is of the cyanotic type, the blood from the systemic veins and pulmonary veins mix within the single ventricle and ejected to both aorta and pulmonary artery. Since there is no pulmonary stenosis, blood flow will be excessive to the pulmonary circulation since pulmonary vascular resistance is significantly less in the pulmonary circulation rather than the systemic circulation.

Excessive pulmonary blood flow will bring back large volume of pulmonary venous return which will dilute the systemic venous return, thus making the oxygen saturation of blood in the single ventricle and consequently in the aorta high, in this case in the low 90s. The single S2 in this child is due to transposition of the great arteries with the pulmonary valve posterior, making its closure sound inaudible.

After initial management using diuretics and inotropic support to control congestive heart failure, the child was taken to the operating room where a band was placed over the main pulmonary artery to restrict pulmonary blood flow. This will be followed at about 3–6 months of age with a cardiac catheterization procedure to study pulmonary vascular resistance to ensure that they are within normal limits, followed by a Glenn shunt and ligation of the main pulmonary artery at about 3–6 months of age. Fontan procedure is completed by connecting inferior vena cava to the pulmonary arterial circulation through an intra-atrial baffle or extracardiac conduit.

Chapter 22
Complex Cyanotic Congenital Heart Disease: The Heterotaxy Syndromes

Shannon M. Buckvold, Jacquelyn Busse, and Joan F. Hoffman

Key Facts

- The hallmark feature of heterotaxy is abnormal positioning of internal organs, including liver, spleen, intestines, venae cavae, atria, ventricles, and great arteries.
- Clinical presentation varies significantly as cardiac anatomy ranges from normal to severely anomalous.
- Bilateral sidedness in heterotaxy indicates duplication of the right or left side of the body, thus loosing to a certain extent the normal asymmetry of the viscera.
- In bilateral right sidedness there is asplenia, while in bilateral left sidedness there is polysplenia. In either case, functional asplenia is common.
- Cyanosis is a frequent feature in most cases of heterotaxy.

Definition

Heterotaxy syndromes are characterized by abnormal left–right positioning with consequent malformations of the usually asymmetric organs: heart, liver, intestines and spleen.

J.F. Hoffman (✉)
Department of Pediatrics, Rush University Medical Center, 1653 W. Congress Parkway, Suite 770 Jones, Chicago, IL, 60612, USA
e-mail: joan_hoffman@rush.edu

Ra-id Abdulla (ed.), *Heart Diseases in Children: A Pediatrician's Guide*,
DOI 10.1007/978-1-4419-7994-0_22, © Springer Science+Business Media, LLC 2011

Incidence

Heterotaxy syndromes are rare, comprising only 1% of congenital heart disease in newborns. Right isomerism is more common in males while left isomerism tends to affect females.

Pathology

During the second and third weeks of embryonic development, normal left–right positioning is established. Disruptions to this process result in a variety of patterns of abnormal positioning and organ malformation:

- *Levocardia with abdominal situs inversus*: Normal cardiac position (left-sided) and structure with abdominal organs in a mirror-image arrangement.
- *Dextrocardia with abdominal situs solitus*: Cardiac apex abnormally positioned to the right with normal cardiac structure and normal abdominal organ arrangement.
- *Dextrocardia with situs inversus*: Cardiac apex to the right with normal cardiac structure and abdominal mirror-image arrangement (Fig. 22.1).
- *Dextrocardia with atrioventricular discordance, ventricular arterial discordance, and abdominal situs solitus*: Multiple cardiac defects including the cardiac apex to the right, right atrium connected to left ventricle connected to pulmonary artery, left atrium connected to right ventricle connected to aorta, (described as l-looped ventricles, l-transposition of the great arteries, or corrected transposition of the great arteries), and normal abdominal organ arrangement.
- *Total absence of asymmetry along the left–right axis*: thoracic and abdominal organ symmetry, or bilateral sidedness, where one side is mirrored on the other.

Though considerable overlap exists between the two categories, right and left isomerism are often broadly described in this way:

Right isomerism *or* bilateral right-sidedness *or* Asplenia syndrome:

- Bilateral right atrial appendages
- Bilateral three-lobed right lungs with bilateral right-bronchial anatomy
- Midline liver with gallbladder
- Intestinal malrotation
- Absent spleen

Left Isomerism *or* Bilateral Left-Sidedness *or* Polysplenia Syndrome:

- Bilateral left atrial appendages
- Bilateral two-lobed left lungs with bilateral left-bronchial anatomy
- Midline liver with occasional absent gallbladder (extrahepatic biliary atresia)
- Intestinal malrotation
- Multiple spleens, often appearing as a cluster of grapes attached to the greater curvature of the stomach

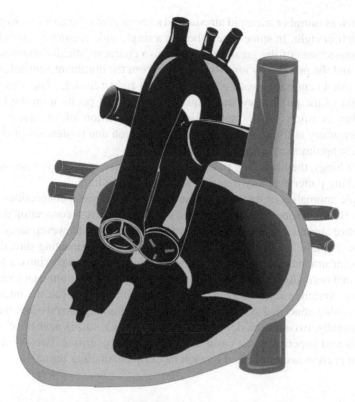

Fig. 22.1 Anatomy of dextrocardia, situs inversus, l-transposition of the great vessels with VSD, and pulmonary stenosis. The single ventricle is of left ventricular morphology and the outlet chamber is small with no inlet (atrioventricular valve). Blood reaches the outlet chamber through the VSD. In addition, this patient has pulmonary stenosis

With few exceptions, complex cardiac malformations accompany the heterotaxy syndromes.

Cardiac Defects Associated with Right Isomerism

More than left isomerism, right isomerism is often associated with severe abnormalities of intracardiac anatomy, great artery connections, and systemic and pulmonary venous drainage.

The most common cardiac defect in right isomerism includes dextrocardia, a common atrium and a common atrioventricular (AV) valve with severe malalignment. This leads to one ventricle (usually the right-sided ventricle) receiving all of the common AV valve flow and the other ventricle (usually the left-sided ventricle) receiving no common AV valve flow and therefore becoming hypoplastic. There are many variations described, but most include significant abnormalities of the AV valves, such as mitral or tricuspid atresia, and some degree or ventricular hypoplasia, whether left or right. In some cases, there is a single indeterminate ventricle.

The connections of the great arteries are also characteristically abnormal. Both the aorta and the pulmonary artery often arise from the dominant ventricle (usually the right-sided ventricle) creating a double-outlet right ventricle. The aorta is often to the right of the pulmonary artery instead of its usual position on the left. This relationship is often called malposition or transposition of the great arteries. Pulmonary artery outflow obstruction is also common due to stenosis or even atresia of the subpulmonary area and pulmonary artery.

In both lungs, the branching pattern of the pulmonary arteries is consistent with the branching pattern usually found in the normal right lung.

Multiple anomalies of the systemic and pulmonary venous connections are also common. Bilateral superior vena cavae are often present, each connecting directly to its respective atrium. The inferior vena cava is usually intact. However, since the liver is midline, hepatic venous drainage is usually bilateral, connecting directly to the respective atrium under which each hepatic lobe lies. The coronary sinus, a left-sided structure that normally courses in the left AV groove, is absent. Pulmonary veins often connect to a systemic vein, either the bilateral superior venae cavae, the inferior vena cava, or another abnormal systemic vein, instead of draining directly into the heart.

Additionally, two sinus nodes are often present, each sitting near the connection of the bilateral superior venae cavae to their respective atrium. Two AV nodes are also often present and connected to each other by conduction tissue.

Cardiac Defects Associated with Left Isomerism

Left isomerism is associated with less severe abnormalities of intracardiac anatomy, great artery connections, and systemic and pulmonary venous drainage. In fact, a normal heart or only minimal malformation may be present in some cases.

Cardiac features of left atrial isomerism are less consistent and more widely variable than the cardiac features of right isomerism. Abnormalities of the atrial septum are frequent, with a common atrium present in about 35% of patients. A common AV valve is present in nearly half, though many are only associated with a primum septal defect and not associated with an AV canal type ventricular septal defect. Two good-sized ventricles are frequently present, but may be malpositioned, often with some type of ventricular septal defect. The great arteries usually arise from the appropriate ventricle. Double-outlet right ventricle, transposed great arteries, pulmonary stenosis, and pulmonary atresia do occur, but with less frequency than in right atrial isomerism.

Conversely, the anomalies of systemic and pulmonary venous connections are more consistent in left isomerism than in right. Interruption of the inferior vena cava is frequently present. A dilated azygous vein drains venous return from systemic veins below the diaphragm to the superior vena cava, which may be left-sided. Pulmonary venous drainage is often divided, with the right pulmonary veins draining to the right-sided atrium and the left-pulmonary veins draining to the left-sided atrium.

In left isomerism, the sinus node is hypoplastic and abnormally located. Though the AV node is present, discontinuity between the AV node and the ventricular conduction tissues confers a substantial risk of heart block, which can spontaneously develop in either fetal or postnatal life.

Pathophysiology

Due to the wide variety of lesions that can be associated with heterotaxy syndromes, there are a wide range of clinical manifestations. The specific combination of cardiac defects determines the pathophysiology. In general, there is often complete mixing of systemic and pulmonary venous blood at the atrial level, with consequent reduction in systemic arterial oxygenation. Cyanosis is further intensified when pulmonary blood flow is reduced secondary to obstructed pulmonary outflow and/ or obstructed anomalous pulmonary venous return. In cases of severe pulmonary stenosis and pulmonary atresia, pulmonary blood flow is provided by the ductus arteriosus. Ductal closure in this circumstance can cause life-threatening cyanosis in the newborn period. Furthermore, following surgical intervention, ductal closure can lead to coarctation or isolation of the left pulmonary artery at the former ductal insertion site, which significantly compromises single ventricle palliation.

Due to the complex nature of the defects, many heterotaxy infants have what is functionally equivalent to single ventricle physiology and require a single ventricle approach to surgical correction. This may be the case even with two good-sized ventricles, usually secondary to uncorrectable types of anomalous systemic or pulmonary venous drainage. If unobstructed pulmonary blood flow is present, pulmonary overcirculation and progression to congestive heart failure may develop.

Clinical Manifestations

Right Isomerism

In the majority of newborns, Cyanosis is present at birth secondary to variable combinations of complete mixing of systemic and pulmonary venous blood, pulmonary outflow obstruction, ductal constriction, and obstructed pulmonary venous return. With ductal closure or progressive obstruction to pulmonary venous return, worsening hypoxemia can lead to profound metabolic acidosis and cardiovascular failure.

The cardiac examination varies significantly depending on the combination of cardiac malformations:

- Precordium may be variably active. A thrill may suggest significant pulmonary stenosis.
- Heart tones may be right-sided, emphasizing the importance of auscultation of the entire chest in a newborn.

- S1 may be obscured by a systolic regurgitant murmur of common AV valve insufficiency.
- S2 may be loud and single if the great vessels are malpositioned or transposed such that the aorta is anterior to the pulmonary artery, thereby obscuring the pulmonary valve closure. S2 will also be single if pulmonary atresia is present.
- A harsh, 3–4/6 systolic ejection murmur of pulmonary stenosis may be present.
- A 2/6 systolic ductal murmur may be appreciated. Ductal murmurs are not yet continuous in the newborn. A continuous murmur would suggest aortopulmonary collateral supply or supplementation of pulmonary blood flow.
- Femoral pulses will be diminished if the defect includes coarctation of the aorta.

The abdominal examination may be notable for a midline liver. Occasionally, jaundice is noted. Bilious emesis secondary to intestinal malrotation may occur. Splenic dysfunction may result in erythrocyte inclusions such as Howell–Jolly bodies, which can be seen on a complete blood count.

Left Isomerism

If heart block occurs in utero, the infant may be born with hydrops fetalis. Spontaneous complete heart block in the newborn period can cause symptoms of heart failure and decreased cardiac output. This may present clinically with respiratory distress (secondary to pulmonary edema and pleural effusions), irritability, lethargy, poor feeding, and renal insufficiency.

Mild cyanosis is often present at birth secondary to a combination of complete mixing of the systemic and pulmonary venous return and some degree of pulmonary outflow obstruction.

As with right isomerism, the cardiac examination varies significantly depending on the combination of cardiac malformations:

- Precordium may be variably active. A thrill may suggest significant pulmonary stenosis.
- Heart tones may be right-sided, as dextrocardia occurs in left isomerism as well.
- S2 may be loud and single if the great vessels are malpositioned or transposed such that the aorta is anterior to the pulmonary artery, thereby obscuring the pulmonary valve closure.
- A 2–3 holosystolic murmur of ventricular septal defect may be appreciated once pulmonary vascular resistance declines, allowing significant left to right flow.
- A harsh, 2–4/6 systolic ejection murmur of pulmonary stenosis may be present.
- A 2/6 systolic ductal murmur may be appreciated. Ductal murmurs are not yet continuous in the newborn period. A continuous murmur would suggest aortopulmonary collateral supply or supplementation of pulmonary blood flow.

Respiratory distress may develop due to pulmonary overcirculation and congestive heart failure. Decreased cardiac output may result in irritability, lethargy, poor feeding, and renal insufficiency.

Abdominal examination may be notable for a midline liver, although the liver is more likely to be lateralized to the left or the right in left isomerism. Extrahepatic biliary atresia may present as jaundice. Gastrointestinal symptoms, particularly bilious emesis secondary to intestinal malrotation, may dominate the clinical presentation. As with right isomerism, Howell–Jolly bodies due to splenic dysfunction may be present on complete blood count, even in the presence of multiple spleens.

Diagnosis

Chest radiography: Dextrocardia may be present and should raise concern for heterotaxy in a sick newborn. Cardiomegaly may be present if there is significant common AV valve regurgitation. Pulmonary vascular markings may be diminished if pulmonary outflow obstruction exists causing decreased pulmonary blood flow. Pulmonary venous congestion and pulmonary edema may be noted with pulmonary venous obstruction. Pulmonary venous obstruction should be suspected if an interval change in lung fields from dark to white coincides with the initiation of prostaglandin or pulmonary vasodilators. Increased pulmonary vascularity may be demonstrated in left isomerism. Bronchial anatomy may help differentiate between left and right isomerism with right isomerism having bilateral short bronchi and left isomerism having bilateral long bronchi. A midline liver or abnormally positioned gastric bubble may also be evident.

Electrocardiography: P wave axis may be abnormal (−30 to −90°), reflecting the malposition of the sinus node, particularly in left isomerism. Sick sinus syndrome may also be present in left isomerism. In right atrial isomerism, two different P wave morphologies may be present, with intrinsic pacemaker rhythm alternating between the two sinus nodes. If a common AV valve is present, a superior frontal QRS axis of −30 to −90° will be present. Variable degrees of right, left, or combined ventricular hypertrophy are demonstrated.

Echocardiography: 2D, Doppler, and color Doppler echocardiography studies are diagnostic in most cases and are needed to delineate the pattern of blood flow and whether the systemic and pulmonary systems are connected in series or in parallel. Specifically, echocardiography will detail cardiac position and direction of the apex, systemic venous connections, pulmonary venous connections, atrial situs, the atrial septum, connection of the atria to the ventricles, ventricular position, components, size, and relationship to surrounding structures, ventricular outflow tracts, connection of the great arteries to the ventricles, and the morphology and pattern of flow in the ductus arteriosus. The short axis abdominal view is used to describe visceral situs.

Cardiac catheterization: Diagnostic cardiac catheterization is rarely necessary in the newborn period except in unusual cases when echocardiography is unable to define the systemic and pulmonary venous connections. However, cardiac catheterization may be used for therapeutic purposes when intervention is needed to maintain pulmonary blood flow. An interventional cardiologist may place a ductal stent or a right ventricular outflow stent. Cardiac catheterization is also used for hemodynamic and angiographic assessment in patients with single ventricle physiology prior to surgical palliation.

Other diagnostic modalities: Magnetic resonance imaging can provide additional anatomic and hemodynamic information, and is particularly useful in defining vascular anatomy and volumetric assessment of the ventricles when a two ventricular repair is being considered. Abdominal ultrasound and hematologic smear are routinely performed to evaluate for presence of a spleen and evidence of splenic function. Finally, all heterotaxy infants warrant diagnostic evaluation for intestinal malrotation, as they have significant risk for developing volvulus, intestinal obstruction and ischemia, and threatened bowel viability.

Treatment

For the newborn who presents with severe cyanosis and cardiovascular compromise, prompt medical stabilization and initiation of prostaglandin infusion are indicated, followed by urgent pediatric cardiology consultation and echocardiography evaluation. If hypoxemia and/or shock seem to worsen following prostaglandin initiation, obstructed pulmonary veins must be considered, as the improved pulmonary blood flow may have unmasked a pulmonary venous obstruction. If obstructed pulmonary veins are suspected, urgent surgical intervention is indicated.

Following medical stabilization and complete diagnostic evaluation in the intensive care unit, an individualized surgical plan can be formulated. For newborns with cyanosis and restricted pulmonary blood flow, an artificial systemic to pulmonary shunt is often required. While some heterotaxy infants may ultimately be good candidates for a biventricular repair, many infants, particularly those with right isomerism, will only be candidates for single ventricle palliation (the Norwood procedure). Single ventricle palliation involves utilizing the stronger ventricle to provide active systemic blood flow while relying on passive venous return to the lungs to provide pulmonary blood flow. This is a multistep surgical repair usually completed by about 2 years of age. (See section "Treatment" of Chap. 23 for complete details of a single ventricle repair.)

Amoxicillin or penicillin prophylaxis against encapsulated organisms is indicated in functionally asplenic patients. Additionally, children should be provided the routine series of *H. influenzae* vaccines and pneumococcal conjugate vaccines (PCV7), as well as the polysaccharide 23 pneumococcal vaccine at 24 months and again 3–5 years later. Meningococcal vaccination should be provided following the second birthday.

Infective endocarditis prophylaxis is indicated for these patients, particularly for single ventricle palliation of the cyanotic lesions.

Prognosis

Nonoperative right isomerism patients may have up to a 95% mortality risk in the first year. The risks incurred with surgery are moderately increased for heterotaxy patients compared to other congenital heart diseases due to the complexity of the lesions. Palliated patients still have a 50% 5-year mortality rate due in large part to infection and sepsis risk from asplenia, but also due to complications from congenital heart disease and intestinal malrotation.

Nonoperative left isomerism patients have a much lower mortality risk in the first year – only 32% – with a 5-year mortality rate of about 50%. Left isomerism lesions are often more amenable to surgical correction.

Many heterotaxy infants will require long-term cardiac medications to control excessive pulmonary blood flow and to reduce cardiac dysfunction and AV valve regurgitation. Furosemide is a commonly prescribed diuretic and carries with it the risk of hypokalemia, hypocalcemia, osteopenia, and hypercalciuria with calcium oxalate urinary stones. Furosemide-associated hearing loss is more commonly associated with rapid intravenous administration of the medication. Angiotensin-converting enzyme (ACE) inhibitors such as captopril and enalapril are often used to decrease systemic vascular afterload. Caution should be exercised in prescribing or advising ibuprofen to any infant or child receiving ACE inhibitors as there is a risk of precipitating acute renal failure.

Patients are also at risk for long-term complications due to their intestinal abnor-malities, including intermittent partial volvulus associated with intestinal malrotation and an increased risk of sepsis due to translocation of abdominal microorganisms.

Case Scenarios

Case 1

A full-term newborn infant is born precipitously in a community hospital. Following good initial respiratory effort, the infant exhibits severe cyanosis. A stat pediatric consult is obtained. The responding pediatrician places an endotracheal tube and an umbilical venous line to stabilize the infant. The infant's color improves and the vital signs stabilize: pulse 148, blood pressure 73/37, oxygen saturation 92% while ventilated with 100% oxygen. Cardiac examination is significant for a single S2 and no murmur. Liver edge is not palpable. A stat chest radiograph raises the suspicion of heterotaxy syndrome. Prostaglandin infusion is initiated, with profound worsening hypoxemia. Transport is arranged to a tertiary care center, where a chest X-ray, ECG, and echocardiogram were performed.

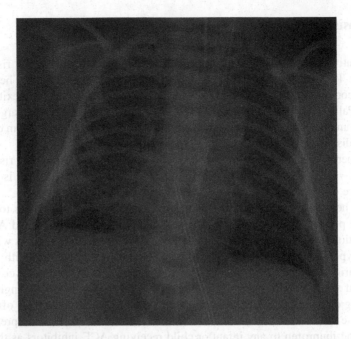

Fig. 22.2 Chest X-ray in AP view: cardiac apex is to the right (dextrocardia). Bilateral increase in pulmonary vascular markings suggestive of pulmonary edema. The umbilical venous line courses up the left spine and terminates in the heart indicating abnormal anatomy of inferior vena cava

CXR (Fig. 22.2): The cardiac silhouette is notable for dextrocardia. There is diffuse pulmonary edema. Bronchial anatomy cannot be determined. The gastric bubble and liver appear midline. The umbilical venous line courses up the left spine and terminates in the heart. (Endotracheal tube; umbilical, arterial, and venous lines; and nasogastric tube all terminate in appropriate positions for given anatomy.)

Discussion

This infant has heterotaxy syndrome, characterized by right atrial isomerism, pulmonary atresia (and therefore no murmur) and obstructed total anomalous pulmonary venous return. Following the first few breaths, inflation of the lungs leads to a decrease in pulmonary vascular resistance and a brisk increase in pulmonary blood flow. When pulmonary venous return is obstructed, the increase in pulmonary blood flow exacerbates the pulmonary edema. Following initiation of prostaglandin infusion, the duct will dilate and further augment pulmonary blood flow, further potentiating pulmonary venous obstruction. CXR findings of pulmonary edema may lag behind the profound hypoxemia that sometimes results. The ECG in this patient reflects myocardial ischemia from cyanosis (Fig. 22.3). Emergent surgical intervention is indicated.

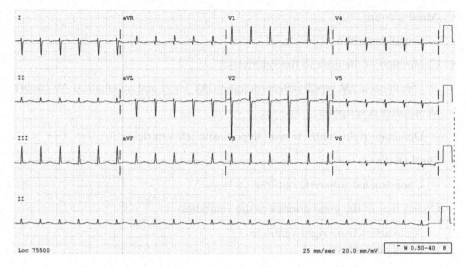

Fig. 22.3 ECG: P waves are absent suggesting junctional rhythm. The QRS axis is +130°, which can be normal in a newborn. There is lack of R wave progression in the precordial leads, where the R wave should become taller and taller from V1 to V6, suggesting right ventricular dominance or dextrocardia. Diffuse T wave flattening indicates a repolarization abnormality and is suggestive of ischemia

Patients who are born without prenatal diagnosis can have a dramatic presentation of right atrial isomerism, secondary to significantly obstructed pulmonary outflow and/or pulmonary venous obstruction. This infant underwent segmental cardiac evaluation by echocardiography, which found:

- Cardiac position and direction of apex:
  - Dextrocardia with apex to the right
- Systemic venous connections:
  - Bilateral superior vena cava
  - Absent coronary sinus
  - Inferior vena cava to right-sided atrium
  - Bilateral hepatic venous connections
- Pulmonary venous connections:
  - Total anomalous pulmonary venous return to a systemic vein below the diaphragm
- Atrial situs:
  - Right atrial appendage isomerism – bilateral broad-based triangular atrial appendages

- Atrial septum:
  - Common atrium
- Connection of the atria to the ventricles:
  - Unbalanced AV septal defect (common AV valve and unbalanced AV canal)
- Ventricular description:
  - Dominant right ventricle with hypoplastic left ventricle
- Outflow tracts:
  - Unobstructed subaortic outflow
- Connection of the great arteries to the ventricles:
  - Aorta arises from right ventricle
  - Pulmonary atresia
- Ductus arteriosus:
  - Open with large caliber

Case 2

A 1-month-old baby boy presents to the office for a routine well-baby exam. He was born by spontaneous vaginal delivery at 41-5/7 weeks and had incomplete prenatal care. Apgar scores were 8 and 8 at 1 and 5 min. Birth weight was 4,035 g. Discharge weight was 3,995 g. The infant is breast fed with formula supplementation. Mother has noted no feeding problems and generally has no specific concerns. This is the first time the infant has been seen by a physician since birth.

On physical examination, the infant is sleepy, but responsive to light touch. He is pink without jaundice. Vital signs: weight is 3,895 g, respirations are 65/min, and pulse is 164/min. Chest inspection is notable for comfortable tachypnea. Lungs are rhonchorous. On palpation, the cardiac impulse is appreciated on the right. Heart tones are appreciated to be louder in the right chest than in the left. A soft, 2/6 systolic flow murmur is noted both at the right and left sternal border. Femoral pulses are present and equal bilaterally. Abdomen is soft and nontender. Liver edge is not palpable. Skin temperature is cool, with livedo reticularis noted. Capillary refill is 2 s.

A pulse oximeter reading is requested and is 89% on room air. A chest radiograph is obtained:

CXR (Fig. 22.4): The cardiac silhouette is notable for dextrocardia. Pulmonary vascularity is slightly increased, suggesting increased pulmonary blood flow. Bronchial anatomy cannot be determined. The gastic bubble is on the right and the liver is on the left.

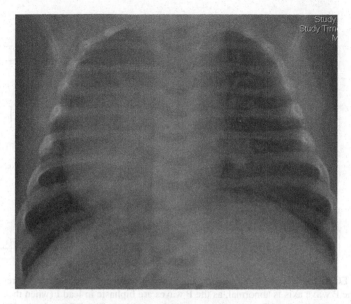

Fig. 22.4 Chest X-ray in AP view: CXR: cardiac apex is rightward indicating dextrocardia, mild increase in prominence of pulmonary vasculature. The gastric bubble is on the right and the liver is on the left indicating situs inversus of abdominal structures

Discussion

The dextrocardia, right-sided gastric bubble, and left-sided liver confirm a condition of abnormal left–right positioning. The differential diagnosis includes:

- Dextrocardia with situs inversus (rightward heart with mirror-image arrangement of the thoracic and abdominal viscera), particularly since bilateral short bronchi cannot be confirmed on chest X-ray. If this were the diagnosis and the patient subsequently developed recurrent pulmonary infections, sinusitis, and bronchiectasis, a diagnosis of Kartagener syndrome should be considered.
- Heterotaxy syndromes of right or left isomerism.

It is the reduced systemic oxygenation, tachypnea, and growth failure which raise the concern for associated intracardiac malformation. Left isomerism more commonly presents with signs and symptoms of increased pulmonary blood flow (tachypnea), growth failure, and signs of congestive heart failure (livedo reticularis suggests increased systemic vascular resistance associated with congestive heart failure). The murmur is a pulmonary flow murmur. This infant was referred to the hospital for cardiology consultation where echocardiogram confirmed left atrial isomerism (Fig. 22.5). Segmental analysis demonstrated:

- Cardiac position and direction of apex:
  - Dextrocardia with apex to the right

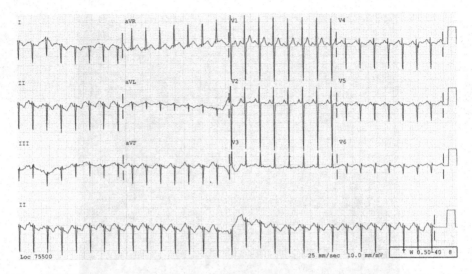

Fig. 22.5 ECG: P waves are followed by QRS waves in every lead confirms a regular atrial rhythm. The P wave axis is abnormal, as the P waves are biphasic in lead I (when they should be upright), and negative in aVL (when they should be positive). The QRS axis is +220, which is interpreted as extreme right axis deviation. There is lack of R wave progression in the precordial leads, where the R wave should become taller and taller from V1 to V6, suggesting right ventricular dominance or dextrocardia

- Systemic venous connections:

    - Left superior vena cava drains to coronary sinus
    - Absent right superior vena cava
    - Interrupted inferior vena cava with azygous continuation to left superior vena cava

- Pulmonary venous connections:

    - Mixed anomalous pulmonary venous return (right veins to right-sided atrium and left veins to left-sided atrium)

- Atrial situs:

    - Left atrial appendage isomerism – bilateral narrow-based and tubular atrial appendages

- Atrial septum:

    - Large secundum and large primum atrial septal defects

- Connection of the atria to the ventricles:

    - Unbalanced AV septal defect (common AV valve and unbalanced AV canal)

- Ventricular description:

    - Dominant right ventricle with hypoplastic left ventricle
    - Double outlet right ventricle

- Outflow tracts:
  - Unobstructed subaortic and subpulmonary outflow
- Connection of the great arteries to the ventricles:
  - Side-by-side relationship of great arteries as they arise from right ventricle
- Ductus arteriosus:
  - Absent

This patient was admitted to the hospital where he underwent medical stabilization with oral diuretics and afterload reduction. He then underwent single ventricle palliation with a pulmonary valvectomy and placement of a systemic-to-pulmonary shunt.

He presented to the office at 4 months of age with lethargy and poor feeding and was found to be responsive, but bradycardic, with a heart rate of 58. EMS was activated and the patient was brought to the hospital. The ECG rhythm strip demonstrated a complete AV block. Since the AV block produced symptoms of lethargy and poor feeding, the infant received an epicardial pacemaker.

Chapter 23
Hypoplastic Left Heart Syndrome

Sawsan Mokhtar M. Awad and Jacquelyn Busse

Key Facts

- Children with HLHS present at 2–4 weeks of age when the ductus arteriosus closes.
- Survival of children with HLHS prior to repair relies on adequate shunting of blood through an ASD and a PDA.
- Presentation often includes evidence of poor cardiac output and, in extreme cases, cardiac shock.
- Poor peripheral pulses and perfusion are the dominant features on physical examination. Murmurs may not be appreciated by auscultation; however, the second heart sound is single.
- Surgical repair is performed in three stages termed Norwood procedure stages I, II, and III. The first stage is typically performed in the neonatal period, stage II at 3–6 months of age, and stage III at 18 months of age.
- Morbidity and mortality from this congenital heart disease continues to be significant when compared to other congenital heart diseases.

Definition

Hypoplastic left heart syndrome is a cyanotic congenital heart disease presenting in the first week of life. Multiple left heart structures are typically involved. The mitral valve is severely stenotic or atretic leading to small or hypoplastic left ventricle and severely stenotic or hypoplastic aortic valve. The ascending aorta tends to be hypoplastic and slightly enlarges towards the aortic arch with a normal

S.M.M. Awad (✉)
Department of Pediatrics, Rush University Medical Center, 1653 W. Congress Parkway, Suite 770 Jones, Chicago, IL 60612, USA
e-mail: sawsan_m_awad@rush.edu

Ra-id Abdulla (ed.), *Heart Diseases in Children: A Pediatrician's Guide*,
DOI 10.1007/978-1-4419-7994-0_23, © Springer Science+Business Media, LLC 2011

descending aorta. Neonates survive this anomaly in the first few days of life due to the presence of a patent foramen ovale (PFO) and ductus arteriosus (PDA). The PFO allows blood returning form the pulmonary veins to shunt to the right atrium while the PDA provides blood flow to the aortic arch through right to left shunting. Blood travels in a retrograde fashion through the aortic arch and all the way back to the ascending aorta to provide blood flow to the coronary arteries. Cardiogenic shock develops as soon as the PDA starts to close depriving cardiac output to the systemic circulation.

Incidence

Hypoplastic left heart syndrome (HLHS) is somewhat rare, comprising only 1.5% of congenital heart diseases. The incidence is less than 0.5 per 1,000 live births with no sex preference.

Pathology

In its extreme, HLHS consists of hypoplasia of the left ventricle with mitral and aortic valve atresia and a hypoplastic aortic arch. Often, the mitral and aortic valves are not completely atretic, but severely hypoplastic. Systemic cardiac output is supplied by the right ventricle through the patent ductus arteriosus (PDA). Infants with HLHS usually do well in utero. In the neonatal period, maintaining the patency of the ductus arteriosus is crucial for survival (Fig. 23.1).

Pathophysiology

With severe hypoplasia of the left heart, there is no forward flow across the aortic valve through the ascending aorta. The systemic circulation relies exclusively on flow through the PDA from the right ventricle. This will feed both the descending and ascending aorta. The blood flows in a retrograde fashion through the ascending aorta to supply the brachiocephalic branches and the coronary arteries.

Blood ejected from the right ventricle supplies the pulmonary artery as well as the systemic circulation. The pulmonary circulation has a lower vascular resistance (about 3 Wood units) compared to the systemic vascular resistance (about 25 Wood units). This significant difference in resistance will favor blood flow into the pulmonary system leading to excessive pulmonary blood flow and eventual pulmonary edema. The comparatively limited blood flow to the systemic circulation will result in poor systemic cardiac output and, in extreme cases, can manifest as cardiogenic shock.

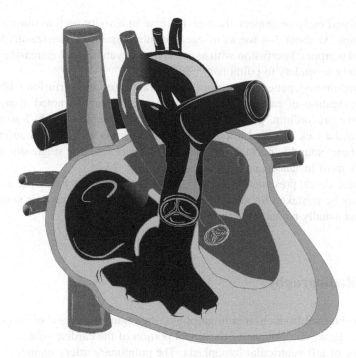

Fig. 23.1 Anatomy of hypoplastic left heart. Left heart structures are hypoplastic or atretic. In view of mitral atresia, the blood in the left atrium shunts across atrial septal defect to the right atrium. Blood flow to the aorta is supplied through the ductus arteriosus

Atrial septal communication has to be present for survival in these patients. Pulmonary venous return to the right atrium cannot flow into the left ventricle due to mitral and/or left ventricular hypoplasia. Therefore, blood will cross through an atrial communication [patent foramen ovale (PFO) or atrial septal defect (ASD)], mix with the systemic venous return and pass through the tricuspid valve into the right ventricle.

The phenomenon of pulmonary edema and cardiogenic shock will become even more pronounced when the ductus arteriosus starts to close around 2–4 weeks of age. Without an adequate right to left shunt, systemic cardiac output will drop and right sided heart failure will develop. The patient will present with severe respiratory distress and poor perfusion evidenced by ashen color, cool extremities, and weak peripheral pulses. Death is imminent unless ductal patency can be maintained, usually with prostaglandin infusion.

Clinical Manifestations

A PDA and an atrial communication such as a PFO or ASD together provide adequate hemodynamic conditions in the first few days of life and thus newborns are often asymptomatic. However, ashen skin discoloration or mottling of the skin may be noted early on, especially with increase in activity such as during feeding or agitation. At about 2–4 weeks of age, patients present with increasing lethargy, decreased peripheral perfusion with ashen color or cyanosis and increasing respiratory distress secondary to pulmonary edema.

On examination, patients have poor peripheral pulses and perfusion with significant prolongation of capillary refill. Hepatomegaly may be noted along with a hyperactive precordium, prominent right ventricular impulse (right lower sternal border), and a lack of apical impulse. Typically there is no thrill. On auscultation, the first heart sound is normal, but the second heart sound is single due to aortic atresia. In most instances, no murmur is heard (Fig. 23.2).

In severe cases, presentation is that of complete circulatory collapse and shock which may be mistaken for sepsis. Patients are cyanotic with poor or nonpalpable pulses and usually no audible murmurs.

Chest Radiography

The data obtained from chest radiography is often nonspecific and of limited use in diagnosis. However, absence of the apical portion of the cardiac silhouette may be suggestive of left ventricular hypoplasia. The pulmonary artery segment is prominent due to increased flow across the main pulmonary artery and PDA. The heart size may be normal or enlarged and the pulmonary vasculature may be normal or increased (Fig. 23.3).

Electrocardiography

Electrocardiography in patients with HLHS shows decreased left ventricular voltage and increased right ventricular voltage. Since a normal newborn's electrocardiography also has increased right ventricular voltage, this finding may be difficult to interpret in this age group (Fig. 23.4).

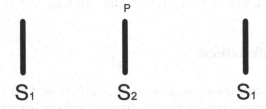

Fig. 23.2 Heart sounds and murmur in HLH. S1: first heart sound, S2: second heart sound, P: pulmonary valve closure. Second heart sound is single due to aortic valve atresia

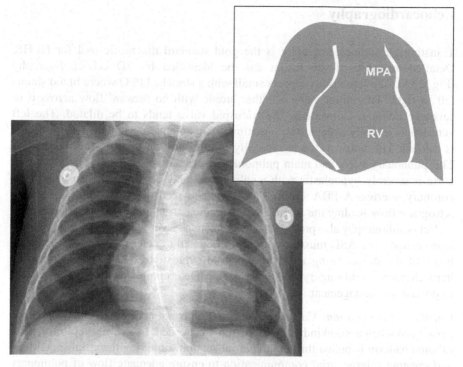

Fig. 23.3 HLH CXR. *MPA* main pulmonary artery, *RV* right ventricle. The apex of the cardiac silhouette is abnormal due to hypoplasia of the left ventricle. Pulmonary artery segment is prominent due to increased flow through the main pulmonary artery and the patent ductus arteriosus

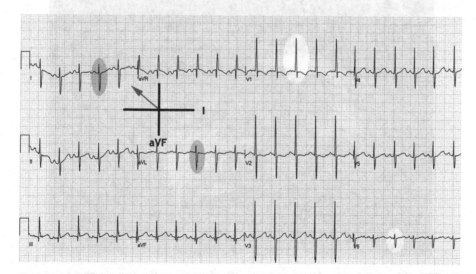

Fig. 23.4 ECG in HLH. Right ventricular hypertrophy: tall R in V1 and deep S in V6. Hypoplasia of left ventricle: small R wave in left chest leads (V6). Right axis deviation due to prominence of right ventricle and hypoplasia of left ventricle

Echocardiography

Transthoracic echocardiography is the gold standard diagnostic tool for HLHS. Detailed anatomy of the lesion can be identified by 2D echocardiography (Fig. 23.5). The left atrium appears small with a stretched PFO where blood shunts left to right. The mitral valve is either atretic with no forward flow across it or severely stenotic. Conversely, the tricuspid valve tends to be dilated. The left ventricle is severely hypoplastic, sometimes with no lumen, while the right ventricle is dilated. The aortic valve is typically atretic with no or little foreword flow. The pulmonary valve and main pulmonary artery are both dilated. The ascending aorta is severely hypoplastic with a caliber that may be no more than that of the coronary arteries. A PDA shunts right to left to feed the descending aorta with retrograde flow feeding the aortic arch, ascending aorta and coronary arteries.

Echocardiography also provides an assessment of severity and need for immediate intervention. The ASD must be carefully evaluated to determine whether enlargement of the defect using a Rashkind atrial septostomy is needed to stabilize hemodynamics until surgery can be performed. Determining the size of PDA is also important for management.

Cardiac catheterization: Cardiac catheterization is not needed for diagnosis but is performed when a Rashkind atrial septostomy is needed. In an atrial septostomy, an inflated balloon is pulled through the atrial septum, rupturing the atrial septal wall and creating a large atrial communication to ensure adequate flow of pulmonary venous blood to the right atrium. In many centers, this procedure is performed

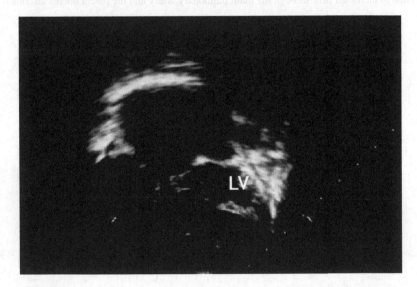

Fig. 23.5 Echocardiography. *LV* left ventricle. 2D echocardiography, four chamber apical view showing hypoplastic left ventricle

using special balloon catheters introduced through the umbilical vein and performed with echo guidance while in the intensive care unit, rather than at the cardiac catheterization laboratory.

Treatment

Initial management in the newborn focuses on correcting metabolic acidosis secondary to poor cardiac output and reestablishing hemodynamic stability. The ASD must be enlarged if it is small and the patency of the ductus must be maintained. Infants known or suspected to have HLHS warrant an urgent echocardiogram and should be started on a prostaglandin infusion immediately.

Many infants present with severe respiratory distress requiring endotracheal intubation and mechanical ventilation. It is important to limit the use of oxygen to that of room air (21%) or less. Using a lower oxygen concentration of 15–18%, called sub-ambient oxygen, causes an intentional hypoxia and helps in maintaining the balance between the pulmonary and systemic circulation. Hypoxia causes pulmonary arterial constriction thus limiting the otherwise excessive pulmonary blood flow and allowing for more flow through the ductus arteriosus to the systemic circulation.

Once hemodynamic stability is achieved and metabolic acidosis is corrected, plans for surgical repair must be made. The most common surgical technique for single ventricle repair is a 3-step repair known as the Norwood procedure. Ultimately, the Norwood procedure results in the right heart structures being used to actively pump blood to the systemic circulation while the systemic venous return bypasses the heart entirely and flows passively to the pulmonary circulation.

Norwood stage I: The first stage of the repair is done shortly after birth. The atretic aorta is reconstructed using the main pulmonary artery augmented with synthetic patch material. The right ventricle becomes committed to pumping blood through the pulmonary valve to the aorta and the systemic circulation. The ductus arteriosus is ligated and is replaced by a more reliable systemic-to-pulmonary arterial shunt to ensure adequate blood flow to the lungs. Two commonly used shunts include the Blalock–Taussig (BT) shunt and the Sano shunt.

Norwood stage II: At about 3–6 months of age, the superior vena cava is connected directly to the pulmonary artery, bypassing the heart. This is called a Glenn shunt and it allows passive flow of systemic venous return from the head and upper extremities to the pulmonary circulation. The BT or Sano shunt is taken down as it is no longer needed. Venous return from the trunk and lower extremities is still flowing from the IVC into the right atrium and mixing with oxygenated blood. Therefore, oxygen saturation will still be low and patients may still have cyanosis.

Norwood stage III: At about 18 months of age, a Fontan procedure is done in which the inferior vena cava is connected directly to the pulmonary circulation. Pulmonary blood flow is now completely dependent on passive venous return to the lungs and there is no longer mixing of oxygenated and deoxygenated blood.

Recently, some centers have replaced the Stage I Norwood procedure with a "hybrid" procedure – hybrid referring to the combined techniques of both surgeons and interventional cardiologists. This procedure is less invasive and involves delaying the repair of the aortic arch until the patient is older. The procedure is performed through a median sternotomy. A stent is placed in the ductus arteriosus to keep it patent without the need for prostaglandin. The right and left pulmonary arteries are banded to prevent overflow into the pulmonary circulation and allow for more blood flow to the systemic circulation. Later, at about 3–6 months of age, the child is taken to the operating room for reconstructing of the aortic arch (completion of stage I Norwood) and a Glenn shunt (Stage II Norwood) is created at the same time. The Fontan is then completed as above around 18 months of age.

Cardiac transplantation is performed in a limited number of centers worldwide. Transplantation eliminates the need for multistaged surgical repair, but comes with other morbidities including complications due to immune suppression, graft rejection, and coronary artery disease.

Prognosis

Hypoplastic left heart syndrome is one of the most severe congenital heart diseases. Children frequently present in critical condition with severe metabolic acidosis and hypoxia. As fetal echocardiography is being done more frequently, many patients are diagnosed in utero allowing more efficient stabilization after birth and avoiding circulatory collapse.

The morbidity and mortality of HLHS continues to be high. Survival after 3-stage repair is low, relative to surgical repair results of other congenital heart diseases. It is believed that not more than 60% of children with this ailment survive up to 5 years of age. Cardiac transplantation has also had limited success with mortality rates comparable to the Norwood approach. There is limited availability of hearts suitable for transplantation in infants and the risk of infection with immune suppression therapy is great. Many children with cardiac transplantation also suffer from coronary artery disease due to increased risk of stenosis of such vessels in transplanted hearts.

Neurological complications associated with HLHS are well documented in the medical literature. Abnormal brain development may actually start in utero due to restricted cerebral blood flow. The catastrophic presentation of cardiorespiratory collapse, as well as the multiple complicated surgeries required, further compound this problem causing developmental delay and, at times, significant neurological impairment.

Case Scenarios

Case 1

A 10-day-old newborn presented to the emergency room with increased irritability, poor feeding and ashen discoloration of the skin for the past 2–3 days. He was born full term via normal vaginal delivery with no history of complications during pregnancy or birth. He was well for the first week of life and has had no fever, vomiting, diarrhea, or any known sick contacts.

On examination, the child appeared to be in moderate to severe respiratory distress with cyanosis and gray skin tone. Capillary refill was more than 3 s with weak pulses in all extremities. Blood pressure was not obtainable. Oxygen saturation was 65% on room air. Mild hepatomegaly was noted and the right ventricular impulse was exaggerated while the apical impulse was not palpable. Auscultation revealed a single second heart sound with no significant murmurs.

The chest X-ray showed a normal sized heart and moderately increased pulmonary vascular markings.

An ECG showed right axis deviation and right ventricular hypertrophy.

Discussion

The presentation of this infant illustrated classic findings of cardiogenic shock. Although sepsis should be a primary consideration, subtle signs suggestive of a cardiac anomaly should be noted. The lack of apical impulse, single second heart sound, and significant oxygen desaturation beyond what is typically seen with sepsis, particularly in the absences of pulmonary disease findings on the chest X-ray, should prompt immediate investigation into cardiac causes.

Other left sided obstructive lesions may also present with cardiac shock with a few notable differences. Subaortic obstruction due to ventricular septal hypertrophy will have a significant and harsh systolic ejection murmur and evidence of left ventricular hypertrophy on examination and electrocardiography. Critical aortic stenosis will also have a harsh systolic murmur. Severe coarctation of the aorta and interrupted aortic arch will have strong brachial arterial pulses with weak femoral pulses.

Echocardiography should be done urgently in any case in which significant congenital heart disease is a possibility. Echocardiography will delineate the cardiac pathology as well as assess the size of any atrial communication and the patency of the ductus arteriosus.

This child must be admitted to an intensive care unit for stabilization including fluid resuscitation, correction of metabolic acidosis, and initiation of prostaglandin infusion to maintain patency of the ductus arteriosus. The latter should be instituted even before diagnosis is confirmed as it will restore cardiac output and hasten stabilization.

Rashkind atrial septostomy must be performed if the atrial communication is restrictive. Stage I surgical repair (either Norwood of hybrid) can be delayed for a few days until the patient is clinically stable.

As discussed, complete repair will require two additional procedures, typically performed at around 6 and 18 months of age.

Case 2

A 32-year-old female at 38 weeks gestation presented in labor to a community hospital. The mother had several fetal echocardiographic evaluations showing HLHS. Delivery was planned at a tertiary care center, but labor progressed rapidly and she came to the nearest hospital. Delivery was uneventful and resulted in a 3,300 g infant male. The infant appeared to be stable at delivery with an oxygen saturation of 85% on room air. Vital signs and physical examination were otherwise unremarkable.

Communication with the pediatric cardiologist at the tertiary care center confirmed the diagnosis on record. Prostaglandin infusion was initiated and the infant was kept on room air.

The patient was transported to the tertiary care center in stable condition with no evidence of respiratory distress or metabolic acidosis. Echocardiography confirmed HLHS with a wide PDA and a small to moderate ASD. In view of the adequate atrial communication, it was felt that a Rashkind atrial septostomy was not necessary.

A few hours after arrival, the child was noted to have apnea, a known complication of prostaglandin infusion, and elective endotracheal intubation was performed. Mechanical ventilation was used with no supplemental oxygen. A slightly elevated pCO_2 was sought to achieve mild pulmonary vasoconstriction to limit blood flow to the lungs and promote flow to the systemic circulation.

As previously discussed with parents, the child underwent a Norwood stage I surgical procedure at 1 week of life.

Chapter 24
Ebstein's Anomaly

Russell Robert Cross and Ra-id Abdulla

Key Facts

- Ebstein's anomaly of the tricuspid valve causes apical displacement of the effective orifice of the tricuspid valve resulting in large right atrium and smaller right ventricle.
- Ebstein's anomaly is associated with bypass tracts between the right atrium and ventricle which may precipitate supraventricular tachycardia.
- Hemodynamic effects of the abnormal tricuspid valve vary from mild to severe. In mild cases there are limited or no symptoms and signs. In severe cases the tricuspid valve is severely regurgitant and the right ventricular outflow tract is obstructed. These changes will lead to high right atrial pressure and right to left shunting at the foramen ovale leading to cyanosis.
- Surgical repair of tricuspid valve is reserved to severe cases.
- Patients with small right ventricle may eventually require Fontan procedure.

Definition

Ebstein's anomaly is a congenital heart disease affecting the tricuspid valve. In its milder form, the tricuspid valve is mildly displaced towards the apex with mild regurgitation and no stenosis. These patients are usually asymptomatic. On the other hand, significant displacement of the tricuspid valve leaflets results in severe tricuspid valve regurgitation and lack of forward flow of blood in the right ventricular outflow tract due to obstruction by the abnormal tricuspid valve. Patients in the

R.R. Cross (✉)
Department of Cardiology, Children's National Medical Center, 111 Michigan Avenue,
NW Washington, DC 20010, USA
e-mail: rcross@cnmc.org

Ra-id Abdulla (ed.), *Heart Diseases in Children: A Pediatrician's Guide*,
DOI 10.1007/978-1-4419-7994-0_24, © Springer Science+Business Media, LLC 2011

severe format of the disease develop significant escape of blood from the right atrium into the left atrium through right to left shunting, thus resulting in cyanosis. Patient with Ebstein's anomaly are also known to have abnormal atrioventricular bridging of conductive tissue leading to preexcitaiton and tachyrhythmia.

Incidence

Ebstein's anomaly is rare, occurring in approximately 0.5% of patients with congenital heart disease, and with an overall occurrence of 1 in 20,000 live births. Most cases occur sporadically and with equal occurrence between male and female. A small number of familial cases suggest that there could be a genetic linkage, but there is currently no specific mutation identified. There is some evidence to suggest an increased risk for Ebstein's anomaly in the off-spring of women who are exposed to lithium during pregnancy, but this relationship has been disputed.

Pathology

It is primarily the septal and posterior leaflets of the tricuspid valve that are affected in Ebstein's anomaly. The leaflets tend to have redundant tissue with short chordae and accessory attachments to the right ventricular septal surface, resulting in tethering of the leaflets to the septum. The anterior leaflet of the tricuspid valve is less affected. The tethering of the septal and posterior leaflets result in apical displacement of the tricuspid valve's effective orifice into the right ventricular body so that the effective orifice no longer resides at the normal level of the atrio-ventricular groove. The true valve annulus (the "hinge points"), remains at the normal level.

The apical displacement of the tricuspid valve results in an "atrialized" portion of the right ventricle, that is, part of the volume of the anatomic right ventricle becomes physiologically a component of the right atrium. This results in a physiologic right atrium that is larger than normal. Additionally, the wall of the atrialized portion of the right ventricle is thin, consistent with the lower pressures of the atrial chamber (Fig. 24.1).

Pathophysiology

The tricuspid valve abnormalities seen in Ebstein's anomaly create varying degrees of tricuspid insufficiency, right atrial enlargement, and right ventricular outflow tract obstruction. In milder forms of the disease, the tricuspid valve is not substantially displaced apically into the right ventricle. These patients usually have minimal tricuspid insufficiency and tend to have little in the way of symptoms.

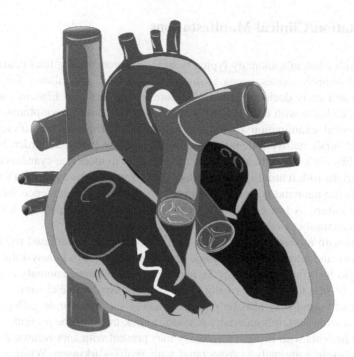

Fig. 24.1 Anatomy of Ebstein malformation. The tricuspid valve is apically displaced causing the right ventricle to be small and the right atrium to enlarge. Severe tricuspid regurgitation (*white arrow*) may cause the right atrium to further enlarge

In more moderate forms of Ebstein's anomaly, the tricuspid valve leaflets are positioned lower in the right ventricle resulting in greater degrees of tricuspid insufficiency. Along with the tricuspid insufficiency there is increased right atrial enlargement. These individuals also may have right-to-left shunting of deoxygenated blood at the level of the atrial septum through a patent foramen ovale or an atrial septal defect. The right to left shunting is a result of the tricuspid insufficiency and associated higher right atrial pressures, this results in cyanosis.

Neonatal physiology in the more severe forms of Ebstein's anomaly is dominated by severe tricuspid insufficiency and inability to create forward flow across the right ventricular outflow tract. The severe tricuspid insufficiency results in even greater right atrial enlargement, and makes it difficult for the right ventricle to create forward flow out the pulmonary artery. In some cases, the abnormal tricuspid valve leaflets can create a physical obstruction to flow across the right ventricular outflow tract. These patients can be profoundly cyanotic with low cardiac output, often are dependent on a patent ductus arteriosus (PDA) to provide pulmonary blood flow, and may have ventilation difficulties secondary to cardiomegally. The situation may improve as pulmonary vascular resistance drops in the first several days of life, allowing more forward flow out the pulmonary artery.

Presentation/Clinical Manifestations

Infants with Ebstein's anomaly typically have an unremarkable fetal course. Fetal echocardiography makes prenatal diagnosis possible, and allows for medical planning and early decision making in more severe forms of Ebstein's anomaly. Newborn children with mild Ebstein's anomaly often have no symptoms, but may have physical examination findings consistent with tricuspid insufficiency – a somewhat harsh, holosystolic murmur along the left lower sternal border. Moderate cases of Ebstein's anomaly are associated with mild to moderate cyanosis resulting from the right-to-left atrial shunting, while more severe forms of Ebstein's anomaly present in the neonatal period with significant cyanosis and evidence for congestive heart failure. A low cardiac output state may also exist in patients with severe Ebstein's anomaly, resulting in poor perfusion and acidosis.

Infants with moderate to severe Ebstein's anomaly have increased right precordial activity and may have a right-sided heave. In addition to a holosystolic murmur of tricuspid insufficiency (Fig. 24.2), neonates with Ebstein's anomaly may have a widely split first heart sound owing to delay in tricuspid valve closure. A third or fourth heart sound may also be present, creating the "quadruple gallop rhythm" associated with Ebstein's anomaly. A systolic click may also be present.

Older patients with Ebstein's anomaly may present with supraventricular tachycardia. Ebstein's anomaly is associated with Wolff–Parkinson–White syndrome (a type of electrical bypass tract) in 10–20% of patients. Additionally, patients with Ebstein's anomaly may present later in life with symptoms of fatigue and exercise intolerance as a result of worsening heart failure associated with progressive tricuspid insufficiency and cardiac enlargement.

Chest Radiography

The chest X-ray in Ebstein's anomaly is most notable for cardiomegally, the degree of which is related to the severity of tricuspid insufficiency. In severe forms of Ebstein's anomaly, the cardiac silhouette can fill the entire chest width on AP chest X-ray. There may also be normal to decreased pulmonary vascular markings and a prominent right atrium (Fig. 24.3).

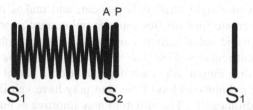

$$S_1 \qquad S_2 \qquad S_1$$

Fig. 24.2 Heart sounds and murmur in Ebstein malformation. S1: first heart sound, S2: second heart sound, A: aortic valve closure, P: pulmonary valve closure. Severe tricuspid regurgitation may be audible as a holosystolic murmur heard best over the left lower sternal border

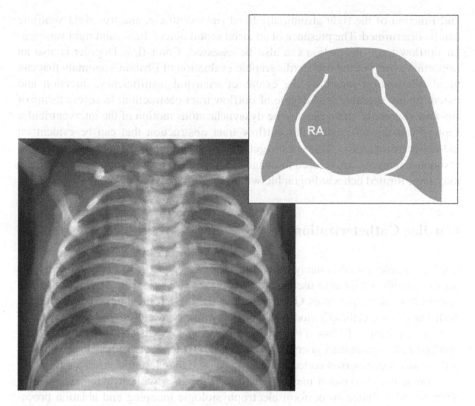

Fig. 24.3 RA: right atrium. Cardiomegaly secondary to severely dilated right atrium

Electrocardiography

The predominant finding on EKG is right atrial enlargement, characterized by tall P waves in lead II greater than 2 mm. The QRS axis is typically rightward or normal. A right ventricular conduction delay is often present, which is characterized by incomplete or complete right-bundle-branch block with an rSR′ pattern in V1.

Patients with Wolff–Parkinson–White may exhibit the typical shortened PR interval with slurring of the R-wave upstroke when in normal sinus rhythm, or may present in SVT with a narrow complex tachycardia. Additionally, atrial flutter or fibrillation may be evident in patients with significant right atrial enlargement.

Echocardiography

The anatomy of Ebstein's anomaly can usually be well delineated by 2D-echocardiography. Anatomic details of the tricuspid valve, its attachments, and the extent of displacement into the right ventricle can be evaluated. Likewise, the size and function of the right atrium, atrialized right ventricle, and true right ventricle can be determined. The presence of an atrial septal defect, PDA, and right ventricular outflow tract obstruction can also be assessed. Color flow Doppler is also an important aspect of the echocardiographic evaluation of Ebstein's anomaly that can yield information regarding the extent of tricuspid insufficiency, direction and extent of any shunting, and degree of outflow tract obstruction. In severe forms of Ebstein's anomaly, there can also be dyssynchronous motion of the interventricular septum causing left ventricular outflow tract obstruction that can be evident on 2D-echocardiography. Transesophageal echocardiography or cardiac magnetic resonance imaging can be used to image older patients with Ebstein's anomaly who may have limited echocardiographic windows.

Cardiac Catheterization

Cardiac catheterization is rarely needed to diagnose or assess patients with Ebstein's anomaly. However, it can be useful in rare cases to measure right atrial, right ventricular, or pulmonary artery pressures. Quantification of right-to-left shunting and cardiac output performed in the catheterization laboratory may also be useful in the management of more severe forms of Ebstein's anomaly. Angiographic evaluation of right ventricular outflow tract or pulmonary artery obstruction can be helpful, particularly in cases where interventional catheterization techniques can be used to relieve the obstruction.

Cardiac catheterization may be performed in cases with arrhythmias, such as SVT or atrial flutter, to perform electrophysiologic mapping and ablation procedures. It is of historical significance to note that the simultaneous measurement of pressure and intracardiac electrocardiogram in the atrialized portion of the right ventricle demonstrates atrial pressures with ventricular electrical tracings. This fact was used in the past to assist in the diagnosis of Ebstein's anomaly.

Treatment/Management

There is a wide variability in the medical management of Ebstein's anomaly that correlates with the severity of the heart disease. In the cyanotic newborn with mild to moderate Ebstein's anomaly, close observation and clinical support may be all that is needed until the normal drop in pulmonary vascular resistance occurs. As the pulmonary vascular resistance decreases, there is increasing forward flow through the right ventricle resulting in less cyanosis secondary to atrial level shunting. These patients often benefit from oxygen to stimulate lowering of the pulmonary vascular resistance, and in some cases, the use of prostaglandin E_1 to maintain ductal patency may be required to ensure adequate pulmonary blood flow.

Infants with mild Ebstein's anomaly may remain completely asymptomatic and require no medical management. Those with more severe forms of Ebstein's anomaly experience congestive heart failure symptoms and benefit from anticongestive therapy with diuretics, and may also require inotropic support if there is significant compromise in cardiac output.

Patients with associated Wolff–Parkinson–White syndrome can be managed conservatively, but if they experience supraventricular tachycardia then appropriate antiarrhythmic medications should be started or the patient should be considered for electrophysiology study and ablation therapy. Other patients may require medical management or ablative therapy for SVT or atrial flutter/fibrillation as a result of atrial enlargement.

Surgical management of Ebstein's anomaly is also variable and dictated by the degree of cyanosis or heart failure. Patients with cyanosis and right ventricular outflow tract obstruction may benefit from interventional catheterization or surgery to relieve the obstruction. In more severe obstruction or those with complete pulmonary atresia, a systemic to pulmonary arterial shunt (Blalock–Taussig, or BT shunt) may be performed. These patients would then usually be considered for a Glenn cavopulmonary anastomosis at several months of age. Newborns with significant tricuspid insufficiency pose a particularly difficult surgical challenge. Patients have undergone varying types of tricuspid valve repairs in the newborn period, but usually with only limited success. Older patients with progressive tricuspid insufficiency may benefit from tricuspid valve repair or replacement. Indications for surgery include progressive cyanosis, worsening heart failure, arrhythmias, and paradoxical emboli due to right-to-left atrial shunting.

Long-term Follow-up

Children with significant tricuspid insufficiency require long-term anticongestive therapy with diuretics and possibly digoxin. However, those patients with mild degrees of tricuspid insufficiency may remain asymptomatic and require no treatment in the early years. It is not uncommon, however, for these patients to develop worsening congestive heart failure or cyanosis due to progressive tricuspid insufficiency during the second or third decade of life. These patients would then need to be treated medically for the heart failure symptoms and surgical repair or replacement of the tricuspid valve should be considered. Patients should be followed closely for the evidence of cyanosis, increasing shortness of breath, increasing fatigue, or for the evidence of arrhythmias.

Prognosis

The prognosis of Ebstein's anomaly is directly related to the severity of the valve abnormality and degree of tricuspid insufficiency. It is estimated that the overall mortality rate in the first year of life is around 20%. The average life expectancy for early survivors is 20 years, but there are ample reports of patients with milder forms of Ebstein's anomaly who live much longer.

Case Scenarios

Case 1

About 6 h after an uncomplicated delivery, it is noted that a full term female infant appears to be cyanotic. Pulse oximetry reveals a room air oxygen saturation of 82%. On examination, the baby's heart rate is 170 bpm, respiratory rate 65 per min, and BP 85/60 mmHg in both the upper and lower extremities. There are no dysmorphic features and the baby is tachypneic with mild distress. Lungs are clear to auscultation. Heart examination reveals increased right precordial activity with a right-sided heave. There is a 3/6 systolic regurgitant murmur of tricuspid insufficiency heard along the left lower sternal border and a wide split first heart sound is heard. There is also an audible systolic click. Her liver is palpable 4–5 cm below the right sternal border and pulses are weak.

Chest X-ray demonstrates a markedly enlarged cardiac silhouette and the lung fields are dark, consistent with diminished pulmonary blood flow. There is right atrial enlargement, a rightward QRS axis, and an rSR' pattern in V1 on electrocardiogram.

An echocardiogram is obtained and shows severe apical displacement of the tricuspid valve into the right ventricle, and there is severe tricuspid valve insufficiency. The right atrium is moderately enlarged and a small atrial septal defect is present. Doppler color flow demonstrates right to left shunting across the ASD. The left heart is normal with good function. A small PDA is present with left to right shunting into the pulmonary artery, but no antigrade flow can be identified across the pulmonary valve.

This newborn has severe Ebstein's anomaly with severe tricuspid valve insufficiency. The right ventricle is unable to produce adequate pressure to overcome the high pulmonary vascular resistance in this newborn. As the PDA closes, pulmonary blood flow through the left to right shunting PDA decreases. There is also right to left shunting of deoxygenated blood across the atrial septum secondary to the tricuspid insufficiency and high right atrial pressures. This also contributes to cyanosis. Immediate treatment for this newborn child is to start prostaglandin E_1 in hopes of reopening the PDA in order to increase pulmonary blood flow. The baby needs to be followed over the following days as the pulmonary vascular resistance drops to determine if forward pulmonary blood flow across the small right ventricle improves. The baby can most likely be tried off the prostaglandin E_1 in 3–4 days to determine if there is adequate pulmonary blood flow after the pulmonary vascular resistance has decreased. If it is not possible to wean the child off prostaglandins, then plans for a surgically placed systemic to pulmonary arterial shunt should be considered to replace PDA. In severe cases, the child may eventually require a univentricular repair (Fontan procedure), however, this is unlikely.

Case 2

A 14-year-old male is seen in the emergency room with narrow complex tachycardia at 220 bpm. He first noted the rapid heart beat while playing basketball with his friends. His past medical history is unremarkable, although his mother had been told in the past that he had a faint murmur. She has also noted that he has been more easily tired over the last few months. Because he is hemodynamically stable, he is treated with adenosine 0.2 mg/kg by rapid bolus push. Following conversion to normal sinus rhythm, an ECG is obtained which shows a 3 mm p-wave in lead II (right atrial enlargement), right axis deviation, a short PR interval, and early depolarization consistent with Wolff–Parkinson–White.

Chest X-ray demonstrates a mildly enlarged cardiac silhouette, but is otherwise normal. On examination now, his heart rate is 75 bpm, respiratory rate 14 per min, and blood pressure 115/80. He is acyanotic and in no distress. Lungs are clear to auscultation. Cardiac exam reveals mildly increased right precordial activity, regular rhythm, and normal first and second heart sounds. There is a 2/6 systolic regurgitant murmur at the left lower sternal border and a systolic click is present. His liver edge is palpable 3 cm below the right costal margin, and he is well perfused with 2+ pulses in all extremities.

An echocardiogram is obtained and shows moderate tricuspid insufficiency associated with mild apical displacement of the tricuspid valve toward the cardiac apex. The right atrium is also moderately enlarged and the right ventricular function is mildly depressed. The remainder of the echocardiogram is normal.

This teenager presented with supraventricular tachycardia as a result of Wolff–Parkinson–White type bypass tract associated with mild to moderate Ebstein's anomaly. He most likely had mild tricuspid insufficiency in the past, but it is now worsened secondary to diminished function due to the supraventricular tachycardia. Immediate treatment could include initiation of diuretics for the treatment of mild heart failure. The heart failure symptoms most likely improve with good arrhythmia control, but he needs to be followed in the future for the progression of tricuspid insufficiency and potential worsening heart failure. Management of Wolff–Parkinson–White syndrome may include medical therapy, but more likely an electrophysiology study with potential ablation of the bypass tract is warranted.

Chapter 25
Vascular Rings

Ra-id Abdulla

Key Facts

- Children with respiratory symptoms should be suspected to have vascular ring if:
  - Symptoms start early in life
  - Dominant clinical features are stridor and upper airway noises
  - Children are noted to assume an arched back and extended neck position
  - Chest X-ray shows evidence of right aortic arch
- Double aortic arch present early in life, while right aortic arch with aberrant left subclavian artery present later in infancy.
- Treatment of vascular ring is surgical to relief the constricting circle of vascular and ligamentum structures around the esophagus and trachea.

Definition

Vascular ring occurs when the great arteries or their branches assume an abnormal anatomy leading to the formation of a ring of vessels surrounding and constricting the esophagus and trachea. Symptoms due to this anomaly may not manifest till later in infancy. Three types of vascular abnormalities are most common, these are: (1) double aortic arch, (2) right aortic arch with aberrant left subclavian artery, and (3) pulmonary sling. The latter abnormality: pulmonary sling does not form a ring around the esophagus and trachea, but rather a sling around the trachea. Other rare abnormalities of the great vessels and their branches (Table 25.1) may lead to compression of the trachea and esophagus; however, these are extremely rare. In

---

Ra-id Abdulla (✉)
Center for Congenital and Structural Heart Diseases, Rush University Medical Center,
1653 West Congress Parkway, Room 763 Jones, Chicago, IL 60612, USA
e-mail: rabdulla@rush.edu

Ra-id Abdulla (ed.), *Heart Diseases in Children: A Pediatrician's Guide*,
DOI 10.1007/978-1-4419-7994-0_25, © Springer Science+Business Media, LLC 2011

Table 25.1 Abnormalities of great vessels and their branches leading to vascular rings compressing the tracheobronchial tree and esophagus

Left aortic arch with right descending aorta and right ductus arteriosus

Right aortic arch with left descending aorta and left ductus arteriosus

Right aortic arch with mirror image branching and left ductus arteriosus

very rare instances, even a patent ductus arteriosus when tortuous and large may lead to airway compression and obstruction. This chapter focuses on the three most common causes of tracheal and esophageal compression.

Incidence

Vascular ring is a rare congenital heart defect constituting less than 1% of all congenital heart diseases. Double aortic arch and right aortic arch with aberrant left subclavian artery with left-sided ductus arteriosus (or ligamentum) constitute 95% of all such vascular rings. The term ligamentum refers to the fibrous band resulting from a closed ductus arteriosus. All other vascular ring anomalies are extremely rare. Abnormality of the aortic arch is typically an isolated lesion, right aortic arch with aberrant left subclavian artery with left-sided ductus arteriosus tends to be an isolated lesion, however, may be found in association with tetralogy of Fallot. Right aortic arch with mirror image branching and left-sided ductus arteriosus (or ligamentum) does not constitute a vascular ring since it does not encircle the esophagus and trachea and occurs almost exclusively in association with other congenital heart diseases (typically tetralogy of Fallot).

Pathology

Vascular rings encircle the esophagus and trachea through a series of abnormally situated vascular structures. This causes stricture of the esophagus and trachea leading to upper gastrointestinal and/or upper respiratory symptoms and signs.

Double aortic arch: This anomaly is easy to understand as the aortic arch maintains its double aortic arch formation from early embryological developmental phases. The ascending aorta bifurcates into two arches which course from the anterior ascending aorta toward the posterior descending aorta on either side of the midline structures of trachea and esophagus, thus encircling them (Fig. 25.1). Each aortic arch gives rise to the carotid and subclavian arteries for that side.

Right aortic arch with aberrant left subclavian artery with left-sided ductus arteriosus : In this association of vascular anomalies, the course of the aortic arch from the anterior and somewhat midline ascending aorta to the right and not to the left. The first branch of the aortic arch should be the left subclavian artery, then

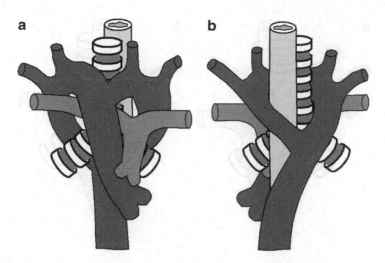

Fig. 25.1 (a) Anterior view and (b) posterior view. Double aortic arch: The ascending aorta bifurcates into two arches which course from the anterior ascending aorta toward the posterior descending aorta on either side of the midline structures of trachea and esophagus, thus encircling them

the left carotid artery before the arch heads rightward, however, in this anomaly; the left subclavian artery does not emerge from where it is expected as the first branch but much later from the distal part of the distal aortic arch. Therefore, the first branch is the left carotid artery, followed by the right carotid artery and then the right subclavian artery. The left subclavian artery emerges from the Diverticulum of Kommerell, a slightly larger blood vessel which emerges from the distal right-sided aortic arch, the Diverticulum of Kommerell courses to the left, crossing the midline behind the esophagus and then giving rise to the left subclavian artery and the ductus arteriosus. The ductus arteriosus continues leftward till it joins the base of the left pulmonary artery (Fig. 25.2). The encircling vascular vessels around the esophagus and trachea are composed of the following:

- Anteriorly by the ascending aorta.
- Rightward by the right-sided aortic arch.
- Posteriorly by the Diverticulum of Kommerell.
- Leftward by the left-sided ductus arteriosus as it travels from the Diverticulum of Kommerell to the base of left pulmonary artery. The latter is anchored to the heart anteriorly through the main pulmonary artery, thus completing the vascular ring.

Vascular sling: This anomaly is technically not a ring since it does not encircle the trachea and esophagus. Instead, the left pulmonary artery which normally emerges from the main pulmonary artery arises from the proximal right pulmonary artery, just right of the tracheobronchial bifurcation. The left pulmonary artery courses leftward behind the distal trachea and in front of the esophagus to reach the left lung hilum (Fig. 25.3). This course compresses the right main bronchus and/or distal trachea.

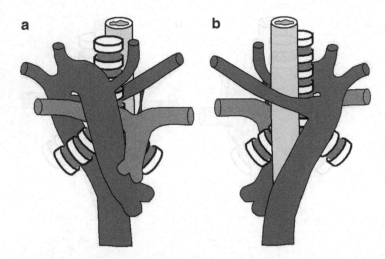

Fig. 25.2 (a) Anterior view and (b) posterior view. Right aortic arch with aberrant left subclavian artery with left-sided ductus arteriosus. The esophagus and trachea are encircled by the ascending aorta, aortic arch, diverticulum of Kommerell, and the ductus arteriosus

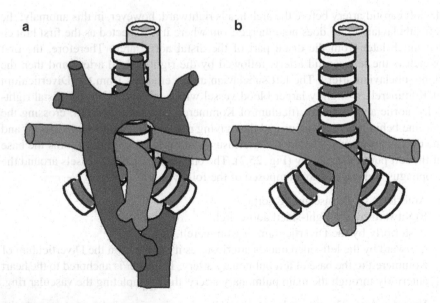

Fig. 25.3 (a) Aortic arch included and (b) aortic arch removed. Vascular sling: The left pulmonary artery emerges in an anomalous fashion from the right pulmonary artery then courses leftward behind the distal trachea and in front of the esophagus to reach the left lung hilum

Pathophysiology

The exact anatomical features of vascular rings are typically difficult to imagine as it involves understanding of the spacial anatomy of great vessels and their branches as they encircle the esophagus and trachea. On the other hand, the pathophysiological changes they cause are more straightforward. Vessels arranged in an abnormal fashion, completing a circle around the trachea and esophagus eventually cause constriction of these tubular structures (esophagus and trachea) leading to difficulty in air flow through the trachea leading to stridor. Pathological constriction of the trachea eventually interferes with normal processes of breathing and clearing secretions from the lower respiratory tract leading to superimposed infections. Constriction of esophagus occurs in most cases; however, symptoms of feeding difficulties tend to be less prominent than respiratory symptoms.

Clinical Manifestations

The dominant symptoms relate to tracheal constriction. Stridor, dyspnea, barking cough, and repeated chest infections are typical. Children are frequently misdiagnosed with reactive airway disease. Respiratory symptoms worsen with feeding and apnea lasting for few seconds may be noted. Patients with double aortic arch present early in infancy as the constriction caused by the double aortic arch is worse. Children with right aortic arch with aberrant left subclavian artery may present later in childhood.

Dysphagia is a complaint of older children since it cannot be verbalized by infants; however, worsening respiratory symptoms is more prominent in infants.

On examination, stridor, wheezing, and upper airway noises are prominent. Children may assume a back arching, neck extending position to keep trachea patent. Intermittent cyanosis may be present.

Chest Radiography

The chest X-ray may give a hint to vascular abnormality through observing a right aortic arch. The cardiac silhouette shape and size is otherwise normal. Pulmonary infection when present may also be noted. Barium swallow (Fig. 25.4) may show compression of the esophagus suggestive of abnormal formation of great arteries.

Fig. 25.4 Barium swallow: indentation of the esophagus indicates compression of the esophagus as a result of an abnormal vascular structure compressing the esophagus as well as the trachea. The findings in this image are highly suggestive, though not diagnostic of vascular ring. Further imaging, such as CT scan, with contrast or MRI provide details of abnormal vascular structures to confirm diagnosis

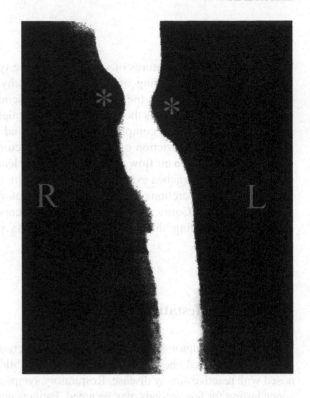

Table 25.2 Findings of Barium swallow

Double aortic arch
Esophagus show indentations on the right and left sides of the esophagus, the right indentation tends to be slightly higher
Right aortic arch with aberrant left subclavian artery and left-sided ductus arteriosus
The esophagus is indented posteriorly and the indentation has an inclination which ascends from right to left
Pulmonary sling
The esophagus is indented anteriorly at the level of tracheal bifurcation

The specific appearance of esophageal compression may hint to the specific type of vascular ring (Table 25.2).

Electrocardiography

This is normal in children with vascular ring as abnormal vascular arrangement does not impact the cardiovascular hemodynamics.

Echocardiography

Echocardiography is a valuable tool in assessing vascular anomalies, however, it may be challenging and requires advanced expertise to perform and interpret. It is not unusual in many such cases that a poorly performed echocardiography misinterpreted as normal causes delay of diagnosis. Therefore, if clinical presentation is suggestive of vascular ring, repeat echocardiography at a center equipped to perform advanced echocardiography is indicated and if findings are not clear MRI or CT scan with angiography should be performed.

The first clue to a vascular ring is the presence of a right aortic arch. In double aortic arch, the echocardiographer first notices that there is a right aortic arch with only two brachiocephalic branches, closer examination shows another aortic arch, to the left and again with only two brachiocephalic branches. The right aortic arch tends to be larger than the left aortic arch. A challenge to diagnosing double aortic arch is when the left aortic arch is atretic since it is not visible by echocardiography without blood coursing through it.

Right aortic arch with aberrant left subclavian artery and left-sided ductus arteriosus is suspected when the aortic arch is noted to be rightward with the first branch being the left carotid artery (rather than the left subclavian artery). Examination of the distal arch shows a branch which starts of as being somewhat large, coursing from right to left, then becoming smaller in caliber to give the left subclavian artery. The larger first portion of this artery reflects the fact that it starts as the diverticulum of Kommerell which gives off the ductus arteriosus, then the subclavian artery.

MRI and CT Scan with Angiography

These test modalities show the vascular anatomy and their relationship to the trachea and esophagus. The capability of producing 3D images of the vascular anatomy, upper airway, and esophagus is truly spectacular in providing accurate diagnosis. MRI is less invasive than CT scan as it does not expose the child to radiation and should be performed whenever possible.

Management

Management of these anomalies is surgical to relief compression of the upper airway structures. Double aortic arch is relieved through ligation and resection of one of the aortic arches, typically the left as it tends to be smaller. The ductus arteriosus or ligamentum must be resected in cases of right aortic arch with aberrant left subclavian artery. In the rare cases of pulmonary sling, the left pulmonary artery is resected at its base and reimplanted from the distal main pulmonary artery, thus relieving the pressure over the right main bronchus and distal trachea.

Clinical Scenarios

Case 1

A 3-month-old girl, product of full term gestation presents to a pediatrician's office because of respiratory distress and bouts of cyanosis noted during feeding. The mother believes that the child has always had these respiratory symptoms, exacerbated by agitation and feeding with worsening of symptoms over the past 2 weeks.

On examination, the child has audible stridor and upper airway noises. Visible intercostal and subcostal retractions are noted. Heart rate is 110 bpm, regular. Respiratory rate is 60/min. Oxygen saturation is 95% with dip into the high 80s when agitated. Physical examination is unremarkable other than the evidence of moderate respiratory distress.

Respiratory distress in this infant could be caused by several etiologies, including:

- Gastroesophageal (GE) reflux and aspiration
- Reactive airway disease
- Tracheoesophageal fistula
- Infectious bronchopulmonary diseases, viral, or bacterial
- Vascular ring

Physical examination is not significantly helpful in any of these diseases. Chest X-ray is helpful first step in this child's management. This showed normal cardiac silhouette, no evidence of bronchopulmonary pathology and a suggestion of a right aortic arch.

GE reflux and infection pulmonary disease as well as tracheoesophageal fistula should all have evidence of parenchymal disease, not noted in this child. The right aortic arch is suggestive of a vascular ring due to double aortic arch or right aortic arch with aberrant left subclavian artery.

Barium swallow showed indentation of the esophagus on either side. This is typical of double aortic arch. Echocardiography confirmed the diagnosis of double aortic arch, the right aortic arch was dominant, therefore surgery was performed though a left thoracotomy and the left aortic arch was ligated and resected. The child's symptoms improved significantly postoperatively and complete resolution of symptoms was noted in a follow-up visit 3 months later.

Case 2

A 10-month-old boy presented to the emergency room due to exacerbation of respiratory distress. The child is suspected to have reactive airway disease and was admitted three times over the past 4 months for increasing respiratory distress associated with wheezing.

On examination, the child appeared to be in moderate respiratory distress, he sat down on mother's lap with slightly extended neck with no cyanosis. Heart rate was 100 bpm, regular. Respiratory rate was 50/min. Oxygen saturation was 95%. Blood pressure in right upper extremity was 90/55 mmHg. Upper airway noises, stridor, and wheezing were noticeable. Cardiac auscultation was within normal limits, no significant Hepatomegaly was detected.

Chest X-ray was not significant for any pulmonary disease, cardiac silhouette was normal in size and there was evidence of right aortic arch.

In view of stridor, repeated previous hospitalization and atypical features for reactive airway disease bronchoscopy was performed which showed a pulsatile mass constricting the posterior and left aspects of the tracheal lumen. Vascular ring was suspected.

Echocardiography was not informative because of poor echo window and lack of child's cooperation; however, right aortic arch was confirmed. MRI with 3D reconstruction confirmed the diagnosis of right aortic arch with aberrant left subclavian artery and left-sided ligamentum connecting the diverticulum of Kommerell to the base of the left pulmonary artery.

Surgery was performed through a lateral thoracotomy and the ligamentum was resected causing relief of tracheal compression. The child's symptoms improved, however, did not completely resolve except after 4–6 months. Delayed resolution is to be expected in view of anatomical changes of the trachea due to prolonged compression.

Chapter 26
Congenital Abnormalities of Coronary Arteries

Russell Robert Cross and Daniel E. Felten

Key Facts

- Congenital coronary artery anomalies are due to abnormal origin. Two types of abnormal origin are recognized:

  - Abnormal origin from pulmonary artery instead of the aorta (ALCAPA) results in myocardial ischemia and dilated cardiomyopathy like clinical presentation in early infancy.
  - Abnormal origin of coronary artery from wrong coronary sinus within the aortic root, particularly the left coronary artery from right coronary sinus may result in acute compromise of coronary blood perfusion associated with exercise which may present as sudden death.

- All infants presenting with dilated cardiomyopathy must be investigated for ALCAPA. Although echocardiography is helpful in making this diagnosis, cardiac catheterization and angiography may be needed to ensure normal origin of coronary arteries.
- Electrocardiography may be diagnostic in abnormal origin of left coronary artery from pulmonary artery. Wide Q-waves may be noted in the left and lateral precordial leads (I, aVL, V4, V5, and V6).
- A somewhat similar electrocardiography may be seen in normal children when wrong technique is used in performing electrocardiography. If the right and left limb leads are reversed, Q-waves will be noted in leads I and aVL, however, not V4, V5, and V6. In addition, the P waves assume an abnormal axis with wrong lead placement.
- Treatment of abnormal origin of coronary arteries is surgical.

(continued)

R.R. Cross (✉)
Department of Cardiology, Children's National Medical Center, 111 Michigan Avenue, NW Washington, DC 20010, USA
e-mail: rcross@cnme.org

Ra-id Abdulla (ed.), *Heart Diseases in Children: A Pediatrician's Guide*,
DOI 10.1007/978-1-4419-7994-0_26, © Springer Science+Business Media, LLC 2011

Key Facts (continued)

- Abnormal origin of left main coronary artery from the pulmonary artery is corrected by reimplanting anomalous coronary artery into the aorta, or creating a baffle to direct blood flow from the aortic root to the coronary artery originating from the pulmonary artery (Takeuchi procedure).
- Abnormal origin of left coronary artery from right coronary sinus can be surgically corrected by widening the opening (unroofing) of left main coronary artery if it is of the intramural type to prevent collapse of orifice when both aorta and pulmonary arteries are distended during exercise.

Definition

In the normal coronary distribution, a single right coronary artery arises from the right aortic sinus and a separate left main coronary artery arises from the left aortic sinus and then divides into the left anterior descending (LAD) and left circumflex coronary arteries. There are many different coronary artery abnormalities, but they can generally be divided into two main groups that influence timing and type of symptoms at presentation: coronary arteries arising from the pulmonary artery or coronary arteries arising from the wrong aortic sinus. The former group is nearly always symptomatic and presents early in life with symptoms of dilated cardiomyopathy. On the other hand, anomalies in the latter are often asymptomatic, but may present catastrophically as sudden death in teenagers.

Incidence

It is estimated that 2–5% of individuals in the general population have a coronary artery anomaly, but of these, only a fraction are clinically significant. On the other hand, it is variously estimated that 10–20% of sudden death in teenagers and young adults is the result of an anomalous coronary. This makes identification of the rare clinically significant coronary artery anomaly important but challenging.

Pathology

Coronary Arteries Arising from the Wrong Aortic Sinus

Anomalies of coronary arteries involving branching off the wrong main artery, for example, the circumflex branching off right coronary instead of left coronary, have essentially no potential for becoming pathologic and is not discussed further. On the other hand, abnormalities of the origin of the coronary arteries where the artery is originating from the wrong aortic sinus have the potential to become clinically significant. When both coronary arteries arise from a single coronary sinus, there are multiple possible paths the artery may take to get to the correct side of the heart, and the path the artery takes determines whether the anomaly becomes significant. For example, if both left and right coronary arteries arise from the right coronary sinus, the left coronary may pass behind the aorta, in front of the right ventricular outflow tract (RVOT), or within the ventricular septum below the RVOT to supply the left side of the heart. These abnormalities are not considered pathologic unless the anomalous artery takes a path between the two great vessels.

If the coronary artery arises from the wrong aortic sinus and does pass between the aorta and the RVOT, this abnormality can be clinically significant and has been associated with sudden death. The most significant of these is when the left main coronary or LAD coronary artery arises from the right aortic sinus or right coronary artery and then passes between the aorta and RVOT. In reverse, the right coronary artery can arise from the left aortic sinus or left coronary artery and then course between the two great vessels. When a coronary artery arises anomalously from the wrong sinus, the proximal portion of the coronary may course through the wall of the aorta rather than leaving as a separate vessel. These coronaries are termed intramural and have particular surgical implications (Fig. 26.1a–e).

Coronary Arteries Arising from the Pulmonary Artery

By far the most common coronary anomaly involving origin from a vessel other than the aorta is anomalous origin of the left main coronary artery from the pulmonary artery (ALCAPA). In this anomaly, the left main coronary artery arises from the pulmonary artery and then divides into the normal LAD and left circumflex coronary arteries to supply the left heart. Other more rare forms of anomalous origin of branch coronary arteries from the pulmonary artery have been identified, including LAD, left circumflex, and right coronary arteries from the pulmonary artery (Fig. 26.2).

Pathophysiology

The pathophysiology of anomalous coronary artery from the wrong sinus and anomalous coronary from the pulmonary artery are quite different and lead to entirely different presentations.

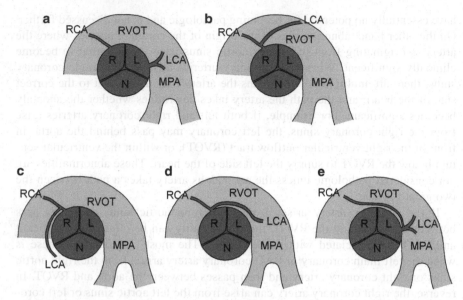

Fig. 26.1 *RVOT* right ventricular outflow tract, *MPA* main pulmonary artery, *L* lofet coronary sinus, *R* right coronary sinus, *N* noncoronary sinus, *LCA* left coronary artery, *RCA* right coronary sinus. Abnormal coronary sinus connection: coronary arteries in normal circumstances originate from their respective coronary sinuses. The right coronary artery emerges from the right coronary sinus and the left main coronary artery originates from the left coronary sinus. Left main coronary artery bifurcates shortly after its take off from the cleft coronary sinus to the left anterior descending (LAD) artery and the circumflex coronary artery. Coronary arteries may originate from the wrong coronary sinus; many different variations of this abnormality are recognized. (**a**) Normal coronary arteries origin. (**b**) Left main coronary artery from right coronary sinus. In this illustration, the left main coronary artery courses leftward anterior to the right ventricular outflow tract. This is clinically insignificant. (**c**) Left main coronary artery from right coronary sinus. In this illustration, the left main coronary artery courses leftward posterior to the aorta. This is clinically insignificant. (**d**) Left main coronary artery from right coronary sinus. In this illustration, the left main coronary artery courses leftward between the aorta and the right ventricular outflow tract. This may cause coronary insufficiency. (**e**) Right coronary artery from left coronary sinus. In this illustration, the right coronary artery courses rightward between the aorta and the right ventricular outflow tract. This may cause coronary insufficiency

In anomalous coronary artery from the wrong sinus, the most clinically significant abnormality occurs when the abnormal course of a major coronary artery passes between the two great vessels. Individuals with this anomaly are at risk for sudden death during exercise. Presumably, the course of the artery between the great vessels causes a portion of the heart to become ischemic during periods of high cardiac output; however, the exact mechanism of ischemia is debated. It has been proposed that the coronary artery may be compressed or stretched by engorged great vessels. Others have theorized that the abnormal origin and course of the coronary artery creates abnormal flow patterns during exercise. Regardless of

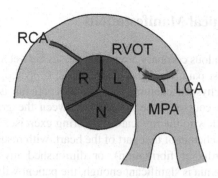

Fig. 26.2 *RVOT* right ventricular outflow tract, *MPA* main pulmonary artery, *L* left coronary sinus, *R* right coronary sinus, *N* noncoronary sinus, *LCA* left coronary artery, *RCA* right coronary sinus. *Arrow* indicates retrograde flow from left coronary artery into main pulmonary artery creating a left to right shunt and coronary steal. Left main coronary artery originates from main pulmonary artery. Low pulmonary arterial pressure causes coronary blood flow to reach the left main coronary artery in a retrograde fashion from the right coronary artery blood supply then escape into the main pulmonary artery casting coronary blood flow "steal"

mechanism, the presumed clinical effect in these cases is that relative ischemia results in ventricular arrhythmias or electromechanical dissociation. Autopsy results in patients with a coronary artery arising from the incorrect sinus do not show significant scar in the heart muscle in the vast majority of cases. These results suggest that the presumed ischemic effect is brought on suddenly. A coronary artery that arises from the wrong sinus but does not pass between the aorta and RVOT does not have a similar ischemic risk.

In the case of anomalous left coronary arising from the pulmonary artery, oxygen supply to the myocardium is compromised due to both delivery of deoxygenated blood and decreased perfusion pressures. During fetal life, the coronary blood supplied from the anomalous pulmonary connection is at high pressure and is appropriately saturated so that myocardial perfusion is normal. At birth, the blood in the pulmonary artery quickly becomes desaturated and pressure drops dramatically. Accordingly, both pressure and oxygenation of the blood in the left coronary artery decreases causing inadequate oxygen delivery to the myocardium. Over time, in an attempt to increase oxygen delivery, the left coronary vessels dilate and collaterals form to the right coronary system, which arises normally from the aorta. However, since the left coronary arises from the low-pressure pulmonary artery and the right coronary from the high-pressure aorta, collateral flow from the right coronary system passes into the left coronary system and then retrogrades through the left main coronary artery to the pulmonary artery. These collaterals effectively bypass the myocardial tissue and create a pulmonary artery steal from the coronary artery with resultant ischemia of the left ventricular myocardium, which leads to progressive left ventricular dysfunction and dilation in most cases.

Presentation/Clinical Manifestations

Patients with an anomalous coronary artery that passes between the two great vessels may present with chest pain, dizziness, palpitations, or syncope during or immediately after exercise. Physical examination in these patients is usually normal. As mentioned above, the course of the coronary between the great vessels results in diminished coronary flow to the myocardium during exercise. This diminished flow can result in relative ischemia of that part of the heart, with resultant pain, ventricular arrhythmias (tachycardia or fibrillation), or diminished myocardial contractility. Ultimately, if the ischemia is significant enough, the patient will experience a sudden and dramatic drop in cardiac output. In some cases, the first presentation of these symptoms is sudden death. However, the majority of patients experience symptoms during exercise that lead them to seek medical attention. It should also be noted that many of the victims of sudden death have been athletes, so it is important that all individuals being evaluated for participation in sports be asked about the history of chest pain, dizziness, palpitations, syncope, or other symptoms associated with exercise. Those individuals who have a positive history should undergo further evaluation for potential anomalous coronary artery. It is interesting to note that there are patients who present with anomalous coronary between the great vessels as an incidental finding, apparently having had no previous symptoms. It is unclear why individuals with the same anatomic abnormalities can have such disparate outcomes.

The presentation of anomalous left coronary artery arising from the pulmonary artery is quite different. Symptoms typically develop within the first 2–3 months of age, corresponding with the normal fall in pulmonary vascular resistance and resultant reversal of flow from the left coronary into the pulmonary artery. About this time, some infants with ALCAPA are noted to have sudden episodes of crying and irritation associated with feeding. They may also be noted to have transient respiratory distress, appear pale and sweaty, and may appear syncopal. It is thought that these symptoms are related to myocardial ischemia and associated angina. Other patients with ALCAPA present with signs and symptoms of congestive heart failure as a result of dilated cardiomyopathy. Signs and symptoms include the failure to thrive, tachypnea, lethargy, tachycardia, and diaphoresis. On examination, these patients may have poor perfusion, a murmur of mitral insufficiency, a gallop rhythm, or hepatomegaly. The majority of infants with ALCAPA present with significant heart failure requiring intervention, or present with sudden death. A small number of individuals improve with time and escape diagnosis as an infant. They may have transient shortness of breath and chest pain with exercise and continue to be at risk for sudden death.

Chest Radiography

Plain film X-rays are not useful in the diagnosis of an anomalous coronary artery arising from the wrong aortic sinus. Patients with anomalous origin of the left coronary artery from the pulmonary artery have X-ray findings consistent with dilated cardiomyopathy, namely, cardiomegaly with left atrial and ventricular enlargement, and associated pulmonary edema. Hepatomegaly may also be appreciated on routine chest X-ray.

Electrocardiography

The resting ECG in patients with anomalous coronary artery passing between the great vessels is most likely normal, but it may demonstrate evidence of prior infarction with Q-waves corresponding to the affected coronary distribution. Evidence of chamber enlargement and arrhythmias may also be noted. On the other hand, patients with ALCAPA typically present with evidence of left ventricular hypertrophy with strain and abnormal R-wave progression. Wide Q-waves in the left and lateral precordial leads (I, aVL, V4, V5, and V6) are evidence for infarction of the left ventricular myocardium that is frequently seen in ALCAPA.

Echocardiography

Echocardiography is the mainstay for the diagnosis of anomalous coronary arteries. An echocardiogram is recommended for all patients who present with syncope or chest pain associated with exercise to evaluate for the possibility of anomalous coronary arteries, as well as other cardiac abnormalities. Attention should be paid to identify the proximal coronary origins and to evaluate for the potential of a coronary artery passing between the aorta and RVOT. It is important that Doppler color flow interrogation of the coronary arteries also be performed. Color flow can help to demonstrate the origins of the coronary arteries from the aortic sinuses and can also help to show a coronary artery passing between the two great vessels. In the case of an ALCAPA, color flow demonstrates reversal of the direction of coronary blood flow as a result of the coronary steal from the left coronary to the pulmonary artery. The coronary flow can also be identified by Doppler color flow in the pulmonary artery as an abnormal diastolic flow signal at the point where the anomalous coronary artery enters. Echocardiography can also demonstrate other important findings in patients with anomalous coronary arteries, including ventricular size and function, the presence of atrioventricular valve insufficiency, and the presence of other congenital heart disease. In older patients or patients with poor echocardiographic windows, transesophageal echocardiography or cardiac MRI or CT may also be used to evaluate the coronary artery anatomy and cardiac function.

Cardiac Catheterization

Cardiac catheterization is typically only used in the diagnosis of anomalous coronary artery when other imaging modalities are inconclusive. Coronary angiography may help in demonstrating the anomalous origin of a coronary artery, but proving an intramural course of a coronary artery can be difficult. Hemodynamic evaluation performed at cardiac catheterization can be useful in the management of certain patients with anomalous coronary arteries to evaluate cardiac output, filling pressures, and measurement of shunts, but in most cases these measurement are not necessary.

Treatment/Management

The treatment of an anomalous coronary passing between the great vessels or of anomalous origin of the left coronary from the pulmonary artery is predominately surgical. In the case of an anomalous coronary passing between the great vessels, surgical reimplantation of the abnormal coronary into the correct sinus can sometimes be performed if the anomalous coronary artery arises as a separate origin from the abnormal sinus. In cases where a portion of the anomalous coronary courses in the wall of the aorta, the coronary may be "unroofed" such that the intramural portion of the coronary is opened to the lumen of the aorta so as to widen the origin and minimize tension or compression effects that may result from the coronary passing between the two great vessels.

In the case of anomalous left coronary from the pulmonary artery, several surgical approaches have been used historically. If adequate collaterals have formed, one straightforward approach is to ligate the anomalous origin from the pulmonary artery to eliminate the pulmonary–coronary steal. This procedure has also been performed in association with a bypass graft to augment coronary flow if collaterals were not sufficient. Currently, however, the most accepted approach is direct excision and reimplantation of the anomalous coronary from the pulmonary artery into the aorta. In some cases, reimplantation cannot be performed without kinking the coronary. In these cases, an aortopulmonary window can be created and a baffle placed in the pulmonary artery to tunnel coronary flow from the aorta (Takeuchi procedure). It is generally accepted that surgical intervention should be undertaken in these patients at the time of presentation. Patients with significant cardiac dysfunction or heart failure may require acute medical management of these symptoms before proceeding to surgery.

Long-Term Follow-Up and Prognosis

It remains unclear as to what extent surgical intervention in cases of anomalous coronary passing between the great vessels minimizes the risk of sudden death. It is widely felt, though, that surgical intervention should be undertaken in any patient with the finding of an anomalous left coronary between the great vessels. The finding of an anomalous right coronary passing between the great vessels is more controversial, but surgical intervention is frequently undertaken, particularly in patients who are symptomatic in any way. Patients with a coronary arising from the pulmonary artery generally have significant improvement in their ventricular function following coronary reimplantation, with some eventually returning to normal myocardial function. However, patients with significant myocardial injury at presentation often continue to have cardiac dysfunction and remain at increased risk for cardiac issues, including sudden death. Following surgical intervention for anomalous coronary arteries, some may benefit from medical therapy to improve cardiac function, such as diuretics and afterload-reducing agents.

Patients undergoing surgical intervention should have long-term follow-up to evaluate cardiac function and rhythm, and potential myocardial perfusion abnormalities. They typically undergo stress testing when old enough, and may have coronary angiography performed in the first decade to evaluate for coronary stenosis. Patients who experience myocardial infarction are at increased risk for lethal arrhythmias and may be candidates for automatic implanted cardiac defibrillators.

Case Scenarios

Case 1

History. A 16-year-old male collapses suddenly while playing soccer at school. The coach and the team trainer immediately evaluate the teenager and find him to be unresponsive and with short gasping breaths. No pulse can be found, so CPR is started and paramedics are called. On arrival to the field, paramedics find that the young man is in ventricular fibrillation. He is successfully defibrillated and following resumption of normal sinus rhythm, the patient is intubated and is then transported to the local emergency room. On arrival to the ER, the patient is still unconscious and a quick echocardiogram shows that there is poor cardiac function; the decision is made to place him on extracorporeal support. When the young man's father arrives at the hospital, he tells the doctors that his son has commented on a couple of episodes of chest pain and dizziness while playing soccer in the past, but that the symptoms had always gone away after he stopped playing. He had never been evaluated for these symptoms. Upon questioning, the father denies any family history of congenital heart disease, arrhythmia, syncope, or sudden death.

Physical examination. Intubated, on mechanical ventilation as well as inotropic and extracorporeal support, but is well perfused. Lungs are clear with saturation 98%. Heart rate is 102 bpm and precordial activity is somewhat hyperactive. On auscultation, a 3/6 systolic regurgitant murmur is heard at the apex and a gallop rhythm is present. Central pulses are 1+ in both upper and lower extremities.

Investigative studies. Chest X-ray shows a normal cardiac silhouette and clear lung fields. His ECG demonstrates normal sinus rhythm with Q-waves in leads I, aVL, V4, and V5. There are also inverted T-waves in the left precordial leads, but ventricular voltages are normal. CBC, BMP, and toxicology screen were all within normal limits.

Differential diagnosis. Sudden collapse in an otherwise healthy teenager is most likely due to a primary cardiac arrest. Some causes include hypertrophic cardio-myopathy, anomalous coronary artery (likely arising from the wrong sinus and passing between the great vessels), valvular abnormality, dilated cardiomyopathy, or arrhythmia due to conduction abnormality or potentially electrolyte abnormality or substance use. If there were history of trauma immediately preceding the arrest, commotio cordis would also be considered.

Assessment. The finding on history that the patient had episodes of chest pain and dizziness suggests some sort of an ischemic process, which makes an anomalous coro-nary artery more likely in this case. The normal chest X-ray and ECG showing acute changes further supports the diagnosis of anomalous coronary artery. A normal X-ray makes dilated cardiomyopathy unlikely, and since there is no hypertrophy noted in ECG, hypertrophic cardiomyopathy is also unlikely. Basic labs would rule out an electrolyte abnormality, and the negative toxicology screen is helpful to rule out drugs of abuse (e.g., cocaine or amphetamines). However, if there were serious concern for substance abuse, specific test would have to be done. Regardless, an echocardiogram is indicated to assess the coronaries and to evaluate for any other congenital defect.

Detailed echocardiogram demonstrates a mildly dilated left ventricle that has moderately decreased function, most notably in the anterior left ventricular free wall and anterior ventricular septum. There is no congenital heart disease, but mod-erate mitral valve insufficiency is present. Examination of the coronary arteries reveals an anomalous LAD coronary artery originating from the right aortic sinus and coursing between the aorta and RVOT. The proximal portion of the LAD coro-nary is demonstrated to be in the wall of the aorta using Doppler color flow.

Diagnosis and management. This young man has anomalous origin of the LAD coronary artery from the right aortic sinus with a proximal intramural course. He has suffered a myocardial infarction of the left ventricular wall and anterior septum. Once he is stabilized on extracorporeal support, he is taken to the operating room and undergoes an unroofing procedure of the intramural portion of the proximal LAD coronary artery. Following the operation, he is able to be weaned from extra-corporeal support, but remains with diminished left ventricular function and mitral insufficiency for which he is treated with diuretics and afterload-reducing agents. After recuperation, the patient will be followed closely for the evaluation of his cardiac function and rhythm status.

Case 2

History. A 10-week-old female infant is seen in the emergency room because of poor feeding and lethargy. Upon questioning, her mother reports several episodes of uncontrollable crying during feeds. She also notes that her baby looks somewhat gray and sweaty during these episodes. She has had a previous child who had significant reflux, but does not think that this is the same thing. The baby was born full term with no perinatal complications and had been well until about 1 week ago.

Her mother had several routine obstetric ultrasounds during the pregnancy and she was always reassured that her baby was "normal."

Examination. The baby is ill appearing and somewhat thin. She is moderately tachypneic and has a dusky appearance. Her respiratory rate is 70 per minute, HR 160 bpm, pulse ox 96% on room air, and blood pressure is 70/45 in the right arm and 75/45 in the right leg. Auscultation of her lungs reveals fine crackles throughout. She has an active precordium with an obvious heave. Cardiac evaluation shows a regular rate and rhythm with a normal S1 and prominent but normally split S2.A 3/6 systolic regurgitant murmur is heard at the apex, and a gallop rhythm is present. Her liver edge is palpable at her umbilicus and she has 1+ to 2+ pulses in all extremities. While she is responsive, she appears very tired.

Initial studies. Chest X-ray demonstrates a severely enlarged cardiac silhouette and increased interstitial markings. An ECG shows sinus tachycardia with significant left ventricular hypertrophy demonstrated by large R-waves in V5 and V6. There are also flipped T-waves in leads V4–V6 indicating left ventricular strain.

Differential diagnosis. This patient presents with signs and symptoms of congestive heart failure at 7 weeks. The most likely structural lesions to present at 7 weeks include those with left to right shunting via a large VSD, either alone or in combination with other anomalies that do not cause cyanosis, aortic or mitral valve regurgitation, ALCAPA, aortic stenosis, or coarctation. Additionally, this patient could have a dilated cardiomyopathy due to a number of etiologies, such as viral myocarditis or metabolic abnormality.

Assessment. Because her blood pressure is equal in both arms, coarctation is unlikely, and without a diastolic murmur, aortic regurgitation is also unlikely. However, it is difficult to narrow the differential diagnosis much further based on the initial studies. Therefore, an echocardiogram must be done to evaluate this patient's heart failure.

The echocardiogram demonstrates a severely dilated and poorly functioning left ventricle, but no congenital heart disease. There is also severe mitral valve insufficiency and moderate left atrial enlargement. Examination of the coronary arteries reveals that the left coronary artery is originating from the proximal main pulmonary artery. Doppler color flow interrogation of the left coronary demonstrates reversal of flow toward the pulmonary artery as well as a diastolic flow jet into the MPA where the coronary originates.

Diagnosis and management. As in most cases, echocardiography is sufficient to make the diagnosis of anomalous left coronary artery from the pulmonary artery in this child. Immediate management would include intensive care observation with the initiation of diuretics and inotropes to treat heart failure. She would be scheduled for surgery on an urgent basis to undergo reimplantation of the left coronary artery into the aortic root. Following surgery, she would continue to be treated with diuretic and inotropic therapy pending improvement in her cardiac function. Improvement, if it occurs, would be expected in the first few weeks following repair.

Part III
Acquired Heart Diseases in Children

Chapter 27
Rheumatic Fever and Rheumatic Heart Disease

Sawsan Mokhtar M. Awad and Daniel E. Felten

Key Facts

- Rheumatic Heart disease is the second most common cause, after Kawasaki disease, of acquired heart diseases in children.
- Rheumatic fever is precipitated by GAS pharyngitis and not other types of GAS infections.
- Pharyngitis with GAS causes T-cell and B-cell lymphocytes to produce antibodies presumably against some antigenic component of the bacteria that cross-react with an antigen on myocytes or cardiac valve tissue.
- Diagnosis is made when there is history of GAS pharyngitis and presence of Jones criteria. Two major criteria, or one major criterion and two minor criteria are required to make the diagnosis.
- Major criteria of Jones are: carditis, polyarthritis, chorea, erythema marginatum, and subcutaneous nodules.
- Minor criteria of Jones are: fever, polyarthralgia, elevated ESR, ECG findings (prolonged PR interval), elevated ASO titer, positive throat culture of group A beta hemolytic streptococci, positive rapid antigen test for group A streptococci and recent scarlet fever.
- Treatment includes eradication of any residual GAS bacteria and the use of anti-inflammatory agents (aspirin with or without steroids). Long-term prophylaxis with antibiotics is done to prevent recurrence.

Definition

Rheumatic fever is an acute inflammatory illness that occurs after Group A Streptococcal (GAS) pharyngitis. While rheumatic heart disease is the development of inflammatory changes to cardiac valves and myocardium leading to pathological

---

D.E. Felten (✉)
Department of Pediatrics, Rush University Medical Center, 1645 W. Jackson,
Suite 200, Chicago, IL 60612, USA
e-mail: Daniel_felten@rush.edu

Ra-id Abdulla (ed.), *Heart Diseases in Children: A Pediatrician's Guide*,
DOI 10.1007/978-1-4419-7994-0_27, © Springer Science+Business Media, LLC 2011

changes of the cardiac valves, especially the mitral and aortic valves leading initially to regurgitation and potentially in the subsequent months or years to stenosis of affected valves.

Incidence

The overall incidence of rheumatic fever and rheumatic heart disease is estimated to be 150 in 100,000 of the population in developing countries and less than 1 in 100,000 of the population in developed countries. Rheumatic fever was the most common cause of acquired heart disease in the USA; however, incidence sharply declined following the advent of penicillin. It has since been replaced by complications of Kawasaki disease as the most common acquired heart disease in children.

Pathology

Rheumatic fever is an acute inflammatory illness that occurs 2–4 weeks after Group A Streptococcal (GAS) pharyngitis. It is thought that immune globulins produced against certain streptococcal antigens cross-react with antigens on cells in individuals with genetic predisposition to rheumatic fever. These immune globulins cause damage to tissues throughout the body, including heart, joints, brain, and skin. Other GAS infections, such as cellulitis or pneumonia, do not stimulate formation of these cross-reactive antibodies; therefore, rheumatic fever is precipitated by GAS pharyngitis and not other types of GAS infections.

Pathophysiology

The exact pathophysiology is unknown, but it is clear that Group A, beta-hemolytic streptococcal infections of the pharynx stimulate T-cell and B-cell lymphocytes to produce antibodies presumably against some antigenic component of the bacteria that cross-react with an antigen on myocytes or cardiac valve tissue. There is a latent period of 2–4 weeks between the acute illness (sore throat and fever) and the development of carditis and cardiac valve damage. The mitral valve is most commonly affected, followed by the aortic valve, and damage caused by the cross-reactive antibodies leads to valvular insufficiency and later stenosis. In addition to injury that occurs during the acute episode of rheumatic fever, future episodes of GAS pharyngitis stimulate the production of antibodies directed against myocytes from memory B-cells, which leads to progressive cardiac valve damage.

Clinical Manifestations

The Jones Criteria have been revised numerous times and are designed to be guidelines for diagnosis. To establish diagnosis, there must be evidence of a GAS infection and either two major criteria or one major and two minor criteria. Major criteria in order of occurrence are:

- Arthritis: Migratory polyarthritis involving large joints, such as the knees, ankles, and elbows. Joints become swollen, red, warm, and painful without permanent damage.
- Carditis: Tachycardia and apical systolic murmur of mitral regurgitation are the most common presenting features of rheumatic carditis. The mitral regurgitation murmur is a holosystolic murmur best heard at the apex with short mid-diastolic apical murmur secondary to increased flow across the mitral valve (functional mitral stenosis). Congestive heart failure may develop in a small number of patients presenting with rheumatic carditis. The presentation is similar to congestive heart failure of any other cause with dyspnea, hepatomegaly, congested neck veins, ascites, and chest pain if pericarditis develops.
- Chorea: Sydenham's chorea is characterized by purposeless choreiform movements that are aggravated by stress and disappear during sleep. The chorea is less common in adolescents and not seen in adults with rheumatic fever and almost never present simultaneously with arthritis. The presence of Sydenham's chorea is sufficient to make the diagnosis of rheumatic fever even if it is the only manifestation noted.
- Erythema marginatum: Irregular, geometric, circinate, marginate, nonitchy red rash over the torso that is evanescent.
- Subcutaneous nodules: Firm nodules over the extensor surfaces and the hard bony areas of upper and lower extremities and the back. These nodules develop at sites of trauma to the bony surfaces in patients who have active disease.

Minor manifestations include fever, arthralgia, long PR interval, and elevated acute phase reactant.

Chest Radiography

Chest radiography findings vary according to the clinical presentation. Cardiomegaly and increased broncho-vascular markings reflecting pulmonary venous congestion may be noted.

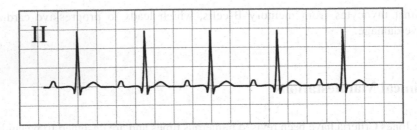

Fig. 27.1 PR interval measured from the beginning of the P wave deflection to the beginning of the QRS complex deflection. Normal PR interval varies with age; normal PR duration in a young child is up to 0.15 s (or just below 4 *small squares*). PR interval in adults is up to 0.2 s (or 5 *small squares*). The PR interval in the example shown here is 0.28 s

Electrocardiography

Nonspecific changes may be present. The most common finding in patients with rheumatic fever is prolonged PR interval (Fig. 27.1), made shorter by atropine. Occasionally, intermittent 2:1 atrioventricular block or rarely complete heart block may be seen. Nonspecific T wave changes may be present.

Echocardiography

Transthoracic echocardiography is a valuable tool for assessing the degree of valve regurgitation and for follow-up of rheumatic valvular lesions. It is of great value in diagnosis and grading of pericardial effusion, and if needed, pericardiocentesis may be performed at the bedside under echocardiography guidance.

The mitral valve is most commonly involved. Valve leaflets may appear thickened by 2D echocardiography. Color Doppler is used to assess the extent of mitral regurgitation, which is initially the result of mitral valve leaflet disease. However, in moderate to severe mitral regurgitation, the left ventricle and atrium dilate over time resulting in mitral valve annulus dilation and worsening mitral regurgitation. Mitral stenosis is a late manifestation of rheumatic fever and not seen during the acute phase of illness. The aortic valve may be involved, and echocardiography would demonstrate thickening of aortic valve cusps with regurgitation. Unlike the mitral valve, aortic valve stenosis is not noted as a complication of rheumatic fever. The pulmonary and tricuspid valves may be involved, but this is not common.

Cardiac Catheterization

Cardiac catheterization is seldom needed in the diagnosis of cases of rheumatic heart disease.

Treatment

Treatment plan should include:

Eradication of the Current Infection: best achieved by Penicillin treatment. IM injection of benzathine penicillin 600,000–900,000 U for children and 1,200,000 U for adults may be used.

Anti-inflammation: best achieved by salicylates. Steroids are reserved for severe cases particularly associated with carditis. Aspirin 100 mg/kg/day divided Q4 hours for 1 week, then reduce to 75 mg/kg/day for 4 weeks, then taper over 2 weeks. In significant carditis (significant valve pathology, congestive heart failure), use steroids (prednisone 2 mg/kg/day) instead of aspirin for 2 weeks, then taper steroids over 2 weeks. Start aspirin after 2 weeks of steroids at 75 mg/kg/day.

Treatment of Congestive Heart Failure: most cases of mild heart failure respond well to steroid therapy and bed rest. If the patient has moderate to severe congestive heart failure, digoxin Lasix and afterload reducing agents may be needed for treatment.

Treatment of Sydenham Chorea: long-term antimicrobial prophylaxis and haloperidol treatment.

Prophylaxis: to prevent further streptococcal infection. Intramuscular injection of 1.2 million units of benzathine benzylpenicillin every 3–4 weeks is the highly recommended method of prophylaxis. Erythromycin 250 mg PO BID can be used for patients who are allergic to penicillin would be better.
Length of prophylaxis may be one of the following:

- Ten years after the last episode of rheumatic fever or to adulthood, whichever is longer.
- Indefinitely in those patients with established heart disease and those with frequent exposure to streptococcal infection.

Case Scenarios

Case 1

History: A 16-year-old female presented to her primary care physician with history of sore throat for the past few days. Fever, malaise, and joints pain were also noted. The patient initially described diffuse joint pain, but after careful questioning, she states that there was severe bilateral knee pain and she was unable to stand. Pain was prominent toward the end of the day. She denied any joint swelling, or redness or rash.

Physical Examination: The patient's throat was red with enlarged tonsils. There was no rash or noticeable swelling of the knee joints. There were no other joint swellings or redness. Cardiac examination revealed normal S1, S2 split and varied with respiration. A grade 2/6 systolic murmur at the left upper sternal border was detected by auscultation with no radiation. The murmur decreased with standing and increased in intensity with lying down.

Investigative Studies: Throat swab for rapid strep was performed; this was negative, however, throat swab for culture was sent and results were positive for GAS infection.

Management: Rheumatic fever was suspected; therefore, penicillin was prescribed to eradicate acute infection and was advised to start long-term prophylaxis for rheumatic fever. A cardiology consult was obtained for further evaluation.

Evaluation by the pediatric cardiologist revealed similar findings through history and physical examination. Electrocardiography was within normal limits. Echocardiography revealed normal cardiac structure and function with no evidence of mitral or aortic valve disease.

Discussion: History and physical examination in this patient do not support rheumatic fever. Although GAS pharyngitis was established in this patient, there is lack of any of the major criteria of Jones. Joint pain alone without evidence of inflammation, such as swelling, redness, tenderness, etc., is a minor, rather than a major criterion. The heart murmur noted in this patient is consistent with an innocent heart murmur rather than a pathological murmur. The pediatric cardiologist may have chosen not to obtain an echocardiogram; however, echocardiogram may be worthwhile in cases where clinical presentation is not clear or when the cardiologist desires to document normality to avoid mislabeling a healthy child with a chronic illness. It is important to appreciate that a normal echocardiogram does not rule out rheumatic fever without cardiac involvement.

Case 2

History: A 16-year-old female was referred to the cardiology clinic by her primary care physician. She had history of sore throat and fever 3 weeks ago. Over the past few days, she has had joint pain and swelling and has felt progressively tired. She first noted joint pain, swelling, and redness in her right knee that resolved just as she began experiencing similar symptoms in the left knee.

Physical Exam: There was noticeable redness and swelling of the left knee joint. The right knee appeared to be within normal limits. Cardiac examination revealed distant S1 and S2 with a 3/6 holosystolic murmur heard best over the apical region; in addition, a 1–2/4 diastolic murmur was heard over the apical region. Abdominal examination revealed mild hepatomegaly.

Investigative Studies: 12-lead ECG showed prolonged PR interval. Transthoracic echocardiography revealed dilated left ventricle with mildly decreased systolic function. The mitral valve leaflets were thickened with moderate to severe regurgitation. Trivial aortic regurgitation was noted. In addition, mild to moderate pericardial effusion was present.

Diagnosis and Discussion: This patient manifested two major Jones criteria: polyarthritis and carditis, thus satisfying criteria for the diagnosis of rheumatic fever and rheumatic heart disease. The time lapse between sore throat and the onset of the symptoms is consistent with the diagnosis of rheumatic fever. The migratory nature of polyarthritis in this patient is consistent with rheumatic fever. Carditis in this patient involves a valve lesion (mitral regurgitation), myocardial affliction (poor myocardial function), and pericardial disease (pericardial effusion). Progressive fatigue and enlarged liver are manifestations of heart failure.

This young lady should be admitted to the hospital for bed rest and monitoring and for the management of pancarditis. She should receive penicillin to eradicate the streptococcal infection and be started on anti-inflammatory therapy with aspirin to reduce arthritis and carditis. Anti-inflammatory therapy may also include steroids in this case due to the severity of carditis. If heart failure does not improve, diuretics and inotropic agents may be used. Once the patient recovers from the acute phase, she should be started on antibiotic prophylaxis, preferably with IM penicillin every 3–4 weeks. Prophylaxis should continue for a minimum of 10 years or longer if there is evidence of permanent cardiac disease.

Chapter 28
Kawasaki Disease

Rami Kharouf and Daniel E. Felten

Key Facts
• Kawasaki disease (KD) is more common in Japanese population and those of Japanese descent. Incidence is higher in males than females.
• Etiology of KD continues to be unclear, there is evidence supporting both genetic and environmental factors.
• Diagnosis of KD is made when there is fever of at least 5 days duration, plus bilateral, nonpurulent conjunctivitis, polymorphous skin rash, mucous membrane changes, erythema of palms and soles; edema of hands and feet; periungual and perineal desquamation and unilateral cervical lymphadenopathy.
• Echocardiography may show coronary artery dilation and aneurysm, pericardial effusion, poor myocardial function, and aortic and/or mitral regurgitation.
• Treatment of KD for the acute phase includes IVIG infusion and high dose aspirin. Long-term therapy includes low dose (antiplatelet) aspirin and in some cases warfarin to prevent clot formation within dilated coronary arteries.

Definition

Kawasaki disease (KD) is an inflammatory disease of unknown etiology involving blood vessels anywhere in the body, not limited to the coronary arteries. Since its description by Kawasaki et al. in 1967, KD has become more widely recognized and is now the most common acquired cardiovascular disease in children, surpassing rheumatic fever in western countries.

R. Kharouf (✉)
Department of Pediatric Cardiology, Mary Washington Hospital,
6804 Omega Ct, Fredericksburg, VA 22407, USA
e-mail: ramikha@hotmail.com

Ra-id Abdulla (ed.), *Heart Diseases in Children: A Pediatrician's Guide*,
DOI 10.1007/978-1-4419-7994-0_28, © Springer Science+Business Media, LLC 2011

Incidence

KD primarily affects young children; 80% of cases occur in children between 6 months and 5 years of age, with a peak incidence between 11 and 12 months. KD can affect infants younger than 6 months and children over 5 years of age. Rare cases of adult affliction by KD have been reported in the medical literature. It is more common in boys than in girls with a ratio of 1.3–1.7:1. The annual incidence varies between countries and ethnic groups. The highest incidence of KD is reported in Japan where annual incidence has increased substantially from 108/100,000 in 1996 to 185/100,000 in 2005–2006 among children below 5 years of age. In the USA, the reported incidence is between 9 and 19/100,000/year. People of Japanese ethnicity living outside of Japan have a higher incidence of KD than the average in the country in which they reside, but not as high as the rate in Japan. Incidence of KD in a sibling of a patient with KD is 1%, and 9% in a twin of a patient with KD. The higher rate among people of Japanese ethnicity and within siblings and twins suggests both genetic and environmental factors in the pathophysiology of this disease.

Etiology

Although many etiologic mechanisms have been proposed for KD, no single causative agent has been proven. The epidemiologic features of the disease suggest an infectious agent(s), which is supported by temporal (winter and early spring) and spatial clustering of cases as well as sharing some clinical features with inflammatory diseases that have well established underlying infectious causes (e.g. scarlet fever and Group A Streptococcal infections). However, no conclusive evidence has linked KD to a specific infectious agent.

Other potential etiologies of KD include drugs, toxins, chemicals like carpet cleaning solutions, and heavy metals. Although studies showed temporal relationships between exposure to some of these agents and development of KD, none has been proven to cause KD. More recent theories suggested a toxin-mediated syndrome similar to toxic shock syndrome and the possible role of superantigens induced by certain viral or bacterial agents.

Pathology

KD causes an acute, diffuse vasculitis that predominantly affects medium-sized blood vessels. Coronary artery involvement is common and leads to much of the morbidity and mortality; however, other arteries like axillary, femoral, iliac, and renal arteries can be involved as well. KD can also cause inflammation of any organ, as well as the myocardium, endocardium (including aortic and mitral valves) and pericardium. The acute inflammation of the coronary arteries can lead to thrombus formation and myocardial infarction. Moreover, the inflammatory changes can weaken the structure of the coronary vessels and lead to dilation and ultimately aneurysm formation. On the other hand, during the healing phase of KD, the vessels may become progressively fibrotic and develop stenosis over time. These areas of stenosis can also cause myocardial infarction.

Clinical Manifestations

The key characteristic of KD is fever greater than 5 days. The fever is usually high and remittent and does not typically completely respond to antipyretics. It usually lasts 1–2 weeks with a mean duration of 12 days in untreated patients, but it may last up to 30 days. KD should be considered in any patient with prolonged fever not otherwise attributable to another cause (Table 28.1).

The criteria for complete or typical KD include the presence of fever for ≥5 days with four out of the following five criteria:

- Changes in the extremities: these include erythema of the palms and soles and/ or painful induration of the hands and feet in the acute phase of the disease. This is more common in infants than in older children. Desquamation around the fingers and toes (periungual desquamation) usually follows at a later stage in the second or third week of illness. Later (1–2 months after onset), deep transverse grooves in the nails (Beau's lines) may be noted.
- Exanthema: an erythematous rash usually appears in the first 5 days of fever onset, and is commonly a diffuse maculopapular rash involving the trunk and extremities. However, the rash may be scarlatiniform, morbilliform, or urticarial; infants may have an evanescent rash involving the intertriginous areas particularly the perineum.

Table 28.1 Criteria for diagnosis of Kawasaki disease

Fever of at least 5 days duration
At least 4 of the following 5 clinical manifestations
  Bilateral, nonpurulent conjunctivitis
  Exanthem: polymorphous skin rash
  Enanthem: mucous membrane changes: red, dry, and cracked lips; strawberry tongue; pharyngeal erythema
  Changes in the extremities: erythema of palms and soles; edema of hands and feet; periungual and perineal desquamation
  Cervical lymphadenopathy: unilateral and >1.5 cm in diameter
Exclusion of diseases with similar presentation
Patients with fever and fewer than four principal clinical features can be diagnosed with
  Kawasaki disease if coronary artery disease is detected by echocardiography or if they have suggestive laboratory findings

• Conjunctivitis: bilateral, nonpurulent conjunctivitis involving the bulbar conjunctivae and sparing the palpebral conjunctiva and the limbus area immediately around the cornea. It usually appears in the acute phase of the disease and lasts 1–2 weeks. Other ophthalmologic involvement like anterior uveitis, which occurs in up to 83% of cases, is usually asymptomatic.
• Oral changes: these include changes involving the lips and oral mucosa. These take the form of red, cracked, and fissured lips, strawberry tongue with prominent fusiform papillae and diffuse oral and/or pharyngeal erythema. Pharyngeal exudates are not part of the clinical picture.
• Lymphadenopathy: this is the least consistent feature and occurs in 50–75% of the cases. It typically involves the anterior cervical lymph nodes and is unilateral and with a size of ≥1.5 cm in diameter.

In addition to the above criteria, other diagnoses with similar presentation should be excluded. The differential diagnosis of KD includes scarlet fever, EBV infection, adenovirus infection, and staphylococcal scalded skin syndrome, drug reactions and Stevens–Johnson syndrome.

Atypical (incomplete) KD refers to cases of KD that do not fulfill ≥4 diagnostic criteria. This is more common in infants who are at higher risk of coronary artery complications. Patients with fever greater than 5 days, two or three classic symptoms, and have either supporting laboratory abnormalities or evidence of coronary artery dilation, or aneurysm formation on echocardiogram should be diagnosed with atypical KD and treated accordingly.

A number of other systems are usually affected in KD. These are not part of the diagnostic criteria, but are helpful in making the diagnosis. Children with KD are usually irritable as compared to children with other febrile illnesses. Meningismus with CSF monocytic pleocytosis is not unusual and may be mistaken for viral meningitis. Occasionally, there is transient sensorineural hearing loss and rarely facial nerve palsy. Arthralgia or arthritis involving small and large weight-bearing joints may occur in the first week of illness. Gastrointestinal manifestations including diarrhea, vomiting, and abdominal pain occur in about one-third of the patients. Hepatic involvement is usually asymptomatic, but is detected by elevated transaminases. Hydrops of the gallbladder is less common, occurring in 15% of patients in the first 2 weeks from onset.

Erythema and induration at the site of a previous BCG vaccine is frequently described in countries where the vaccine is used like Japan and the UK. Rare manifestations include testicular swelling, pulmonary infiltrates, and pleural effusions.

Cardiac manifestations: Cardiac involvement is the main cause of acute morbidity and mortality, and is the principal long-term complication of KD. Physical examination of the heart may reveal the presence of flow murmur related to fever and anemia or a murmur of mitral regurgitation. Approximately 50% of patients have mild myocarditis evidenced by sinus tachycardia. Signs of congestive heart failure, such as gallop rhythm, are occasionally seen and indicate more significant myocardial involvement. The most significant cardiac manifestation of KD is involvement of the coronary arteries. The coronary arteries are involved in 18–24% of patients with untreated KD, but involvement decreases to 4–8% if intravenous immunoglobulin (IVIG) is given within the first 10 days of illness. As mentioned above, the coronary arteries may become inflamed as part of the acute phase of KD. This inflammation may cause acute morbidity or mortality, such as thrombus formation or acute MI, or may lead to complications up to 6–8 weeks from onset of fever. Coronary artery dilatation or ectasia is the most common complication from the acute inflammation. Approximately 8% of untreated patients develop aneurysmal dilatation and only about 1% develop giant aneurysms (>8 mm in diameter). Risk factors for coronary artery involvement include male sex, infants below 1 year of age, and fever of >10 days duration.

Laboratory Investigations

Markers of acute inflammation are usually increased in patients with KD but are not essential for the diagnosis. The ESR is elevated in 2/3 of patients and is usually significantly elevated >50 mm/h. The C-reactive protein is elevated in almost half of the patients. A complete blood count may show neutrophilic leukocytosis, with white blood cell count >15,000 in more than half of the patients, nonspecific anemia, or thrombocytosis. However, thrombocytosis, which is described as a marker of KD, is usually not seen until the second week of the disease and is not helpful in making the diagnosis in the acute stage. Other nonspecific laboratory findings include mild to moderate elevation of the liver transaminases (40%), low serum albumin level, sterile pyuria (33%), and aseptic meningitis (up to 50%).

Imaging and Studies

Chest X-ray may show the nonspecific findings of pulmonary infiltrates or cardiomegaly, but is typically normal. Electrocardiogram changes in KD include nonspecific changes like prolonged PR interval and nonspecific ST-T wave changes and sinus tachycardia. Although echocardiography is helpful in the management of patients with KD, there should be no delay in the treatment based on its result. An initial echocardiogram should be performed as soon as the diagnosis of KD is suspected and repeated 2 weeks after fever onset. Coronary artery involvement is seen in about 25% of untreated cases of KD, and pericardial effusion is seen in approximately 30% of cases. Coronary artery dilatation or aneurysm noted on echocardiogram is diagnostic for KD in the presence of other characteristic features. However, coronary artery involvement may develop as late as 6–8 weeks after the onset, so a follow-up echocardiogram is necessary around that time. If the echocardiogram is normal at 6–8 weeks, a follow-up echocardiogram beyond 8 weeks is optional.

Treatments

The standard therapy of KD is IVIG 2 g/kg over 10- to 12-h period, and an anti-inflammatory dose of aspirin of 30–100 mg/kg/day. A second and even a third dose of IVIG may be given for persistent fever within 36–48 h of the initial dose, but 90% of patients' defervesce within 48 h of the first dose. Once the patient is afebrile, the dose of aspirin is decreased to 3–5 mg/kg/day. This dose of aspirin is given until a repeat echocardiogram at 6–8 weeks of illness shows no coronary artery dilatation. Patients with coronary artery abnormalities require long-term treatment with aspirin and possibly other anticoagulants such as warfarin in cases of giant aneurysm of coronary arteries to prevent thromboembolism.

Follow Up and Prognosis

Prior to the introduction of IVIG, the mortality rate of the acute stage of the disease was approximately 2%, which was thought to be due to thrombosis or rupture of coronary artery aneurysms. If IVIG is given within the first 10 days of illness, mortality is significantly less. A high percentage of patients who develop coronary artery abnormalities show resolution of these abnormalities within 2–5 years, depending on the severity of the initial changes. There are reports of increased risk of early arteriosclerosis in patients with history of KD, even if the initial coronary artery changes have resolved. Long-term follow-up for these patients may be needed.

Case Scenarios

Case 1

History. A 15-month-old child is brought to the emergency room for evaluation. She had fever for the last 9 days. She was seen by her pediatrician a week ago and sent home on antipyretics with a diagnosis of a viral infection. Today her parents report that she has been more irritable than usual. Her fever was 103.5 last night and did not respond to acetaminophen. She had new onset skin rash 2 days ago with a bad diaper rash. Her mother mentions that she had pink eyes. She has been feeding less than usual and her crying is not consolable.

Physical exam. Temperature 101.8 F, despite antipyretic 2 h ago. She is very irritable, even when carried by her mother. HR is 168 bpm, RR 40, BP 98/52, Oxygen saturation 99%. She is well perfused. HEENT evaluation shows mild conjunctivitis with no discharge. Her lips are cracked and red. She had pharyngeal erythema with no exudates. Her tongue is red. She has a diffuse maculopapular rash with peeling in the diaper area. Hand and feet show erythema with no swelling.

Investigative studies. CBC shows a white count of 13,000, platelet count of 379,000, and Hb of 10.2 g/dL. PCR for RSV, influenza A and B, and parainfluenza, are all negative. Urinalysis shows 10–20 WBC/HPF, otherwise normal. A comprehensive panel comes back significant for AST of 119 and ALT of 235. ESR is elevated at 79 mm/h. Blood and urine cultures are pending. Her CXR shows no focal abnormality. You order an ECG and an Echocardiogram.

Differential diagnosis. Due to length of fever and constellation of findings, this patient most likely has KD. A viral syndrome, EBV for example, could be a cause of prolonged fever, irritability, and some of the laboratory abnormalities, but would not account for all findings. Scarlet fever could also cause many of these signs and symptoms, but the rash is not classical nor is there any preceding sore throat reported. Moreover, scarlet fever is very rare in this age group.

Diagnosis and management. This is a typical case of KD, with the initial presentation in the first few days of illness mistaken for a viral infection. The manifestations may not be all present at the same time, but appear sequentially. The presence of fever for 9 days, with the other clinical criteria and no obvious infectious cause is supported by the laboratory investigations. A high ESR is typical of KD, but is unlikely to be related to viral infections. An echocardiogram will help in looking for coronary artery involvement, but is not essential to make the diagnosis and should not delay starting treatment.

Treatment should be initiated once diagnosis is suspected with IVIG at dose of 2 g/kg and Aspirin at 80 mg/kg/day in four divided doses. The child defervesces the following day and becomes consolable. Initial echocardiogram is normal so she is discharged home after 3 days on Aspirin at 3 mg/kg/day with no recurrence of fever and with a follow-up echocardiogram in 2 weeks.

Case 2

History. An 8-month-old infant presents with 6 days of fever with no focus of infection. He had a skin rash earlier on day of presentation which disappeared by the time you saw him. He is described as being irritable and tachypneic. He had bilateral conjunctivitis.

Physical examination. The patient has nonexudative bilateral conjunctivitis and mild pharyngeal and oral erythema with some cracking of the lips. The patient has no skin rash or lymphadenopathy, and the rest of the exam is unremarkable. There is no focus for an infection.

Investigational studies. CBC shows a white cell count of 17,000 with left shift and high band count, hemoglobin level of 9.5 g/dL, and a platelet count of 350,000. A bag urine specimen shows 20 WBC/HPF, with no red cells and trace protein. CRP was elevated at 35 mg/dL and ESR level of 89 mm/h. A lumbar puncture was done, and examination of the CSF reveals white cells of 27/mm^3, normal protein, and two RBCs. You send rapid antigen for viruses, blood, CSF, and urine cultures and start him on antibiotics.

Differential diagnosis. Given the elevated WBC with elevated band count, and WBCs in the CSF, infection should be high on the list of potential etiologies. The CSF is suggestive of viral meningitis given the elevated WBC, but normal protein. However, the prolonged fever, conjunctivitis, pharyngeal and oral erythema, as well as the history of fever should suggest KD as a possible etiology as well. The laboratory findings help to support that diagnosis.

Assessment. The presence of prolonged fever, 2–3 classic symptoms of KD and the supporting lab results – elevated ESR and CRP, WBCs in the urine and CSF without other signs of bacterial infection (sterile pyuria and aseptic meningitis), mildly elevated WBC with left shift, and anemia – point to atypical KD. Since symptoms have persisted for 6 days, it would be reasonable to treat immediately; however, it could also be argued that waiting for results of blood and CSF cultures or viral PCR would also be reasonable as there is no proven additional benefit to treating early as long as IVIG is given by day 10. Ordering an echocardiogram at this point is indicated since findings consistent with KD would clinch the diagnosis. The echocardiogram in this patient shows a small pericardial effusion, mitral regurgitation, mildly dilated right and left anterior descending coronary arteries, and normal ventricular function.

Diagnosis and management. These findings on echocardiogram are consistent with KD and are diagnostic in the presence of the other symptoms discussed above. The patient is given 2 g/kg of IVIG and started on high dose aspirin, and he defervesces. However, 24-h later the fever recurs, and a second dose of IVIG is given. After the second dose, the fever resolves and does not return. He is discharged home on Aspirin with follow-up with cardiology.

Chapter 29
Infective Endocarditis

Rami Kharouf and Laura Torchen

Key Facts

- Infective endocarditis is a rare disease, mostly affecting individuals with underlying cardiac pathology or intracardiac foreign bodies such as central lines.
- Mortality of IE is high, particularly with resistant bacterial agents or fungal infection.
- Patients may develop severe congestive heart failure due to worsening of valvular function.
- Treatment may require multiple antibiotics for a prolonged period of time to eradicate infection.
- Surgical intervention is performed to correct significant valvular disease, embolization, or failure to respond to medical therapy.
- Use of prophylactic antibiotics to prevent IE in patients with congenital heart disease has been recently limited to those with prosthetic valves, unrepaired cyanotic congenital heart disease, residual defects after surgical repair, past history of IE and patients with cardiac transplantation and valvular heart disease.

Definition

Infective endocarditis (IE) is an infection of the endocardial lining of the heart or cardiac vessels, usually affecting abnormal cardiac structure, such as valvular disease, septal defects or after surgical repair of heart disease, particularly in the presence of foreign material such as mechanical valves and patch material. IE can be caused by bacterial or fungal agents.

R. Kharouf (✉)
Department of Pediatric Cardiology, Mary Washington Hospital,
6804 Omega Ct, Fredericksburg, VA 22407, USA
e-mail: ramikha@hotmail.com

Ra-id Abdulla (ed.), *Heart Diseases in Children: A Pediatrician's Guide*,
DOI 10.1007/978-1-4419-7994-0_29, © Springer Science+Business Media, LLC 2011

Incidence

Although IE is a rare disease affecting 0.3 per 100,000 children per year, it is a devastating disease with high morbidity and mortality.

Epidemiology

There has been an increase in the pediatric population at risk for IE with increased survival of repaired congenital heart disease. The risk of IE in the general population is approximately 5/100,000 per year and is higher with increasing age. This risk is much higher in patients with certain cardiac risk factors with an incidence of up to 2,160 cases/100,000 patient-years in the highest risk lesions. The exact risk depends on the specific disease.

Patients with complex cyanotic congenital heart disease and those with cardiac prosthesis and shunts are at highest risk. The most common congenital heart defects involved are ventricular septal defects, patent ductus arteriosus, aortic valve disease, and tetralogy of Fallot. Neonates and infants with such conditions appear to have worse outcomes of IE. There is also an increase in the incidence in neonates with no underlying heart disease, likely related to the increased use of intravascular devices and catheters.

Etiology

The most common infectious agents responsible for IE of a native valve are gram-positive cocci. Although Viridans streptococci continues to be the most common infectious agent responsible for IE overall, *Staphylococcal* species have surpassed the Viridans group in some recent series in adults. *Enterococci* are less common agents in the pediatric age group.

Gram-negative organisms are responsible for <10% of cases, but are more common in certain groups of patients such as neonates and immunocompromised patients. The HACEK group is a group of gram-negative bacilli that includes *Haemophilus*, *Actinobacillus*, *Cardiobacterium*, *Eikenella* and *Kingella* species associated with IE.

Infection of a prosthetic valve early after surgery is most likely to result from Staphylococcal species (*Staphylococcus aureus* and coagulase-negative Staphylococci). Other uncommon microorganisms are fungi which occur in immunocompromised patients, patients on prolonged antibiotic therapy, and neonates. Intravenous drug users are at special risk for fungal endocarditis and right-sided *S. aureus* IE. In about 10% of all cases of IE, a microbiologic agent cannot be identified.

Pathogenesis and Pathophysiology

The infection starts at a site of endothelial damage secondary to a congenital or an acquired lesion. The first step in the pathogenesis of IE is the formation of nonbacterial thrombotic endocarditis, which is an area of denuded endothelium with deposition of fibrin, platelets and red blood cells. States of transient bacteremia may then lead to the adhesion of bacteria to the thrombotic endocarditis via special adhesion molecules present on the bacterial surfaces. The ability of certain bacteria to cause IE more than others is related to these adhesive properties. Subsequently, bacteria proliferate within the nidus of infection and are covered by fibrin which protects the bacteria in this milieu. The bacteria rapidly proliferate inside the vegetations. Most of the bacteria inside the vegetations are in an inactive state which confers additional protection from antibiotics and explains the need for prolonged treatment.

Clinical Manifestations

The most common presenting feature of IE is fever, which tends to be higher in *S. aureus* infections. The associated features of IE are related to acuity of the infection. While subacute cases are more likely to be associated with nonspecific manifestations like myalgias, arthralgias, headache, and general malaise, acute IE typically has a more toxic presentation with higher fevers.

The clinical manifestations of IE can be grouped into those resulting from the infection itself and those secondary to the structural damage incurred on the valves and other cardiac structures. These structural alterations result in manifestations like acute valvular regurgitation, obstruction, congestive heart failure, and heart block. Those manifestations related to the infective process include the clinical manifestations of bacteremia and those due to the separation of vegetations and systemic embolization. Still other features are secondary to immunologic phenomena associated with IE, such as immune complex diseases.

Cardiac manifestations depend on the site of infection:

– Congestive heart failure might be related to acute valvular regurgitation.
– Heart block is related to extension of the infection to the conduction system, usually with aortic valve involvement.

Extracardiac manifestations include the following:

– Neurologic manifestations: these are reported in 20% of cases and are related to an abscess formation, infarct, aseptic meningitis, encephalopathy, or hemorrhage.
– Renal manifestations: these are due to septic emboli to the kidneys or immune complex mediated glomerulonephritis. These manifest as proteinuria, hematuria, pyuria, or abscess formation.

– Neonates are more likely to present with extracardiac infections due to septic embolization that result in osteomyelitis, meningitis, or septic arthritis.

Physical examination may show the classic signs of IE which include the following:

– Janeway lesions: Nontender, flat, macular, blanching violaceous lesions on the palms and soles.
– Osler's nodes: Tender, raised violaceous nodules which are located on the pulps of fingers and toes.
– Roth's spots: Exudative, edematous lesions of the retina.
– Splinter hemorrhages: Nonblanching, linear, reddish-brown lesions under the nails.

Other physical findings include a new regurgitant heart murmur or change in character of an existing heart murmur or signs of CHF. Splenomegaly may be present in subacute disease of several weeks or months duration.

Electrocardiography

This is usually nondiagnostic and nonspecific, showing complications of IE such as heart block with conduction system damage or ischemic changes with embolization into the coronary arteries.

Chest Radiography

This may show the presence of pulmonary infiltrates caused by septic pulmonary emboli from right-sided IE. Pulmonary edema and cardiomegaly may result from congestive heart failure complicating IE.

Echocardiography

This diagnostic modality should be used in cases with at least moderate suspicion of IE. Transthoracic echocardiography is more helpful in children than adults, especially with normal cardiac structure or isolated valvular disease. Transesophageal echocardiography should be used if transthoracic echocardiography is limited and in patients with prosthetic valves.

Findings by echocardiography include valvular vegetations, valvular regurgitations, abscess formation, and rarely rupture of cardiac structures. In addition, vegetations may be noted; these may be attached to cardiac structures or foreign material such as prosthetic valves or central venous catheters.

Diagnostic Criteria

The modified Duke criteria are the mostly widely used for the diagnosis of IE. The diagnosis is classified into definite, possible, and rejected.

Definite endocarditis is defined as one of the following conditions:

- Direct histologic evidence of IE.
- Positive gram stain result or culture of specimen obtained during cardiac surgery or at autopsy.
- Two major criteria.
- One major and three minor criteria.
- Five minor criteria.

Major criteria:

- Microbiologic isolation of the organism in at least two separate blood cultures
- Echocardiographic findings consistent with IE

Minor criteria:

- Predisposition: Congenital heart disease or intravenous drug use
- Fever
- Vascular phenomena: Major arterial emboli, septic pulmonary infarcts, mycotic aneurysm, intracranial hemorrhage, conjunctival hemorrhages, and Janeway lesions
- Immunologic phenomena: glomerulonephritis, Osler's nodes, Roth's spots, and rheumatoid factor
- Microbiological evidence: Positive blood culture but does not meet a major criterion as noted above or serological evidence of active infection with organism consistent with IE

Possible IE includes those cases with one major and one minor criterion or only three minor criteria. Rejected cases include those in which an alternative diagnosis is confirmed or if the fever resolves with a short course of antibiotics of less than 4 days.

Laboratory Investigations

Blood cultures are the most important laboratory tests in the diagnosis of IE and are a component of the major criteria. This criterion requires three blood cultures collected over a 24-h period.

Acute phase reactants are usually elevated in patients with IE. About half of the patients have positive rheumatoid factor or evidence of immune complexes. Anemia may be present and is caused by hemolysis or the presence of chronic infection.

Treatment

Treatment of IE involves antimicrobial therapy, supportive therapy, as well as surgical treatment when indicated. Prolonged therapy is usually required and the specific duration and combination of agents used is determined by the infecting microorganism, the location of the infection, whether it involves a native or a prosthetic valve, and the presence of complications.

It is essential to obtain information about the microbiologic sensitivity to antibiotics and the minimal inhibitory concentrations as this will determine the duration and combination of antibiotics used.

For streptococcal endocarditis, most of which is caused by Viridans group (α-hemolytic group), it is usually sufficient to treat with 4 weeks of IV Penicillin G in uncomplicated cases. For patients allergic to penicillin, vancomycin can be used.

For staphylococcal endocarditis, treatment requires use of a penicillinase-resistant penicillin (like nafcillin) or vancomycin IV for 6 weeks. IE caused by *S. aureus* carries a high mortality rate of 25–40%.

Fungal endocarditis is more commonly seen in immunocompromised hosts, IV drug users, patients on broad-spectrum antibiotics, and those with intravascular devices. The drug of choice is amphotericin B IV for at least 6–8 weeks. A high percentage of these patients need surgical intervention.

Prosthetic valve endocarditis usually requires treatment for at least 6 weeks with IV antibiotics.

Surgical treatment may be required in 25–30% of patients in the acute phase of the disease. Circumstances in which surgical treatment is necessary include patients with recurrent embolization despite antibiotic therapy, those who fail medical therapy, and those with progressive heart failure due to damage of cardiac structures such as with severe valve regurgitation.

Prognosis

Infective endocarditis continues to have significant morbidity and mortality despite advances in medical and surgical treatment. Those with IE caused by *S. aureus* and fungal IE have a higher mortality rate. Untreated, IE is fatal. Mortality rate for viridans streptococcal endocarditis with no significant complications is less than 10%. On the other hand, *Aspergillus* endocarditis after prosthetic valve surgery carries an almost 100% risk of death.

Prognosis is poorer with:

- Resistant organisms
- Underlying cardiac pathology
- Aortic or multiple valve involvement
- Large vegetations
- Polymicrobial bacteremia
- Prosthetic valve infections

- Mycotic aneurysms
- Valve ring abscess
- Major embolic events

Prognosis is better with:

- Right-sided compared to left-sided endocarditis
- Infection with streptococcal viridans
- Absent systemic emboli

Prophylaxis

In recent years, there have been dramatic changes in the recommendations for IE antibiotic prophylaxis before dental and other procedures. The rationale is that there has been no proof that such prophylaxis prevents IE and that only a small percentage of cases of IE is related to such procedures.

The cardiac lesions that are considered high risk for IE and in which prophylaxis is indicated are summarized in Table 29.1. Antibiotic prophylaxis is no longer recommended at the time of gastrointestinal or genitourinary procedures.

Prophylaxis regimens include oral amoxicillin at 50 mg/kg (up to 2 g) or ampicillin 50 mg/kg IV or IM. Alternatives in patients allergic to penicillin include cephalexin 50 mg/kg PO (up to 2 g), clindamycin 20 mg/kg (up to 600 mg), azithromycin or clarithromycin at 15 mg/kg (up to 500 mg).

Case Scenarios

Case 1

History: A 6-year-old girl presents with 2-week history of intermittent fevers. She was initially seen in the first week of illness by her physician and was diagnosed with otitis media. She received oral amoxicillin for a week, but continued to have spikes

Table 29.1 Cardiac conditions associated with the highest risk of adverse outcome from IE for which prophylaxis prior to dental procedures is recommended

Prosthetic cardiac valve

Previous IE

Congenital heart disease

    Unrepaired cyanotic CHD, including palliative shunts and conduits

    Completely repaired CHD with prosthetic material or device, whether placed by surgery or by catheter intervention, during the first 6 months after the procedure

    Repaired CHD with residual defects at the site or adjacent to the site of a prosthetic patch or prosthetic device

Cardiac transplantation recipients who develop cardiac valvulopathy

of fever. In addition she complains of headaches, abdominal pains, and daily fevers with sweating. The patient's mother reports that she appears less active than usual. Her past history is significant for a heart murmur that was thought to be benign.

Physical exam: Physical examination reveals a temperature of 103.1°F, respiratory rate of 24/min, pulse rate of 121 bpm and BP of 93/51 mmHg, and oxygen saturation of 98% on room air. The patient appears pale and ill, but awake. Cardiac examination is significant for regular rate and rhythm with no thrill; normal S1 and narrow splitting of S2. There is a 2/6 systolic ejection murmur at right upper sternal border and 2/4 early diastolic murmur at left midsternal border. The peripheral pulses are bounding. The patient is noted to have extensive dental caries.

Investigative studies: A complete blood count is obtained with a white cell count of 11,000/UL, 80% neutrophils; hemoglobin of 10.5 g/dL and a platelet count of 271,000. ESR is mildly elevated at 35 mm/h. A comprehensive metabolic panel was within normal limits. Chest radiography reveals mild cardiomegaly with no pulmonary infiltrates. A 12-lead ECG is consistent with sinus tachycardia and left ventricular hypertrophy.

Differential diagnosis: This patient is presenting with the complaint of a 2-week history of fever and lethargy. History suggests an infectious process. Her physical examination is significant for systolic and diastolic murmurs. These findings, coupled with the laboratory studies are suggestive of IE and an echocardiogram is necessary to rule out this possibility. These auscultatory findings are most consistent with a stenotic and insufficient aortic valve. Due to the rather insidious onset in this particular patient, Strep viridans would be the most likely infectious etiology, but other causes such as *S. aureus*, fungal pathogens, and gram-negative HACEK organisms must be considered.

Final diagnosis: Due to the presence of fever with heart murmur, three sets of blood cultures are obtained and a transthoracic echocardiogram is performed. The echo shows the presence of a bicuspid aortic valve with a 4-mm vegetation on one of the leaflets and moderate aortic valve regurgitation. Left ventricular dilatation is present with normal systolic function.

Assessment: This case shows the typical presentation of a native valve endocarditis with history of aortic valve stenosis that was not diagnosed previously. Although this patient had no recent dental work, it is the presence of poor oral hygiene and transient states of bacteremia that poses a high risk of IE. Group A *Streptococcus* (Viridans group) continues to be the most common causative agent in this situation. This patient was treated for 6 weeks and did not require immediate surgical therapy, although she does demonstrate the complication of aortic valve regurgitation.

Management: Empiric intravenous antibiotic therapy is initiated based on these findings pending blood culture results. After 24 h, two of the blood cultures grow Viridans streptococci and therapy with IV ampicillin continues for a total 6-week course based on sensitivity of the organism.

Case 2

History: A 2-week-old twin male infant, born prematurely at 28 weeks gestational age, is weaning from mechanical ventilatory support to nasal CPAP when he develops apnea and bradycardia that necessitates re-intubation and mechanical ventilation.

Physical examination: On exam, the patient has a pulse rate of 190/min, RR 70/min, BP 61/28, and oxygen saturation of 94% on 50% FiO2. The patient is intubated, with an umbilical central venous line and a peripheral intravenous line in place. He appears pale with decreased perfusion, but no murmurs on cardiac auscultation. There are no other pertinent physical findings.

Investigative studies: A complete blood count is performed with a white cell count of 31,000 with 66% segmented neutrophils and 18% bands, Hgb of 9.1 g/dL, and a platelet count of 91,000. BUN is 16 and Cr is 0.8 mg/dL. A blood culture is obtained and treatment is initiated with empiric ampicillin and gentamicin. A chest radiograph shows diffuse pulmonary infiltrates.

Differential diagnosis: This case presents a premature infant with a corrected gestational age of 30 weeks who develops apnea and bradycardia while attempting to wean ventilatory support to nasal CPAP. While apnea of prematurity is possible in this case, the findings of the CBC are concerning for infection. In addition, the patient demonstrates acute renal failure based on his BUN and creatinine and the CXR is concerning for pneumonia. Each of these findings are concerning for sepsis.

Final diagnosis: After 24 h, the initial blood culture grows gram-positive cocci and Ampicillin was changed to Vancomycin. Daily blood cultures are obtained and after two days of IV antibiotics, blood culture remains positive for gram-positive cocci. At this time, the identification of the initial blood culture reveals *S. aureus*, resistant to methicillin, but sensitive to Vancomycin. Due to the persistent positive blood cultures, an echocardiogram is performed which shows a mobile 12-mm mass on the atrial septum with small vegetations on both sides of the septum. The patient was treated for 6 weeks with vancomycin. Repeat blood cultures after 4 days of vancomycin were negative.

Assessment: This case emphasizes the increased incidence of IE in a special group of pediatric patients. Premature infants have increased susceptibility due not only to prematurity, but also the increased use of indwelling catheters used for intravenous fluids, nutrition, and monitoring in the intensive care unit. These patients are also at increased risk for gram-negative and fungal endocarditis in addition to *Staphylococcus* species.

Management: Treatment is continued for 6 weeks with vancomycin. Repeat blood cultures after 4 days of vancomycin were negative. This patient does well with prolonged antibiotic therapy and is discharged home without sequelae.

Case 3

History: A 16-year-old female presents with a 3-day history of fevers, chills, headaches, shortness of breath, and chest pain. Her past medical history is significant for the diagnosis of aortic stenosis and regurgitation which necessitated aortic valve replacement with native pulmonary valve and insertion of a homograft pulmonary valve replacement 1 month ago (Ross procedure).

Physical examination: Her physical examination shows a pulse rate of 118/min, respiratory rate of 20/min, BP 91/45 mmHg, oxygen saturation of 89% on room air, and temperature of 102.3°F. She appears ill and pale. Cardiac examination is significant for normal S1 and single S2 with an ejection systolic-early diastolic murmur over the left upper sternal border with no clicks or gallop. Abdominal examination reveals an enlarged liver down to 3 cm below right costal margin.

Investigative studies: A complete blood count is performed with a white blood cell count of 17,400 with 85% segmented neutrophils, Hgb of 11.9 g/dL and platelet count of 150,000. ESR is 30 mm/h and CRP is 28 mg/dL. Liver transaminases and basic metabolic profile are within normal limits.

Differential diagnosis: This case presents a patient with recent valve replacement who subsequently develops a febrile illness with physical examination findings suggestive of pulmonary stenosis and insufficiency with evidence of new congestive heart failure. While IE affecting the pulmonary valve is most likely, pulmonary valve failure unrelated to endocarditis is also a possibility. Myocarditis or pericarditis as a cause for fever and new onset congestive heart failure must also be considered.

Final diagnosis: Transthoracic echocardiogram shows the presence of a large vegetation 1 cm in diameter attached to the pulmonary valve with moderate degree of pulmonary stenosis and insufficiency. The right ventricle is dilated with decreased systolic function. A chest CT scan shows the presence of multiple pulmonary emboli with no abscess formation. Two sets of blood cultures are sent and the patient is started on empiric antibiotic therapy with oxacillin and gentamicin. After 18 h, the blood culture is positive for *S. aureus* with later antibiotic sensitivity testing showing the organism sensitive to methicillin.

Assessment: This case illustrates the late presentation of prosthetic valve endocarditis caused by *S. aureus*. These patients frequently require prolonged antibiotic therapy and often surgical intervention for debridement and replacement of the prosthetic valve. These postoperative infections are thought to be caused by organisms inoculated at time of surgery. The presentation is usually in the first 2–3 months after surgery, but can occur several months after.

Management: The patient continues to have daily positive blood cultures. She develops evidence of pulmonary embolism which requires surgical therapy with replacement of the pulmonary valve. The patient is treated with IV antibiotics for a total duration of 6 weeks with sterilization of blood cultures and clinical improvement.

Chapter 30
Myocarditis

Rami Kharouf and Laura Torchen

Key Facts

- Most cases of myocarditis are thought to be secondary to viral infection; however, in many instances, documentation of viral infection is lacking.
- The most common viruses implicated in myocarditis include Coxsackie virus type B and parvovirus B19.
- Many children present with prodrome of illness which may include lethargy, poor feeding, irritability, respiratory distress, or even sudden collapse and cardiogenic shock.
- Myocarditis leads to poor ventricular function leading to poor cardiac output and pulmonary edema.
- Echocardiography shows dilation and poor function of the left ventricle. Echocardiography cannot differentiate acute myocarditis from dilated cardiomyopathy.
- Myocarditis may eventually lead to dilated cardiomyopathy.
- Treatment is mostly supportive to minimize effects of congestive heart failure.

Definition

Myocarditis is characterized by an inflammatory infiltrate of the myocardium with necrosis/degeneration of the myocytes. It is estimated that 50–80% of pediatric patients with acute presentation of dilated cardiomyopathy have myocarditis as the underlying cause.

R. Kharouf (✉)
Department of Pediatric Cardiology, Mary Washington Hospital, 6804 Omega Ct,
Fredericksburg, VA 22407, USA
e-mail: ramikha@hotmail.com

Ra-id Abdulla (ed.), *Heart Diseases in Children: A Pediatrician's Guide*,
DOI 10.1007/978-1-4419-7994-0_30, © Springer Science+Business Media, LLC 2011

Etiology

The most common cause of myocarditis is viral infection. Coxsackievirus type B and parvovirus B19 are common viral agents implicated in myocarditis. In addition, many other viral causes of myocarditis in children have been identified, including influenza, cytomegalovirus (CMV), herpes simplex virus (HSV) hepatitis C, rubella, varicella, mumps, Epstein–Barr virus, human immunodeficiency virus (HIV), and respiratory syncytial virus.

Besides viruses, myocarditis can be caused by a myriad of other infectious agents like bacteria, rickettsiae, protozoa, and others. In South America, Chagas disease caused by *Trypanosoma cruzi* is the commonest cause.

Myocarditis can also be caused by noninfectious systemic diseases such as systemic lupus erythematosus (SLE), rheumatoid arthritis, rheumatic fever, and scleroderma. Toxicity to medications such as antimicrobials and chemotherapeutic medications such as anthracyclines has been implicated in the cause of myocarditis. Hypersensitivity reactions to certain medications represent a particular type of cardiomyopathy. Finally, in many cases of myocarditis, no underlying cause is identified.

Pathology

The gold standard for diagnosing myocarditis has been the pathological findings on endomyocardial biopsy. The cellular infiltrate is usually lymphocytic, but can also include eosinophils and plasma cells. There is usually variable and patchy myocyte degeneration and necrosis, which sometimes makes biopsy diagnosis difficult. The endocardium and valves are usually spared in viral myocarditis. Other more rare forms of myocarditis are characterized by giant cell infiltrates.

Recently, immunohistochemical staining of biopsies has allowed the identification of viral genomes in the affected cardiac tissues. Other more advanced staining has allowed for the characterization of different immune mediated reactions of the involved myocytes to the causative agents.

Pathophysiology

Most cases of myocarditis are caused by viral infection. Three mechanisms are proposed to lead to the final clinical presentation. Initially there is direct viral invasion of the myocytes. This is followed by activation of the immune system with cytokine formation. Finally, lymphocytes are activated and autoantibody formation ensues. In all stages, direct damage to myocytes and inflammatory reaction leads to loss of myocytes and fibrous tissue formation, thus diminishing the contractility of the myocardium.

Clinical Manifestations

The initial presentation of acute myocarditis in children is variable and depends on the age of the child as well as the rapidity of progression of the disease process itself.

The onset is usually heralded by a viral prodrome consisting of fever, upper respiratory and gastrointestinal symptoms, thought to coincide with the viremic stage of the disease. Infants usually present with nonspecific symptoms of lethargy, poor feeding, irritability, respiratory distress, or even sudden collapse and cardiogenic shock. Older children and adolescents are more likely to have chest pain, easy fatigue and general malaise, exercise intolerance and abdominal pain, or even arrhythmias and syncope. As the course progresses, respiratory symptoms become more prominent.

On physical examination, infants might have pallor and appear dusky in addition to the findings of congestive heart failure signs. Tachycardia is commonly seen in about 2/3 of patients. Respiratory distress is the next most common finding, followed by hepatomegaly and abnormal heart sounds or a heart murmur of mitral regurgitation. Jugular venous distension is more likely in older children, as this is an unreliable sign in the younger age group.

Chest X-Ray

Chest X-ray may show the presence of cardiomegaly and increased pulmonary vascular markings or frank pulmonary edema in almost half of patients (Fig. 30.1).

Electrocardiogram

ECG abnormalities are described in almost 90% of patients. The classic findings include sinus tachycardia, low voltage QRS complexes, and T wave changes. Other ECG findings are T wave inversions, ST segment changes and pathological Q waves. Arrhythmias such as ventricular or supraventricular tachycardia or atrioventricular block can also be seen.

Echocardiography

The typical findings include the presence of a dilated left ventricle with decreased systolic function in most patients (Chap. 4, Fig. 4.4b). Echocardiography may also reveal the presence of mitral valve regurgitation and pericardial effusion.

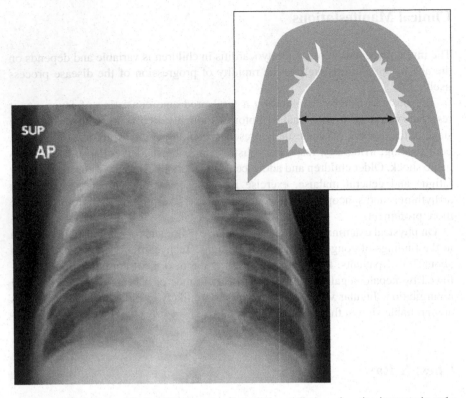

Fig. 30.1 Chest X-ray, AP view. The heart is enlarged; the cardiothoracic ration is approximately 65%. Pulmonary vasculature is prominent due to congested pulmonary venous circulation secondary to poor ventricular function due to myocarditis

Laboratory Investigations

The gold standard for the diagnosis of myocarditis historically has been endomyocardial biopsy. However, this is not routinely done due to the low sensitivity of the procedure (3–63%) and the often patchy involvement of the myocardium. Viral cultures and viral titers can also be performed, but these are nonspecific.

Elevation of the cardiac enzymes especially involving cardiac troponins is positive in about 1/3 of patients. Other nonspecific findings include elevation of ESR and alanine aminotransferase.

Cardiac Catheterization

This is not routinely performed in the workup of patients with myocarditis. The main indication for this procedure is to perform endomyocardial biopsy, which is invasive and has higher complication rate in younger age groups.

Differential Diagnosis

The diagnosis of myocarditis is considered in the differential diagnosis of sudden death, heart failure, shock states, or in asymptomatic ECG changes. It is estimated that about one quarter of pediatric patient cases of dilated cardiomyopathy is caused by acute myocarditis. The differential diagnosis of the presenting manifestations in infants include sepsis, metabolic disturbances, inherited metabolic disorders, mitochondrial myopathies and anomalous origin of the left coronary artery from the pulmonary artery. The differential diagnosis in older children includes idiopathic and inherited cardiomyopathy, chronic tachyarrhythmia, and connective tissue diseases.

Treatment

The mainstay of treatment of myocarditis remains supportive. This includes use of intravenous inotropic support with Dopamine, Dobutamine, and Milrinone. Intravenous after-load reducing agents like sodium nitroprusside are used in the acute intensive care setting. Diuretic therapy is usually used for those patients who present with congestive symptoms and signs.

Oral therapy with afterload reducing agents is used in patients with more stable clinical condition who have persistent left ventricular dysfunction. Angiotensin-converting enzyme inhibitors such as captopril and enalapril, β-adrenergic blockers, and anticoagulant or antiplatelet medications are the main treatment modalities.

Bed rest in the acute stage with close observation is the mainstay of treatment in mild and asymptomatic cases.

Digitalis is avoided during the acute stage of the inflammation due to possible cardiac side effects such as ventricular arrhythmias, although it can be used in the chronic stage of the disease or in those who progress to dilated cardiomyopathy.

Other therapies, such as the use of immunosuppressive therapy and immuno-modulating agents like intravenous immunoglobulin is still controversial. So far studies showed no benefit of steroids or other immunosuppressants in the long-term outcome of the disease. Recent reports on the use of antiviral agents and interferon are encouraging.

Patients who present with fulminant myocarditis or intractable arrhythmias may need mechanical support like extracorporeal membrane oxygenation, ventricular assist devices, or even heart transplantation.

Prognosis

The long-term outcome of patients with acute myocarditis varies by the initial presentation. The best outcome is for patients who present with asymptomatic ECG abnormalities. About 2/3 of pediatric patients with myocarditis recover completely.

Patients who present with acute fulminant myocarditis have the best recovery outcome if they survive the initial acute stage, with full recovery of ventricular function in >90% of patients in one series.

Overall, about 1/2 to 2/3 of pediatric patients with myocarditis show complete recovery, 10% have incomplete recovery and up to 25% either die or require heart transplantation. A higher mortality rate (up to 75%) has been described in newborn infants.

Case Scenarios

Case 1

History: A previously healthy 3-year-old boy is brought to the emergency room because he has been having abdominal pain and vomiting for the last 2 days. His family also noted that he has been less active than usual and looked pale. He had a low-grade fever 3 days ago and has not been eating well.

Physical examination: The patient's physical examination shows that he has mild dehydration. His RR is mildly increased at 36 bpm, HR 155 bpm, Temp 100.4°F, and BP 92/45. He has a 2/6 ejection systolic murmur, with capillary refilling time of 1–2 s. Rales are noted on auscultation. The patient's liver is felt 1.5 cm below right costal margin and the rest of his physical examination is unremarkable.

Investigative studies: His laboratory investigations show normal CBC. His metabolic workup is normal except for a CO_2 of 19 and BUN of 24. An ECG shows sinus tachycardia with nonspecific changes of ST segment and T waves. A chest X-ray reveals cardiomegaly with increased vascular markings.

Differential diagnosis: Based on the information obtained so far, it appears that this child has some degree of heart failure, based on the findings of tachycardia, tachypnea, hepatomegaly, cardiomegaly, and increased vascular markings on chest X-ray. Anemia as a cause for this presentation was ruled out with the normal CBC. Other causes such as endocarditis, myocarditis, or pericarditis must be considered. Undiagnosed congenital heart disease is also a possibility.

Final diagnosis: An echocardiogram is performed which shows dilatation of the left ventricle with decreased systolic function and moderate mitral regurgitation. In the ER the patient is orally rehydrated, but continues to have mild tachypnea and tachycardia. He is admitted to PICU for further management.

Assessment: This case is the typical presentation in this age group. It is usually preceded by a viral prodrome of either upper respiratory tract infection or gastroenteritis. Abdominal pain is common even in the absence of other gastrointestinal symptoms. Pallor and decreased activity are other common manifestations.

Management: This child is treated with intravenous inotropic support and diuretics. He recovers from the acute phase of the disease and is then discharged home on an oral ace inhibitor, aspirin, and a diuretic.

Case 2

History: An 8-month-old infant is brought to the emergency room by ambulance after what is thought to be a brief seizure episode. This infant was previously healthy and was playing at home when she suddenly became limp and unresponsive for a few seconds prior to regaining consciousness. She had a preceding upper respiratory tract infection and low-grade fever 5 days prior to this episode. She has otherwise been well with no change in her activity level or appetite.

Physical examination: On physical exam, the patient is fully awake and alert with mild tachypnea. Temp is 99.2°F, HR 160 bpm, RR 40/min, BP 85/39, and oxygen saturation of 99% in room air. Besides mild nasal congestion, her physical examination is unremarkable.

Investigative studies: Laboratory workup shows mildly elevated white cell count, with lymphocytic predominance. Her electrolytes are normal except for a total CO_2 of 14, with -12 base deficit on the blood gas and an anion gap of 25.

Differential diagnosis: The differential diagnosis remains quite broad at this time. This event represents an ALTE (acute life threatening event) and the differential includes: seizure, arrhythmia, syncope, breath holding spell, and sepsis among other possibilities. The lymphocytic predominance on her CBC may be secondary to her recent URI. However, the anion gap metabolic acidosis is more concerning; causes including hypoperfusion leading to lactic acidosis, diabetic ketoacidosis, and toxic ingestion must be considered.

Final diagnosis: The patient is observed on a cardiorespiratory monitor and rehydrated with IV fluids. During this observation period, she has another episode during which she becomes pale, dusky, and limp. Her cardiac monitor during the episode shows wide complex tachycardia at 240 bpm. Resuscitation is initiated and she is successfully cardioverted to sinus rhythm. The patient is then transferred immediately to a tertiary center. An echocardiogram performed upon arrival to the tertiary care center is significant for dilatation of the left ventricle with decreased systolic function.

Assessment: This is a less common presentation of acute myocarditis presenting with loss of consciousness secondary to ventricular arrhythmias. This represents a more fulminant presentation as it can lead to sudden death. This patient needs management in a pediatric cardiac intensive care with access to cardiovascular mechanical support that may be needed in case of arrhythmia unresponsive to medical therapy. This has a good recovery rate if the child survives the initial presentation.

Management: The patient is followed closely in the PICU. She is maintained on mechanical ventilation with inotropic support and diuretics during the acute phase of her illness. Following her initial rocky course, she is discharged home following a 2-week stay in the PICU.

Chapter 31
Cardiomyopathy

Zahra J. Naheed and Laura Torchen

Key Facts

- Dilated cardiomyopathy is the most common form of cardiomyopathy. It may be an end result of myocarditis. In most instances the etiology is unknown.
- Dilated cardiomyopathy causes poor cardiac output and pulmonary edema. Treatment includes diuretics to reduce preload, inotropic agents to improve cardiac contractility, and vasodilators such as ACE inhibitors to reduce after load.
- Hypertrophic cardiomyopathy is secondary to a genetic disorder.
- Presentation of hypertrophic cardiomyopathy may include arrhythmia, syncope, chest pain, or a heart murmur.
- Treatment of hypertrophic cardiomyopathy involves reduction of left ventricular outflow tract obstruction through negative inotropic agents and control of arrhythmias through drugs or an implanted defibrillator.
- Restrictive cardiomyopathy is a rare form of cardiomyopathy. Symptoms are due to systemic venous congestion and may include edema of GI tract resulting in anorexia and poor absorption.

Definition

Cardiomyopathy is a disease of the myocardium resulting in thickening of the myocardial fibers or fibrosis. Hypertrophic cardiomyopathy is characterized by thickening of the muscular walls of the ventricles, typically involving the ventricular septum. Dilated cardiomyopathy may also cause hypertrophy of the ventricular walls, however due to severe dilation of the ventricular chambers, they appear thin and stretched.

Z.J. Naheed (✉)
Department of Pediatrics, John H. Stroger, Jr. Hospital of Cook County,
5742 N. Chrishana Ave. 15, Chicago, IL 60659, USA
e-mail: amekha2000@yahoo.com

Ra-id Abdulla (ed.), *Heart Diseases in Children: A Pediatrician's Guide*,
DOI 10.1007/978-1-4419-7994-0_31, © Springer Science+Business Media, LLC 2011

Incidence

Cardiomyopathy is a chronic and variably progressive disease of the heart muscle that can present in various forms and in severe cases can lead to heart failure and sudden death. According to the Pediatric Cardiomyopathy Registry, 1 in 100,000 children are diagnosed with symptoms each year, with 30,000 children in the US affected annually if all forms of cardiomyopathy are considered together. However, it has to be noted that many asymptomatic and undiagnosed cases are unaccounted for in this survey. Infants less than a year old are ten times more likely to develop cardiomyopathy compared to children aged 2–18 years. Hypertrophic cardiomyopathy occurs at a rate of 5 per million children.

Pathology

Hypertrophic cardiomyopathy is characterized by abnormal growth and arrangement of muscle fibers, termed muscle disarray. The process starts in the ventricles and in severe cases can involve the wall of the atria. It can be acquired, secondary to a viral infection or chemotherapy, or inherited as an autosomal dominant, autosomal recessive, or X-linked disease such as the Barth Syndrome. Cardiomyopathy could also be secondary to a more generalized metabolic, mitochondrial, or multisystem disorder.

Cardiomyopathy can be mainly divided into two types: ischemic and nonischemic. Pediatric cardiomyopathy is almost exclusively nonischemic which is further divided into four types by the World Health Organization depending on the type of muscle damage:

- Dilated cardiomyopathy (58%)
- Hypertrophic (30%)
- Restrictive (5%)
- Arrhythmogenic Right Ventricular Cardiomyopathy, or ARVC (5%)

Dilated cardiomyopathy is most commonly idiopathic. Other cases are caused by viral infections such as coxsackie virus or HIV, secondary to toxins such as doxorubicin, or related to severe anemia or nutritional deficiencies.

In hypertrophic cardiomyopathy most commonly the left ventricle is the more affected chamber with the septum showing the most growth. The term for this phenomenon is the asymmetric hypertrophic cardiomyopathy. The thickening can sometimes be symmetric or concentric involving the entire left ventricular wall or localized to the apex in rare cases.

ARVC is an extremely rare disorder in children in which the muscles in the right ventricle become disorganized and are replaced with fibrous tissue. After starting as a patchy lesion, the process can gradually spread to involve the entire right ventricle and then to the left ventricle. The disorganization of the cells leads to arrhythmias and poor contractility.

Pathophysiology

Dilated cardiomyopathy leads to dilation and poor contractility of the ventricles. There is progressive mitral and tricuspid regurgitation. Eventually the patient develops signs of CHF and fluid overload.

Hypertrophic cardiomyopathy causes abnormal relaxation of the heart during diastole and secondary obstruction to venous return. In the terminal stages of this disease, the heart resembles those seen in a dilated cardiomyopathy.

In restrictive cardiomyopathy there is normal systolic function but abnormal relaxation. The ventricles turn rigid and show poor flexibility to expand. While the ventricles do not show any enlargement, the atria are grossly enlarged. The blood flow to the heart is restricted.

Clinical Manifestations

Cardiomyopathy is not gender, race, geography or age specific. About 50–60% of children with hypertrophic cardiomyopathy and 20–30% with dilated cardiomyopathy have a family history. Symptoms of hypertrophic cardiomyopathy could first manifest with the spurt of growth during puberty.

The clinical symptoms are very variable and can be absent, mild or severe. The general symptoms, not specific to any single type of cardiomyopathy, include tachypnea, poor feeding, and failure to thrive in infancy and poor exercise tolerance in older children. Gastrointestinal distress like nausea and vomiting can occur. There may be hepatomegaly, pedal edema and crackles in the lungs. Other presenting features may include a murmur, arrhythmias, chest pain and syncope.

In restrictive cardiomyopathy, common presenting symptoms include resting tachypnea, easy fatigability, syncope, chest pain, or dry cough. Cardiomyopathy may be associated with a metabolic disorder which may present with symptoms such as muscle weakness, decreased muscle tone, growth retardation, developmental delays, failure to thrive, or constant vomiting and lethargy. Rarely, there could be a stroke or seizures. There also may be an association with a malformation syndrome with dysmorphic features specific to the syndrome, such as short stature and webbed neck seen in Noonan's syndrome.

Diagnostic Testing

Any suspicion of cardiomyopathy should prompt a consult to the pediatric cardiologist. Echocardiogram is the most widely used and most informative noninvasive test for diagnosing cardiomyopathy (Fig. 31.1). With echocardiogram, the practitioner cannot only specify the type of cardiomyopathy but also determine the degree of dysfunction of the heart muscle. By echo one may

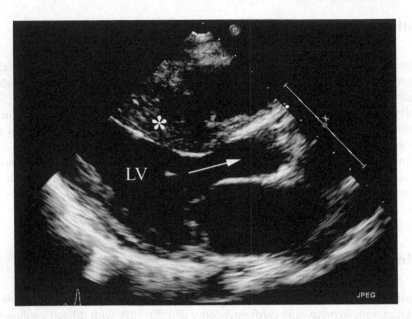

Fig. 31.1 Echocardiography: parasternal long axis: the ventricular septum is severely hypertrophied in an asymmetrical fashion causing narrowing and obstruction of the left ventricular outflow tract. *Asterisk*: interventricular septum, *arrow* indicates path of left ventricular outflow, *LV* left ventricle

measure the wall thickness, ejection fraction, chamber size, degree of obstruction, if any, and regurgitation of the mitral or tricuspid valves. Measurements of the pressures in the ventricles and the great vessels like the pulmonary artery may also be performed. Regular echocardiograms are required to assess the progress of the disease. In addition a chest X-ray, electrocardiogram and a 24–72 h Holter monitor are necessary for evaluation. A chest X-ray may show cardiomegaly or pleural effusion. An abnormal EKG may indicate a carrier status in the absence of symptoms.

In some cases there may be need for more invasive tests like radionuclide ventriculogram or cardiac catheterization. A radionuclide ventriculogram may be the best way to diagnose ARVD. Cardiac catheterization may be necessary in order to perform a muscle biopsy. This helps in evaluating for possible infections of the heart and certain metabolic diseases. Biopsy may also identify the fat in the muscle wall or ventricular structural damage for an ARVD diagnosis.

Certain biochemical, genetic and enzyme deficiency tests are needed before starting the most appropriate medical therapy. It is especially important to get a metabolic screening in children with cardiomyopathy under 4 years of age. This may require additional blood, urine and tissue testing in consultation with specialists such as geneticists or neurologists.

Management

The medical therapy in a child with dilated cardiomyopathy is aimed at accomplishing several goals:

1. Controlling the symptoms of congestive heart failure by using drugs such as ACE inhibitors and diuretics.
2. Improving the contractility by using dopamine and dobutamine in critically ill patients and digoxin orally as maintenance therapy.
3. Treating or preventing arrhythmias with antiarrhythmics such as amiodarone.
4. Preventing blood clots with anticoagulants like aspirin or warfarin.

Treatment specific to a child with hypertrophic cardiomyopathy includes:

1. Control of symptoms related to obstruction with calcium channel blockers or beta blockers like verapamil and propranolol.
2. Improvement of the filling of heart chambers.
3. Prevention of arrhythmias and sudden death with antiarrhythmics like amiodarone or disopyramide.

Patients with associated metabolic disorders may need careful dietary monitoring of fats, avoidance of fasting and possible daily carnitine orally.

Pacemaker implantation may be considered to monitor or stabilize bradycardia. Dual chamber pacing has been shown to decrease outflow obstruction in hypertrophic cardiomyopathy. An automatic internal cardioverter defibrillator is recommended in cases of severe life threatening arrhythmias, syncope, or history of resuscitation from a cardiac arrest.

Myectomy is the surgical removal of part of the thickened septal muscle that blocks the blood flow in hypertrophic cardiomyopathy. Even though it may control symptoms of heart failure secondary to obstruction, studies have not shown that this procedure prevents sudden death from arrhythmias or stops progression of the disease.

Heart transplantation is the last resort when patients reach the end stage of the disease. About 20% of symptomatic infants with cardiomyopathy require a cardiac transplant within the first year of life.

Extracorporeal membrane oxygenation (ECMO) may be used to sustain critical patients until a suitable organ is available. In addition, children greater than 50 kg are eligible for support by a device called "Left Ventricular Assist System" for about 3–12 months.

In addition to the patient, all first degree relatives must be screened with an echocardiogram and an EKG every 1–3 years until age 12 and more frequently up to the age of 21. Those with a family history of cardiomyopathy and no symptoms may continue screening every 5 years thereafter. If a specific genetic diagnosis is made all siblings should be genetically tested to assess their risk.

Prognosis

The overall prognosis depends on the type of cardiomyopathy and the age at first diagnosis. Up to 40% of children with a diagnosis of cardiomyopathy fail medical treatment within first year of diagnosis. Mortality and heart transplant rates are much higher in children with cardiomyopathy as compared to adults. For those children who acquire cardiomyopathy secondary to a viral infection 33% recover, 33% stabilize and 33% experience progression of their disease. Current 5-year survival for children diagnosed with hypertrophic cardiomyopathy is 85–95%, while it is 40–50% with dilated cardiomyopathy. In cases of restrictive cardiomyopathy there is a 2-year survival of 44–50%. Sudden cardiac deaths accounts for 50% of deaths in hypertrophic cardiomyopathy and 28% in restrictive cardiomyopathy.

Case Scenarios

Case 1

History: A 6-month-old girl is suspected of having reactive airway disease. For the past 2 months she has had several visits to the primary care physician for management of shortness of breath and wheezing. Inhaled bronchodilators were prescribed in the past with no significant improvement. Mother brought her because of concern of increasing effort to breathe and poor feeding.

Physical examination: The infant appeared pale and in mild to moderate respiratory distress with visible intercostal and subcostal retractions. There was no cyanosis or jaundice. Heart rate was 165 bpm; respiratory rate was 50/min. The oxygen saturation was 90% while breathing room air. Blood pressure in the right upper extremity was 60/50 mmHg. Peripheral pulses were equally diminished with prolonged capillary refill (3 s). The liver edge was palpated at 4 cm. below right costal margin, and the precordium was hyperactive with a prominent and laterally displaced apical impulse. Auscultation revealed bilateral rales and wheezing. A 3/6 harsh holosystolic murmur was heard over the apical region.

Diagnosis: Chest X-ray showed significant cardiomegaly with prominent pulmonary vasculature markings suggestive of pulmonary edema. Electrocardiography (ECG) showed biventricular enlargement with generalized flattening of T waves.

In view of physical findings on examination, cardiomegaly on chest X-ray, and ECG findings, cardiac pathology was suspected as the cause of the child's symptoms. Referral to a pediatric cardiologist confirmed this suspicion. An echocardiogram was performed which revealed dilated and poorly contracting ventricles with severe mitral regurgitation due to a dilated mitral valve ring. The coronary arterial origin appeared to be normal. Diagnosis of dilated cardiomyopathy was established. Laboratory studies for viral titers were obtained to investigate the possibility of viral myocarditis.

Treatment: the child was initially admitted to the intensive care unit for management of congestive heart failure and monitoring for arrhythmias. Diuretics and intravenous milrinone were used with improved evidence of cardiac output. These medications were transitioned to oral diuretics and an ACE inhibitor (enalapril). Viral myocarditis was ruled out in view of negative inflammatory markers and negative viral titers. Endomyocardial biopsy was performed revealing nonspecific myocardial fibrosis with no evidence of inflammation. The child's oral intake improved after few days and the child was discharged home. At the time of discharge the ventricular function was slightly improved, but continued to be depressed.

Case 2

History: A 2 year old was seen by the primary care physician at 5 years of age because of concern by mother that the child appeared to pass out for few seconds that same morning. Mother states that the child's father died suddenly last year but did not know why since they were separated. The child is otherwise healthy and not on any medications.

Physical examination: Heart rate was 100 bpm, regular. Respiratory rate was 30/min. Blood pressure in the right upper extremity was 110/65 mmHg. Oxygen saturation was 97% while breathing room air. Peripheral pulses were normal with brisk capillary refill. No hepatomegaly was detected. The precordium was hyperactive with a prominent and slightly laterally displaced apical impulse. A harsh 3/6 systolic ejection murmur was heard over the midsternum, no diastolic murmurs were detected.

Diagnosis: In view of the heart murmur, which was not previously appreciated, the child was referred for further evaluation to a pediatric cardiologist. The primary care physician was also concerned to hear of the sudden and unexplained death of the father. Chest X-ray revealed cardiomegaly and electrocardiography showed normal sinus rhythm with evidence of left ventricular hypertrophy. Echocardiography showed asymmetrical septal hypertrophy with left ventricular outflow (LVOT) obstruction. Pressure gradient across the LVOT was 50 mmHg. Diagnosis of hypertrophic cardiomyopathy was made.

Treatment: The child was started on a beta blocker to reduce left ventricular outflow obstruction and potentially minimize ventricular arrhythmias. A 24 Holter monitor was placed to assess for potential abnormal heart rhythm. Genetic counseling of the child and his two other siblings was also sought to determine if the child or his siblings have positive genetic markers for hypertrophic cardiomyopathy. The history of loss of consciousness was discussed with mother as potentially caused by significant arrhythmia or sudden exacerbation of LVOT obstruction. Referral to a pediatric electrophysiologist was arranged for further assessment of arrhythmias and potential need for implanted defibrillator.

Chapter 32
Cardiac Arrhythmias

William J. Bonney and Ra-id Abdulla

Key Facts

- An initial and crucial step in managing any child with a cardiac arrhythmia is to determine the hemodynamic stability of the child. A healthy pink color of skin/mucosa, brisk capillary refill, good peripheral pulses, normal blood pressure, and absence of respiratory distress are all reassuring signs that the hemodynamic status of the child is normal or near normal. Stable hemodynamics suggests that the cardiac output generated by the heart, despite the arrhythmia, is adequate.
- Management of children with stable hemodynamics allow the treating physician to use less invasive measures, such as inserting an intravenous line and using pharmacological agents. Failure to respond to medications will then require more invasive management such as pacemaker insertion in patients with bradycardia or the use of cardioversion in patients with tachyarrhythmias.
- Children with significant bradycardias resulting in hemodynamic instability may require atropine and/or epinephrine to increase the rate of the escape rhythm, particularly in patients who present with complete heart block and slow junctional rhythms. Transcutaneous pacing can be performed with most bedside external defibrillators, although this maneuver is quite painful. Thereafter insertion of pacemaker may be needed.

(continued)

W.J. Bonney (✉)
Division of Cardiology, The Children's Hospital of Philadelphia, 34th and Civic Center Blvd,
Philadelphia, PA, USA
e-mail: bonneyw@email.chop.edu

Ra-id Abdulla (ed.), *Heart Diseases in Children: A Pediatrician's Guide*,
DOI 10.1007/978-1-4419-7994-0_32, © Springer Science+Business Media, LLC 2011

Key Facts (continued)

- Tachyarrhythmias with stable hemodynamics can be treated with pharma-cological agents such as rapid intravenous bolus of adenosine in patients with SVT.
- A wide range of pharmacological agents are available for treating and preventing cardiac tachyarrhythmias. The more commonly used medications include beta-blockers, amiodarone, digoxin, and other agents. The specific type of antiarrhythmic agent, route of administration, and dose depends upon the type of arrhythmia and patient stability. These agents should be prescribed and administered under the supervision of a pediatric cardiologist. Many of these agents are listed in the Appendix section of this book.
- Truly unstable or pulseless tachyarrhythmias should be treated with prompt cardioversion.

Introduction

Abnormal heart rhythms, particularly those causing hemodynamic compromise, are not common in children; however, pediatricians are frequently faced with the responsibility to determine if a heart rhythm is normal in a child. Most of the time this is a straightforward issue, but sometimes because of the child's young age and anxiety, the task becomes more challenging.

Key clinical and electrocardiographic features of each arrhythmia are reviewed along with a basic management plan for each arrhythmia. It is important to remember that while the arrhythmia mechanisms encountered in children are the same as those seen in adults, the incidence of various arrhythmias is quite different in the two groups.

By knowing the patient's age, heart rate, and a brief history, the differential diagnosis can be narrowed substantially even before the first electrocardiogram (ECG) is obtained. It is crucial to remember the importance of the overall condition of the child (i.e. stable vs. unstable). This is the most important piece in the diagnosis and management of any arrhythmia. Children with stable hemodynamics can be observed or treated with oral medications. Unstable patients (delayed capillary refill, poor peripheral pulses, low blood pressure, pallor, and ashen skin discoloration) need urgent care which may include electrical cardioversion, initiation of cardiopulmonary resuscitation (CPR) and intravenous medications.

All rhythm strips in this chapter represent lead II.

Bradyarrhythmias

Sinus Bradycardia

Definition: Slow heart rate due to physiologic slowing of the sinus node. The lower limit of normal for heart rate varies with age (first year of life <100 bpm, 1–4 years <90 bpm, >5 years <60 bpm) (Fig. 32.1).
Recognition clues:

- A P wave precedes every QRS.
- A QRS follows every P wave.
- Normal P waves axis and morphology (upright in leads I and AVF).
- The PR interval is generally less than 200 ms.

Causes: Factors influencing the sinus node, such as vagal stimulation, hypothyroidism, sedative medications, etc. Almost every antiarrhythmic medication causes sinus bradycardia to some degree.
Management: Diagnose and treat the underlying cause of sinus bradycardia. In the case of symptomatic sinus bradycardia due to sinus node dysfunction with or without sinus pauses, atropine or epinephrine can be given to increase the sinus rate.

Ectopic Atrial Rhythm

Definition: A rhythm originating from a nonsinus source in the atrium. This can often be an escape rhythm seen when the sinus rhythm becomes very slow, or an accelerated ectopic atrial rhythm in the range of 70–90 bpm that is "outrunning" the sinus rate (Fig. 32.2).
Recognition clues:

- The P wave morphology is *abnormal* (often inverted in AVF).
- A P wave precedes each QRS.
- A QRS follows each P wave.

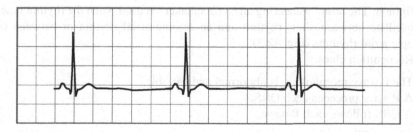

Fig. 32.1 Sinus bradycardia

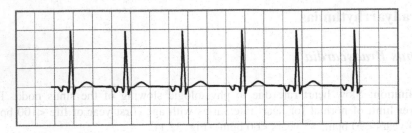

Fig. 32.2 Ectopic atrial rhythm

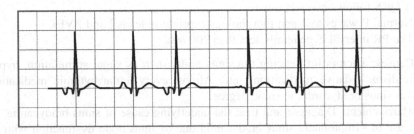

Fig. 32.3 Wandering atrial pacemaker

Causes: This rhythm is usually idiopathic. Rhythms originating from low in the atrium near the coronary sinus are not uncommon.

Management: Ectopic atrial rhythms are generally benign and require no treatment. They are often seen as escape rhythms in patients with injury to the sinus node following surgery for congenital heart disease.

Wandering Atrial Pacemaker

Definition: The term "wandering atrial pacemaker" is used when the rhythm is seen to oscillate between sinus rhythm and an ectopic atrial rhythm or between two ectopic atrial rhythms (Fig. 32.3).

Recognition clues:

- The P wave morphology is abnormal and variable.
- A P wave precedes each QRS.
- A QRS follows each P wave.

Causes: Idiopathic.

Management: This is generally a benign finding that does not require treatment.

Junctional Rhythm

Definition: A rhythm originating from the AV junction with a slow or low-normal heart rate (Figs. 32.4 and 32.5).

Recognition clues:

– P waves are absent or appear after the QRS in the T wave.
– QRS is narrow or identical to baseline sinus QRS morphology.

Causes: Slow junctional rhythms are usually escape rhythms that are seen with slowing of the sinus node rate. Junctional rhythms that slightly exceed the sinus rate (70–90 bpm range) are referred to as "accelerated junctional rhythms."

Management: Generally benign and require no treatment. Very slow junctional rhythms (<50 bpm) may indicate sinus node dysfunction or hypervagal tone.

First Degree AV Block

Definition: Sinus rhythm with a prolonged PR interval (typically greater than 200 ms). The term "First Degree AV Block" is somewhat of a misnomer because every atrial beat conducts to the ventricle, and hence there is delayed AV conduction, but no real AV "block." Regardless, the term is commonly used and accepted (Fig. 32.6).

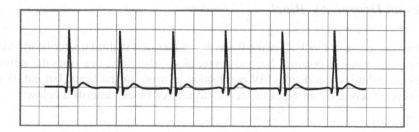

Fig. 32.4 Junctional rhythm

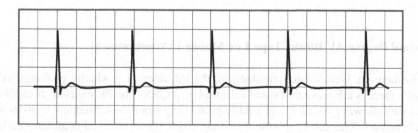

Fig. 32.5 Escape junctional rhythm

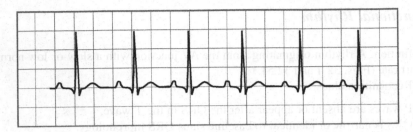

Fig. 32.6 First degree AV block

Recognition clues:

- A P wave precedes every QRS and a QRS follows every P wave.
- The PR interval is greater than 200 ms.

Causes: Anything producing conduction delay between the atrium and the ventricle will prolong the PR interval. Increased vagal tone will prolong conduction through the AV node. Conduction delay in the His–Purkinje system after heart surgery may prolong the PR interval as well. The PR interval is sometimes prolonged in rheumatic fever or Kawasaki disease.

Management: Generally benign and requires no treatment.

Second Degree AV Block

In first degree heart block all of the P waves conduct, and in third degree heart block none of the P waves conduct. Second degree block, therefore, describes the various bradyarrhythmias that display AV conduction on *some* of the beats, but not *all* of the beats. There are four types of second degree AV block, described below:

- Mobitz I
- Mobitz II
- 2:1 AV block.
- High Grade AV block

Second Degree AV Block: Type I or Mobitz I (Wenckebach)

Definition: In Wenckebach conduction, the PR interval gradually prolongs until finally there is a P wave that is not followed by a QRS. The PR interval shortens on the beat following AV block, gradually prolonging again on subsequent beats as the cycle repeats. This can be a normal finding, and is often observed in athletes during sleep. Every individual's AV node has an upper limit of conduction, and Wenckebach phenomenon is observed at this upper limit (Fig. 32.7).

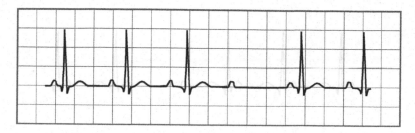

Fig. 32.7 Second degree AV block: Type I or Mobitz I (Wenckebach)

Recognition clues:

– This is an *irregular* rhythm.
– Gradual prolonging of the PR interval until finally a P wave does not conduct.
– The R–R interval between subsequent beats shortens as the PR interval prolongs.

Causes: Increased vagal tone, antiarrhythmic drugs or digoxin, and secondary to injury to the AV node after surgery for congenital heart disease.

Management: This is generally a benign finding that does not require intervention in the absence of symptoms. It is particularly common in well-trained endurance athletes. In symptomatic individuals temporary or permanent pacing may be required.

Second Degree AV Block: Type II or Mobitz II

Definition: Type II AV block does not display any gradual prolonging of the PR interval prior to AV block, rather, the PR interval remains the same and intermittently sinus beats are not conducted. Mobitz II, in contrast with Wenckebach conduction, is considered an abnormal finding (Fig. 32.8).

Recognition clues:

– This is an *irregular* rhythm.
– The PR interval on conducted beats remains constant.

Causes: Mobitz II block is often related to conduction system disease below the level of the AV node in the His bundle or the bundle branches.

Management: Symptomatic bradycardia with second degree heart block is an indication for temporary or permanent pacing. In asymptomatic infants who have undergone surgery for congenital heart disease, second degree heart block is an indication for pacing.

Second Degree AV Block: 2:1 AV Block

Definition: In two-to-one AV block, every other atrial beat does not conduct. Since there is never more than one conducted beat in a row, there is no opportunity to look for gradual prolongation vs. fixed PR intervals and hence, 2:1 AV block may represent Mobitz I or Mobitz II block (Fig. 32.9).

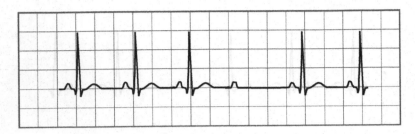

Fig. 32.8 Second degree AV block: Type II or Mobitz II

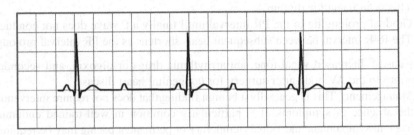

Fig. 32.9 Second degree AV block: 2:1 AV block

Recognition clues:

- This is a *regular* rhythm.
- The PR interval on conducted beats usually remains constant.

    Causes: 2:1 AV block has the same etiology as Mobitz I or Mobitz II block.
    Management: This arrhythmia is treated similarly to other types of second degree AV block.

Second Degree AV Block: High Grade AV Block

Definition: The term "high-grade AV block" applies to the patient with near complete heart block, but clear evidence of occasional conduction (Fig. 32.10).
    Recognition clues:

- Two or more P waves in a row are not followed by a QRS.
- Appears similar to complete heart block except occasional atrial beats have AV conduction.

    Management: Temporary or permanent pacing is indicated in symptomatic individuals.

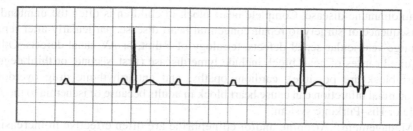

Fig. 32.10 Second degree AV block: high-grade AV block

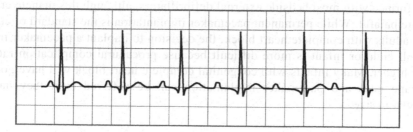

Fig. 32.11 Third degree AV block

Third Degree AV Block

Definition: Complete heart block is when atrial depolarization is not followed by ventricular depolarization due to block of conduction at the AV node. The P wave in these cases are not followed by QRS complexes throughout the rhythm strip (Fig. 32.11).

Recognition clues:

– The QRS rate should be *regular* in complete heart block. The atrial rate is also usually regular. Any irregularity in the ventricular rate should raise suspicion for intermittent AV conduction (second degree block).
– It is impossible to diagnose complete heart block unless there are more P waves than QRS complexes. For example, in a patient with a sinus rate of 60 bpm and accelerated junctional rhythm at 80 bpm, AV conduction cannot be evaluated because the ventricular rate is "outrunning" the atrial rate.
– QRS morphology depends on the escape rhythm in complete heart block. Most patients will have a junctional escape rhythm with regular, narrow QRS complexes. Patients with a ventricular escape rhythm will have wide QRS morphology.

Causes: Complete heart block can be congenital or acquired and is caused by conduction block at the level of the AV node, His bundle, or Purkinje conduction system. In some instances congenital complete heart block is caused by maternal lupus, although many mothers of infants with congenital heart block have no evidence of autoimmune disease. Complete heart block in children is often the unintended consequence of surgery to repair congenital heart disease, particularly after repair of large ventricular septal defects, tetralogy of Fallot, or AV canal defects. Other acquired causes of heart block include lyme disease (first, second, or third degree heart block are possible), cardiomyopathy, and antiarrhythmic drug overdose. Myocardial infarction can cause heart block in adults because of ischemia to the AV node or His–Purkinje system.

Management: Atropine and/or epinephrine are often effective in increasing the rate of the escape rhythm, particularly in patients who present with complete heart block and slow junctional rhythms. Transcutaneous pacing can be performed with most bedside external defibrillators, although this maneuver is quite painful. While permanent pacemaker implantation is the standard of care for adults with complete heart block, the decision to implant a pacemaker in a small child or infant is more difficult because procedural complication rates are higher. Many infants with congenital complete heart block will have good escape rates and pacemaker implantation can be deferred until they have grown in size.

Normal Sinus Rhythm

Definition: The normal cardiac rhythm originates from a collection of cells in the high lateral right atrium knows as the sinus node. Normal sinus rhythm is defined as a rhythm originating from the sinus node with a normal rate and normal AV conduction (Fig. 32.12).

Recognition clues:

- P wave axis is normal.
- A P wave precedes every QRS.
- A QRS follows every P wave.
- The PR interval is normal.

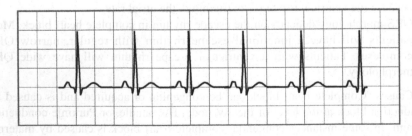

Fig. 32.12 Normal sinus rhythm (NSR)

Tachyarrhythmias

Sinus Tachycardia

Definition: Sinus tachycardia is the most common "arrhythmia" encountered in children, and is defined as normal tachycardia originating from the sinus node. The sinus node is sensitive to catecholamines and achieves maximal rates just above 200 bpm in most children. A rate of 220 bpm is a useful benchmark for differentiating sinus tachycardia from true arrhythmias, although some children (particularly newborns) can achieve sinus rates as high as 230 bpm (Fig. 32.13).
Recognition clues:

– "Warms up and cools down."
– Normal P wave morphology.
– Normal PR interval.
– Usually a regular narrow complex rhythm.
– Patients who have a preexisting wide QRS (i.e. s/p repaired congenital heart disease) will have a wide QRS during sinus tachycardia.

Causes: Pain, agitation, fever, beta agonist medications (such as albuterol), distress, dehydration, etc.
Management: Sinus tachycardia should be considered a normal response to stressors and stimulation rather than an arrhythmia. Once the diagnosis of sinus tachycardia has been confirmed, efforts should be made to diagnose and treat the secondary cause of tachycardia. Antiarrhythmic medications should not be used in patients with sinus tachycardia because they will blunt the body's compensatory response and will decrease cardiac output.

Supraventricular Tachycardia

Second to sinus tachycardia, supraventricular tachycardia (SVT) is by far the most common tachyarrhythmia seen in infants and children. The term

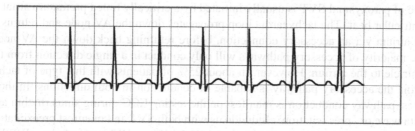

Fig. 32.13 Sinus tachycardia

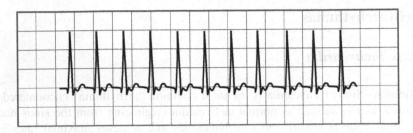

Fig. 32.14 Supraventricular tachycardia (SVT)

Table 32.1 Prevalence of SVT mechanism by age

	Infants (%)	Children (%)	Adolescents (%)
Accessory pathway mediated	80	60	30
AVNRT	10	30	60
Atrial tachycardia, flutter, fibrillation, and others	10	10	10

"supraventricular tachycardia" describes any arrhythmia that originates from above the ventricles or AV junction. AV nodal reentrant tachycardia (AVNRT) and orthodromic reciprocating tachycardia (ORT) account for about 90% of SVT encountered in children. These two arrhythmias have a similar clinical course and are often described with the term "paroxysmal SVT" (PSVT). Less common causes of SVT in children include atrial fibrillation, atrial flutter, ectopic atrial tachycardia, multifocal atrial tachycardia, and others (Fig. 32.14, Table 32.1).

Paroxysmal SVT: WPW and Tachycardia Mediated by an Accessory Pathway

Definition: Circus movement tachycardia (CMT), orthodromic reciprocating tachycardia (ORT), and AV reentrant tachycardia (AVRT) are all synonyms used to describe the most common type of SVT mediated by an accessory pathway. This type of paroxysmal SVT is usually initiated by a critically timed premature atrial or ventricular beat. The tachycardia loop propagates down the AV node and returns to the atrium via an accessory connection, before returning back down the AV node. The majority of accessory pathways will only conduct in a single direction from the ventricle to the atrium. However, in about 25% of patients with this type of tachycardia the accessory pathway is capable of conduction in both directions. In those cases, pathway conduction is manifest on the resting ECG during sinus rhythm as a delta wave or "preexcitation". Individuals with both SVT and manifest preexcitation on their baseline ECG are said to have Wolff–Parkinson–White syndrome (WPW).

Paroxysmal SVT: AV Node Reentrant Tachycardia

Definition: In terms of its clinical presentation, AVNRT is nearly indistinguishable from accessory pathway mediated tachycardia. Electrophysiologically, it is a reentrant arrhythmia that circles within the AV node or peri-AV nodal tissue. This arrhythmia is thought to occur when there are two extensions on the AV node (often referred to as "dual AV node pathways" or "dual AV node physiology"). The tachycardia loop travels down one extension and up the other, completing the reentrant loop.

Paroxysmal SVT recognition clues:

– Classically present as palpitations that start and stop abruptly.
– Usually 200–300 bpm.
– Always regular, usually narrow QRS tachycardia.
– Wide QRS (bundle branch block or SVT with aberrancy) is sometimes observed.
– Bimodal age distribution: most commonly encountered in infants or adolescents, but can be seen in any age group.
– Rarely associated with syncope.
– Patients with WPW syndrome will demonstrate a short PR interval and wide QRS during sinus rhythm (preexcitation).
– Shortness of breath and heart failure symptoms will develop after 12–24 h of continuous SVT.

Causes: Although accessory pathway connections and/or dual AV node physiology are anatomically present from the time of birth, tachycardia usually does not occur until it is initiated by a critically timed premature atrial contraction (PAC) or premature ventricular contraction (PVC). Hence, episodes of tachycardia tend to be relatively infrequent, but are often provoked by exercise or anxiety. Stimulant drugs like caffeine can provoke SVT episodes. Fever and respiratory infections can also provoke episodes, particularly when high doses of beta-agonist inhalants are required to manage the respiratory symptoms.

Management of acute SVT episodes: If given properly, adenosine should terminate any episode of paroxysmal SVT. Once sinus rhythm is restored, the patient is usually started on antiarrhythmic medication to prevent future episodes. While electrical cardioversion will also terminate SVT, it should be remembered that the vast majority of SVT episodes are relatively well tolerated. Cardioversion is only indicated as a first line therapy in the patient who is truly pulseless and appears lifeless.

Long-term management of paroxysmal SVT: Beta-blockers and digoxin are the most commonly used first line drugs for SVT. Verapamil could also be considered for first line therapy in an older patient. Drugs like Sotalol, Propafenone, Flecainide, and Amiodarone are considered when first line agents fail.

The majority of infants with SVT will "outgrow" the arrhythmia by 1 year of age and antiarrhythmic medications can be discontinued. In about one-third of cases, the arrhythmia will return later in life, usually in adolescence.

Catheter ablation is the definitive cure for SVT, and is equally effective for both AVNRT and pathway-mediated SVT. In general, success rates are over 95% with this procedure. Serious complications occur in less than 1% of procedures. Ablation can be considered as a first-line therapy for adolescents with SVT. In younger children (5–10 years old) ablation is also safe and effective, but is generally reserved for children who have frequent tachycardia or have failed medical therapy. While ablation is sometimes performed in infants and toddlers, the risk of complications like vascular compromise and heart block increases. Ablation in very young children is therefore reserved for patients with incessant refractory tachycardia that has not responded to maximal medical therapy.

Ectopic Atrial Tachycardia

Definition: Just as an Ectopic pregnancy occurs outside the normal intrauterine location, ectopic atrial tachycardia is similar to sinus tachycardia except that it occurs in an abnormal atrial location away from the sinus node. It differs from the previously mentioned forms of SVT because the mechanism is abnormal automaticity rather than reentry. Ectopic atrial tachycardia often occurs in short bursts. The rate can accelerate and decelerate (similar to sinus tachycardia) in a "warm up" or "cool down" fashion (Fig. 32.15).

Recognition clues:

- A P wave usually precedes every QRS.
- The PR interval is slightly prolonged (160–200 ms).
- P wave morphology in tachycardia is distinctly different from P wave morphology in sinus rhythm.

Causes:

- Ectopic atrial tachycardias can originate from anywhere in the atria, but most commonly originate near the pulmonary veins in the left atrium, or around the right atrial appendage or crista terminalis in the right atrium.

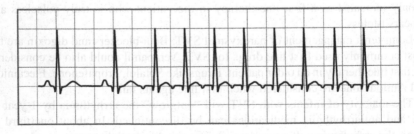

Fig. 32.15 Ectopic atrial tachycardia

- EAT can be provoked by systemic infections, particularly respiratory infections with fever.
- Inotropic medications like epinephrine can exacerbate EAT.

Management: Beta-blockers are first line therapy, although they are not as effective in EAT as in the more typical forms of reentrant PSVT. Second line agents like flecainide or amiodarone may be required. Nonsustained tachycardia may persist despite treatment. In refractory cases catheter ablation is an option.

Atrial Flutter

Definition: Atrial flutter is a reentrant arrhythmia confined to the atrium. In adults and older children, the most typical form has atrial rates of about 300 bpm. In infants, atrial rates can be 400 bpm and above. Ventricular rates will vary, and while 2:1 conduction is the most commonly observed finding in adults (atrial rate of 300 bpm and ventricular rate of 150 bpm), variable conduction can sometimes make this rhythm look irregular. Ultimately, the pulse rate during atrial flutter depends on the robustness of AV nodal conduction (Figs. 32.16 and 32.17).

Scars left in the atrium after surgery to repair congenital heart disease can serve as a substrate for unusual types of atrial flutter. In this setting, the arrhythmia is

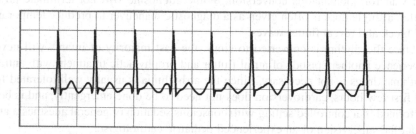

Fig. 32.16 Atrial flutter

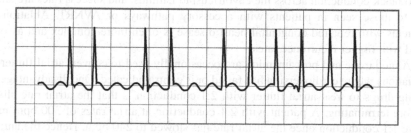

Fig. 32.17 Atrial flutter with variable atrioventricular conduction and irregular heart rhythm

referred to as "intra atrial reentrant tachycardia" (IART), and the atrial rates may be much slower than the 300 bpm seen in typical atrial flutter.

Recognition clues:

- Classically sawtooth pattern, especially in inferior leads.
- Atrial rate is always regular.
- Ventricular rate is usually regular, but may be irregular if there is variable AV conduction.
- Abnormal P wave morphology.
- Incessant behavior, unlike the paroxysmal or episodic types of SVT.
- Atrial rate is unaffected by adenosine.

Causes: In children, "typical" atrial flutter is much less common than other forms of SVT. It is more common in neonates and is often encountered in the newborn nursery. The key electrophysiologic substrate in "typical" atrial flutter is a zone of slow atrial conduction between the tricuspid valve and the inferior vena cava ("the cavotricuspid isthmus"). Conduction travels across this gap and through the atrium in a counterclockwise, or less commonly a clockwise direction. In the patient with repaired congenital heart disease, atriotomy scars may create other areas of slow conduction that serve as a substrate for the arrhythmia.

Management: Atrial flutter in infants is often managed with synchronized cardioversion. If available, transesophageal pacing can sometimes be successful in terminating atrial flutter and avoids the need for cardioversion. Atrial flutter will spontaneously resolve without cardioversion in many cases and often within 24 h. If the patient is tolerating the rhythm, it is reasonable to give digoxin or diltiazem and wait for spontaneous conversion. While adenosine will not terminate atrial flutter, a single dose is often given as a diagnostic maneuver to produce temporary AV block and reveal flutter waves.

Once the rhythm is converted to sinus, the vast majority of infants will never experience another episode of atrial flutter and prophylactic treatment with antiarrhythmic drugs is not necessary. Since the arrhythmia is usually well tolerated for the first few hours, cardioversion does not need to be done emergently, and is best performed in a controlled setting with conscious sedation or general anesthesia and under the supervision of an experienced pediatric cardiologist.

Catheter ablation is offered to older children and adults with atrial flutter, and provides a definitive cure for the arrhythmia. In a "typical" flutter ablation, the goal is to block conduction across the cavotricuspid isthmus, and success rates are similar to those seen in patients with accessory pathways or AVNRT. Ablation in patients with repaired congenital heart disease is often more complex and associated with higher recurrence rates.

Amiodarone and procainamide are occasionally used to convert atrial flutter in situations where cardioversion has failed or is contraindicated. One disadvantage of using drugs to treat atrial flutter with 2:1 conduction is that the atrial rate slows before terminating. A patient with 2:1 conduction at atrial rates of 300 bpm may have 1:1 conduction once the atrial rate has slowed to 240 bpm. Hence the antiarrhythmic drug may actually lead to an increased heart rate. AV nodal blocking agents like diltiazem or digoxin will not terminate atrial flutter, but are useful for controlling ventricular rates until cardioversion is performed.

Management Overview of Tachyarrhythmias

Tachyarrhythmias can be challenging to diagnose in children. The sinus node is capable of achieving rates in the low 200s and occasionally as high as 230 bpm. Sinus tachycardia at rates above 180 bpm is often seen in infants and young children with fever or agitation.

Assessment of vital signs and overall condition is the first and most important step in arrhythmia diagnosis and management. Truly unstable or pulseless tachyarrhythmias should be treated with prompt cardioversion. Otherwise, a proper 12 lead ECG should be obtained prior to administration of adenosine or other antiarrhythmic drugs. Single lead rhythm strips and bedside monitors can be misleading and a 12 lead ECG is the most important tool in choosing the correct diagnosis and management plan.

A fast tachyarrhythmia of any kind will eventually lead to congestive heart failure and decreased myocardial contractility. Patients who present 12–24 h after arrhythmia onset often complain of shortness of breath and fatigue and may have low blood pressure. As in other forms of cardiogenic shock, intravenous fluid boluses may worsen symptoms and should be avoided.

Adenosine is an invaluable tool for the treatment and diagnosis of supraventricular arrhythmias (Table 32.2). Adenosine is a safe medication due to its short half life. It is important to note the following issues when using adenosine:

– Adenosine should be administered through a large bore IV and followed immediately by a large saline flush (5–10 cc depending upon the length of the IV line

Table 32.2 Response of arrhythmias to adenosine

Arrhythmia	Response to adenosine
AVNRT	Terminates abruptly
Accessory pathway mediated SVT (ORT)	Terminates abruptly
Atrial flutter	Atrial rate is unaffected, ventricular rate slows briefly with AV block
Ectopic atrial tachycardia	Gradual slowing and termination followed by gradual reinitiation – two distinct P wave morphologies may be observed with sinus vs. ectopic beats
Sinus tachycardia	Gradual slowing with AV block, followed by gradual reinitiation – P wave morphology should remain unchanged throughout
Ventricular tachycardia	Ventricular rate is unaffected by adenosine, atrial rate may slow to reveal VA dissociation

to the patient). This is best accomplished with the use of a "T" connector that allows the adenosine and the flush to be attached simultaneously so the flush can be given immediately following the adenosine.

- In small infants, the volume of adenosine can be as small as 0.3 ml when only 1 mg is required. It may be helpful to dilute the medication to allow for a larger volume to ensure that all of the medication enters the circulatory system and remains in the IV line.
- Adenosine is rapidly metabolized in the bloodstream, so anything prolonging the transit time to the heart will potentially render the drug ineffective. Adenosine should always be injected into the most central vein that is available with the shortest external IV tubing possible. Despite this, adenosine can be effective when administered through a peripheral IV or even an intraosseous line if a large flush is given.
- Diminished cardiac output slows the velocity of blood through the veins, and hence prolongs adenosine's transit time from the IV to the heart. In patients with heart failure or patients who have developed heart failure from a prolonged tachyarrhythmia, larger doses of adenosine may be required and longer times (up to 20 s) may be observed from the time of injection to the observed effect.
- Atrial fibrillation, sustained or nonsustained, may be observed after a dose of adenosine is given and this may occur in as many as 10% of patients. While this rhythm is relatively well tolerated in most patients, patients with WPW may have rapid AV conduction during atrial fibrillation resulting in rapid ventricular rate.
- Since hemodynamic compromise is an unusual, but possible complication of adenosine administration, a crash cart with an external defibrillator should always be readily available when adenosine is administered.
- Adenosine is a bronchoconstrictor and its administration may cause pain. Its use is cautioned in patients with acute asthma exacerbation. Patients almost always have sinus tachycardia for 1–2 min following adenosine administration, which is possible secondary to pain. Patients with atrial flutter and 2:1 conduction may experience 1:1 conduction during the 1–2 min post-adenosine catecholamine surge with a resulting doubling of the heart rate.

Junctional Ectopic Tachycardia and Accelerated Junctional Rhythms

Definition: Junctional tachycardias are automatic arrhythmias arising from the AV junction. Junctional rhythms that slightly exceed the sinus rate are relatively benign and are referred to as "Accelerated Junctional Rhythms". For faster junctional tachycardias associated with hemodynamic compromise, the term "junctional ectopic tachycardia" (JET) is used. JET is frequently seen in the first 24 h following surgery

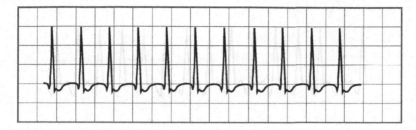

Fig. 32.18 Junctional ectopic tachycardia (JET)

for congenital heart disease. Patients undergoing extensive repair around the AV junction (Tetraolgy of Fallot, VSD repair, AV Canal repair, etc.) are particularly susceptible to JET (Fig. 32.18).

Recognition clues:

- A narrow complex tachycardia with no visible P waves
- Usually regular, but may be irregular.
- Displays "warm-up" and "cool-down" phenomenon.
- Unaffected by adenosine.

Causes: Accelerated junctional rhythms are idiopathic and for the most part benign. JET is most often seen in the postoperative period and may be related to inflammation or surgical trauma relating to the AV node or AV junction. In this setting, the arrhythmia may be exacerbated by fever, pain, inotropic infusions, or anything that provokes endogenous catecholamine release. Outside of the post-operative period, clinically significant JET is extremely rare.

Management: When JET occurs after cardiac surgery, the rhythm can usually be controlled by weaning inotropic medications, controlling fever and pain, and waiting for the arrhythmia to resolve. In severe cases, amiodarone or procainamide are used, sometimes in combination with ice to cool the patient's core temperature.

Ventricular Tachycardia

Definition: In the emergency department or EMS setting, ventricular tachycardia (VT) is most often encountered in older adults with coronary artery disease and/or heart failure and is often thought to be a more malignant or poorly tolerated arrhythmia than SVT. In the pediatric population, ventricular tachycardia usually occurs in children without structural heart disease or ventricular dysfunction. Hence VT is often reasonably well tolerated and may be strikingly similar to SVT in terms of its clinical presentation. Furthermore, SVT in children is often associated with wide QRS or bundle branch block aberrancy which makes it challenging to differentiate VT from SVT with aberrancy. The most reasonable strategy is to *treat all wide complex tachycardia as VT until proven otherwise.* "Monomorphic VT" describes a regular wide complex tachycardia with identical QRS morphology

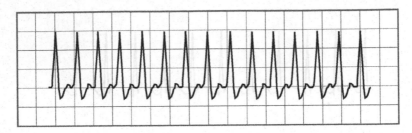

Fig. 32.19 Ventricular tachycardia (VT)

in each beat. "Polymorphic VT" describes an irregular wide complex tachycardia with beat-to-beat variations in the QRS morphology. "Torsade de points" describes polymorphic VT that occurs in the setting of a long QT interval (Fig. 32.19).

Recognition clues:

– Wide QRS tachycardia.
– History of structural heart disease.
– "VA dissociation" is pathognomonic for VT and is seen when the P wave or atrial rate is slower than the ventricular rate during tachycardia.
– Sinus capture or "fusion beats" are also pathognomonic and are seen as occasional narrow QRS beats during wide complex tachycardia.
– QRS duration greater than 130 ms.
– Rates of 160–250 bpm.

Causes: Ventricular tachycardia often occurs in the setting of underlying structural heart diseases, like hypertrophic cardiomyopathy, myocarditis, arrhythmogenic right ventricular dysplasia, cardiac tumors, and congenital heart disease (particularly tetralogy of Fallot or left sided obstructive lesions). Underlying electrical heart diseases like long QT syndrome, catecholaminergic polymorphic VT (CPVT), and Brugada syndrome are all causes of polymorphic VT.

Management: Cardioversion is the treatment of choice for patients who are pulseless or unstable. With rare exceptions, ventricular tachycardia will not respond to adenosine. However, adenosine is safe to give for the patient with VT, and is often given as a diagnostic maneuver to differentiate VT from SVT with aberrancy.

Correction of electrolyte abnormalities, especially in patients with long QT syndrome, is essential. Cardiology consultation is recommended before starting antiarrhythmic drugs for VT in the stable patient. Intravenous procainamide or amiodarone are usually effective first line treatments for VT. Verapamil is generally contraindicated in VT, but is useful in certain situations. In older children with stable monomorphic VT, catheter ablation is the definitive cure for this arrhythmia. In patients with unstable VT or with underlying disease like hypertrophic cardiomyopathy, an implantable cardioverter defibrillator (ICD) is often indicated.

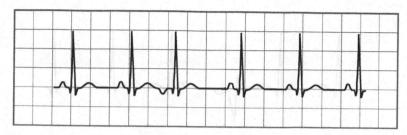

Fig. 32.20 Premature atrial contraction (PAC)

Premature Atrial Contraction

Definition: A single beat originating from a nonsinus location in the atrium that occurs prior to the next expected sinus beat, and is preceded by a premature P wave. Depending on how early the PAC occurs, the P wave will be followed by either a narrow QRS (conducted PAC), a wide QRS (aberrantly conducted PAC), or no QRS (nonconducted PAC) (Fig. 32.20).

Recognition clues:

- A premature P wave is seen.
- The P wave morphology usually differs from the sinus morphology.

Causes:

- Electrolyte disturbances
- Idiopathic
- Misplaced central venous lines or intracardiac devices with the tip in the atrium (typically right atrium)
- Common in newborns
- Inotropic infusions (epinephrine, dopamine, etc.)

Management: PACs are generally well tolerated and benign. Generally no treatment is required.

Premature Ventricular Contraction

Definition: A single wide QRS beat that occurs prior to the next expected sinus beat, and is not preceded by a premature P wave (Fig. 32.21).

Recognition clues:

- Always wide QRS
- Not preceded by a P wave

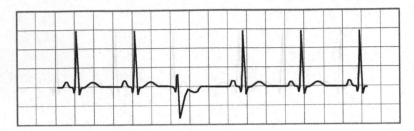

Fig. 32.21 Premature ventricular contraction (PVC)

Causes:

- Electrolyte disturbances
- Idiopathic
- Misplaced central venous lines or intracardiac devices with the tip in the ventricle (typically right ventricle)
- Digoxin toxicity
- Pericarditis and/or myocarditis
- Inotropic infusions (epinephrine, dopamine, etc.)
- Cardiomyopathy

Management: PVCs are generally well tolerated and benign, especially if the QRS morphology is identical with each PVC (monomorphic) indicating that PVCs are originating from a single ventricular focus. Generally no treatment is required. A thorough workup for underlying electrolyte abnormalities or structural heart disease should be performed before deeming the problem benign. Antiarrhythmic drug ingestions should be considered, particularly in toddlers, and one should inquire about bottles of antiarrhythmic drugs in the household.

Case Scenarios

Case 1

A 5-day-old newborn boy was observed in the neonatal ICU for sepsis. Blood cultures have been negative and the antibiotic course will continue for 2 more days. The baby is breathing room air spontaneously and is taking oral feeds well. The nurse noticed a sudden increase in heart rate to 260 bpm. The child appears stable with no change in respiratory rate, blood pressure, or oxygen saturation.

On examination, the capillary refill was slightly prolonged, peripheral pulses were 1+ with rapid heart rate. No hepatomegaly noted, heart sounds indicated tachycardia; murmurs were too difficult to appreciate in view of tachycardia.

The heart rhythm shown here was obtained through lead II ECG monitor.

ECG shows a heart rate of 280 bpm, regular. P waves were difficult to determine, QRS duration was normal. This is consistent with SVT (Fig. 32.22).

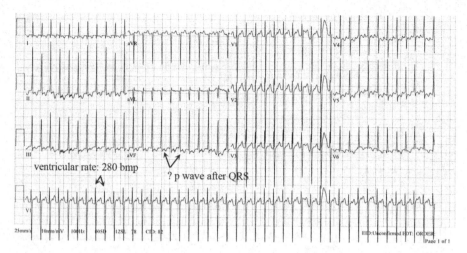

ventricular rate: 280 bmp

? p wave after QRS

Fig. 32.22 SVT. Heart rate is approximately 280 bpm, P waves not clearly seen. Narrow QRS complexes

Adenosine IV bolus was given with sudden break of rapid heart rate to 140 bpm.

CXR and 12-lead ECG should be obtained. ECG was within normal limits with no evidence of Wolff–Parkinson–White syndrome. It is advisable to obtain a pediatric cardiology consult for further assessment and follow-up. An echocardiogram would also be useful because up to 20% of children with SVT also have congenital heart disease. The child should be started on maintenance antiarrhythmic therapy (usually digoxin or propranolol) and monitored in the hospital for 48 h after starting therapy to ensure that tachycardia does not recur. Otherwise tachycardia recurrence is very likely in the first year of life. Also, the parents should be counseled on how to check the infant's heart rate at home because the baby will not be able to communicate the feeling of palpitations in the event of a recurrence.

Case 2

A 2-month-old infant was seen by the primary care physician for a well child care visit. Mother says that the child is doing well; however, she noticed that he tends to sleep more and feed less than her previous child. The baby is a product of full-term gestation. Mom did well during gestation except for rash and joint pain which resolved spontaneously.

On examination, the baby appears well with pink mucosa, no jaundice. Heart rate was 45 bpm, regular, respiratory rate was 45 min and oxygen saturation was 95%. Capillary refill was slightly prolonged and pulses were 1+ throughout all four extremities. Mild hepatomegaly is present. The precordium reveals forceful heart beats; however, bradycardia is again noted through palpation of the chest and auscultation. No added murmurs were detected.

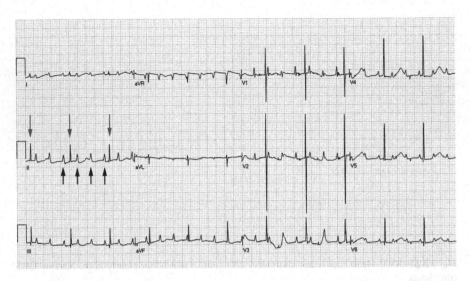

Fig. 32.23 Complete heart block. *Black arrows* point to P waves, while *red arrow* point to QRS complexes. There is no association between the atrial (P waves) and ventricular (QRS waves) rhythms

Twelve-lead ECG performed is shown here, Fig. 32.23. The P waves axis was normal, atrial rate appears to be 150 bpm, while ventricular rate was 66 bpm, there appears to be no correlation between P waves and QRS complexes indicating complete heart block.

Congenital complete heart block is suspected and the mother underwent investigative studies for lupus erythematosus which were positive. The child was admitted to the intensive care unit where he received an implanted pacemaker to improve the heart rate. The mother was advised to undergo fetal echocardiographic evaluations of future pregnancies.

Case 3

Sixteen-year-old athlete presents with palpitations. The young man complains that he experiences irregular heartbeats with occasional "heavy beat." Palpitation is typically experienced while at rest and not during exercise. The young man is a member of the high school football team and is seeking clearance to continue on the team. Patient denies use of any medications, illicit drugs or steroids. He has been healthy with no significant family history.

On examination Heart rate was 65 bpm with occasional irregularity. Respiratory rare was 18/min; oxygen saturation was 97% while breathing room air. Blood pressure in right upper extremity was 110/70 mmHg and in the right lower extremity was 112/67 mmHg. The mucosa was pink with good peripheral pulses and perfusion

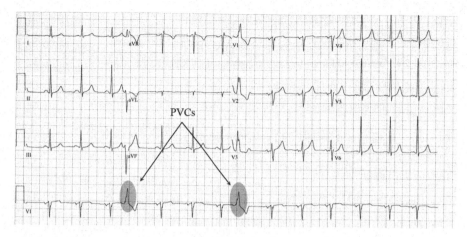

Fig. 32.24 PVC. Premature, wide QRS complexes, not preceded by P waves with compensatory pause after each premature ventricular contraction

and brisk capillary refill. No hepatomegaly. Precordium was quiet with normal right and left ventricular impulses and no palpable thrill. Heart sounds were within normal limits with no added murmurs. Occasional irregularity in heart rhythm was again noted.

Twelve-lead ECG was obtained, shown here, Fig. 32.24. This revealed normal sinus rhythm (upright P wave in leads I and aVF) with normal PR interval, QRS duration, QT and QTc durations. Early, wide QRS complexes are present, not preceded by a P wave. No evidence of chamber hypertrophy. The ECG is consistent with premature ventricular contractions.

The history and physical examination were suggestive of premature atrial or ventricular complexes. ECG confirms the presence of premature ventricular contractions. The fact that these occur during rest and seem to resolve with exercise is reassuring that these PVCs are benign, however, due to the young man's interest in sports, it is worthwhile ensuring that the premature ventricular contractions do not reflect a myocardial disease such as cardiomyopathy.

Echocardiography revealed normal cardiac structure and function. A treadmill stress test was also performed which again shows premature ventricular contractions, with uniform morphology and resolution with exercise, all consistent with benign premature ventricular contractions. Worrisome features of the ventricular premature beats would have included multiform PVCs (different shapes of QRS complexes in the same lead), poor myocardial function or worsening of PVCs with exercise. This young man did not exhibit any of these features and was therefore cleared to participate in sports.

Part IV
Office Cardiology

Chapter 33
Hypertension

Shada Al-Anani and Ra-id Abdulla

Key Facts

- Hypertension should not be diagnosed till blood pressure is repeated 2–3 times to confirm findings.
- When evaluating blood pressure in children, gender, age and height should be taken in consideration.
- Hypertension is when blood pressure measurements are above the 95th percentile for age, gender and height.
- Prehypertension is when blood pressure measurements are between the 90th and the 95th percentile for gender, age, and height.
- Primary hypertension is the most common cause of hypertension in children older than 2 years of age.
- Secondary hypertension must always be ruled out in children prior to making the diagnosis of primary hypertension.
- Primary hypertension is more common in obese children, particularly those with positive family history.

Definition

Hypertension is elevation of systemic blood pressure above the 95th percentile for age and gender. Blood pressure consists of systolic and diastolic measurements. In most instances, both components are elevated, however, occasionally only the systolic blood pressure may be elevated (systolic hypertension).

The importance of detecting hypertension in the pediatric age group is recent. This issue is gaining attention due to the growing epidemic of obesity and concern

---

Ra-id Abdulla (✉)
Center for Congenital and Structural Heart Diseases, Rush University Medical Center,
1653 West Congress Parkway, Room 763 Jones, Chicago, IL 60612, USA
e-mail: rabdulla@rush.edu

Ra-id Abdulla (ed.), *Heart Diseases in Children: A Pediatrician's Guide*,
DOI 10.1007/978-1-4419-7994-0_33, © Springer Science+Business Media, LLC 2011

of future development of cardiovascular risks in these populations of pediatric patients. National health surveys (NHANES I–IV) done between 1963 and 2002 show progressively increasing trends of high blood pressure among children and adolescents for the last decade. Racial and ethnic disparities were also found; Hispanic and Black Americans being the most affected. This should alert pediatricians of the responsibility for early prevention of obesity and subsequently hypertension in an effort to control this trend. The relationship of obesity and hypertension was established through numerous studies and it is now believed that increased body mass index (BMI) in children represents a risk factor for hypertension and cardiovascular disease during adult years. Furthermore, family history of hypertension, diabetes and stroke predict development of hypertension for children as they become adults. These factors emphasize the importance of monitoring childhood obesity as well as exploring risk factors such as family history of cardiovascular risk ailments.

Routine blood pressure screening for 3-year-old children is required during routine pediatric visits. Assessment of blood pressure in younger children is important for patients with risk factors such as congenital heart disease or suspected kidney disease, prolonged neonatal ICU stay, and umbilical arterial catheterization.

Obtaining an accurate measurement of blood pressure is crucial, typically through an automated oscillometric device. Measurements should be confirmed manually if the blood pressure is more than 90th percentile for height or age. In this situation BP should be measured using auscultation with mercury sphygmomanometry or a calibrated aneroid device using the first and the fifth Korotkoff sounds as the systolic and diastolic pressures respectively. An appropriate size cuff bladder 80–100% of the arm conference covering two-thirds of the length of the upper arm should be used to avoid erroneous elevation blood pressure when using smaller cuffs.

The National High Blood Pressure Education Program (NHBPEP) Working Group revised the definition of normal and elevated BP in children in 2004 and updated normal values for systolic and diastolic blood pressure in children and adolescents based on age, gender and height as following:

- Prehypertension is defined as systolic and/or diastolic BP ≥90th percentile, but <95th percentile for age and height.
- Hypertension is defined as either systolic and/or diastolic BP ≥95th percentile or if BP exceeds 120/80 mmHg even if <95th percentile is measured on three or more occasions.

The severity of hypertension is further categorized in two stages:

- Stage 1: BP ranging from 95th percentile to 5 mmHg above the 99th percentile
- Stage 2: BP is higher than 5 mmHg above 99th percentile

Ambulatory 24-h blood pressure monitoring provides a better understanding of the values of BP throughout the day. This method correlates better with end organ damage than one time blood pressure measurement at the physician's office. This is particularly useful to rule out white coat hypertension and nocturnal hypertension.

It can also identify patterns of elevated blood pressure which can be diagnostic in certain types of secondary hypertension and also in follow up of patients with known hypertension.

Types of Hypertension

Two types of hypertension are recognized: primary hypertension and secondary hypertension. The incidence of secondary hypertension is more common in children than in adults, but recent studies have shown that primary/essential hypertension has become increasingly more frequent, increasing from 23% in 1994 to about 50% in another study conducted in 2001; most of these patients had positive family history and a BMI of more than 95th percentile for age. Causes of secondary hypertension include renal parenchymal disease which constitutes the majority of the cases like reflux nephropathy and renovascular diseases (e.g. renal artery stenosis) in 8–10%. Coarctation of the aorta accounts for only 2% of cases. Less common causes are endocrine and central nervous system diseases.

Prevalence

Large survey studies and school based surveys conducted between 2003 and 2006 showed increasing incidence in hypertension amongst children. The prevalence of systolic hypertension on age adjusted rates was found to be 3.3, 4.2, and 4.6% for blacks, whites and Mexican Americans, respectively. This is an increase in prevalence from previous studies by 1% for hypertension and by 2.6% for pre-hypertension. Recent studies show even higher percentages.

An important factor related to hypertension is obesity. Overweight children increased the odds of hypertension up to 2–3 times. Ethnicity was also implicated, even after adjusting for BMI, when comparing Hispanic to white boys, this difference disappeared in females.

Pathophysiology

Essential hypertension is of unknown etiology. Nevertheless, different factors have been implicated including hereditary/genetic alterations, obesity, salt intake, and stress. Genetic factors include renin–angiotensin system, insulin sensitivity, calcium and sodium transport, and reactivity of the smooth muscles of the blood vessels which may explain the polygenic inheritance in familial hypertension.

Secondary hypertension on the other hand is due to identifiable causes, such as:

- Renovascular disease such as renal artery stenosis which leads to stimulation of the rennin secretion from the juxtaglomerular apparatus due to decrease in blood flow in the afferent arteriolar system of the kidney and in turn renin converts angiotensinogen to angiotensin, which has dual effect as a potent vasoconstrictor and as a stimulant to aldosterone secretion which causes water and salt retention.
- Renal parenchymal lesions such as nephritis lead to decreased glomerular filtration rate resulting in salt and water retention. Renal tumors have either mass effect on the renal arterioles (solid tumors or cysts) or loss of biofeedback to renin excretion such as in Wilms' tumor.
- Endocrinopathies may induce hypertension via different mechanisms, hyperthyroidism causes tachycardia and systolic hypertension, hyperparathyroidism and resultant hypercalcemia lead to increase in vascular tone. Primary or secondary mineralocorticoid excess secretion will result in salt and water retention, thus leading to hypertension. Pheochromocytomas secrete catecholamines (epinephrine and norepinephrine) that can give rise to intermittent but most commonly persistent hypertension secondary to inotropic and chronotropic cardiac effects and increased vascular resistance.
- Intracranial lesion may affect the sympathetic flow from the central nervous system and lead to hypertension.

All the implicated mechanisms ultimately lead to increase in cardiac output and/or peripheral vascular resistance and consequently lead to elevated blood pressure.

Diagnosis

Evaluation of patients with hypertension should involve measuring BP two times during the initial visit separated by 2 min. In addition, BP should be measured in the upper right extremity as well as the lower extremity to rule out coarctation of the aorta. Diagnosis cannot be made unless BP is shown to be elevated on three separate occasions (Tables 33.1 and 33.2).

Careful history and physical examination is warranted to identify patients at risk for cardiovascular disease: obesity and family history of premature cardiovascular disease, diabetes, and renal disease. Furthermore, it is essential to look for clues of secondary hypertension during physical examination as well as assessment of end organ damage, evaluation of optic fundi, thyroid gland, and abdominal or carotid bruit.

Initial work up should include complete blood count, serum electrolytes, blood urea nitrogen and creatinine, urinalysis and urine culture, and renal Doppler ultrasound.

All hypertensive patients should undergo two-dimensional echocardiography to evaluate left ventricular hypertrophy. Furthermore, lipid profile and fasting blood glucose level should be assessed for patients with suspected primary hypertension and/or obesity.

Table 33.1 Blood pressure levels for boys by age and height

Age (in years)	Systolic BP (range for each percentile reflects range of height)			Diastolic BP (range for each percentile reflects range of height)		
	50th Percentile	90th Percentile	95th Percentile	50th Percentile	90th Percentile	95th Percentile
1	80–89	94–103	98–106	34–39	49–54	54–58
2	84–92	97–106	101–110	39–44	54–59	59–63
3	86–95	100–109	104–113	44–48	59–63	63–67
4	88–97	102–111	106–115	47–52	62–67	66–71
5	90–98	104–112	108–116	50–55	65–70	69–74
6	91–100	105–113	109–117	53–57	68–72	72–76
7	92–101	106–115	110–119	55–59	70–74	74–78
8	94–102	107–116	111–120	56–61	71–76	75–80
9	95–104	109–118	113–121	57–62	72–77	76–81
10	97–106	111–119	115–123	58–63	73–78	77–82
11	99–107	113–121	117–125	59–63	74–78	78–82
12	101–110	115–123	119–127	59–64	74–79	78–83
13	104–112	117–118	121–130	60–64	75–79	79–83
14	106–115	120–128	124–132	60–65	75–80	80–84
15	109–117	122–131	126–135	61–66	76–81	81–85
16	111–120	125–134	129–137	63–67	78–82	82–87
17	114–122	127–136	131–140	65–70	80–84	84–89

Table 33.2 Blood pressure levels for girls by age and height

Age (in years)	Systolic BP (range for each percentile reflects range of height)			Diastolic BP (range for each percentile reflects range of height)		
	50th Percentile	90th Percentile	95th Percentile	50th Percentile	90th Percentile	95th Percentile
1	83–90	97–103	100–107	38–42	52–56	56–60
2	85–91	98–105	102–109	43–47	57–61	61–65
3	86–93	100–106	104–110	47–51	61–65	65–69
4	88–94	103–109	107–113	50–54	64–68	68–72
5	89–96	104–112	108–116	52–56	66–70	70–74
6	91–98	104–111	108–115	54–58	68–72	72–76
7	93–99	106–113	110–116	55–59	69–73	73–77
8	95–101	108–114	112–118	57–60	71–74	75–78
9	96–103	110–116	114–120	58–61	72–75	76–79
10	98–105	112–118	116–122	59–62	73–76	77–80
11	100–107	114–120	118–124	60–63	74–77	78–81
12	102–109	116–122	119–126	61–64	75–78	79–82
13	104–110	117–124	121–128	62–65	76–79	80–83
14	106–112	119–125	123–129	63–66	77–80	81–84
15	107–113	120–127	124–131	64–67	78–81	82–85
16	108–114	121–128	125–132	64–68	78–82	82–86
17	108–114	122–127	125–131	65–68	78–82	82–86

Adapted from The Fourth Report on the Diagnosis, Evaluation, and Treatment of High Blood Pressure in Children and Adolescents

Screening patients for secondary causes of hypertension should be carefully examined since younger patients and those with more severe hypertension are more likely to have secondary cause for hypertension. The most common cause for secondary hypertension is renal disease. Coarctation of the aorta constitutes one-third of cases of hypertension in the neonatal period, however, only 2% of childhood hypertension. Residual hypertension can also be found in patients post repair of coarctation. Another important reversible secondary hypertension in adolescents is drug abuse and if suspected these patients should undergo drug screening test (Table 33.3).

Table 33.3 Features which may suggest particular etiology of hypertension

Finding on physical examination	Possible etiology
Vital signs	
Tachycardia	Hyperthyroidism, pheochromocytoma, neuroblastoma, primary hypertension
Decreased lower extremity pulses; drop in BP from upper to lower extremities	Coarctation of the aorta
Obesity (high BMI)	Primary hypertension
Inspection	
Skin lesions	
Truncal obesity	Cushing syndrome and insulin resistance syndrome
Moon facies	Cushing syndrome
Enlarged thyroid gland	Hyperthyroidism
Pallor, flushing, and diaphoresis	Pheochromocytoma
Acne, hirsutism, and striae	Cushing syndrome and anabolic steroid abuse
Café au lait spots	Neurofibromatosis
Adenoma sebaceum	Tuberous sclerosis
Malar rash	Systemic lupus erythematosus
Growth retardation	Chronic renal failure
Joint swelling	Systemic lupus erythematosus and collagen vascular disease
Ambiguous/virilization	Adrenal hyperplasia
Palpation	
Palpable kidneys	Polycystic kidney disease, hydronephrosis, multicystic-dysplastic kidney
Mass	Wilms' tumor, neuroblastoma, and pheochromocytoma
Auscultation	
Systolic ejection murmur over back	Coarctation of aorta
Epigastric/flank bruit	Renal artery stenosis
Genetic syndromes	
Turner syndrome: Widely spaced nipples, and webbed neck	Coarctation of aorta
Williams syndrome: Elfin face, friendly disposition, and mental impairment	Peripheral arterial stenosis

Adapted from Flynn JT. *Prog Pediatr Cardiol*. 2001;12:177–188

Rare endocrine disorders causing hypertension includes pheochromocytoma and hyperthyroidism, endogenous or exogenous causes of excess corticosteroids. Severe hypertension with bradycardia can be secondary to increase intracranial pressure. Metabolic disorders/toxic reactions like hypercalcemia and lead poisoning can also produce hypertension.

Treatment

Modification of life style is a crucial aspect of management. Weight reduction, healthy diet, regular exercise, and avoidance of sedentary life style are essential aspects of such modification. Diet should aim to increase fruit and vegetable intake and consume low fat dairy products with reduced saturated fat and decrease in salt intake. These principals are described in the DASH diet (dietary approach to stop hypertension).

The deleterious role of smoking, alcohol intake, drug abuse, anabolic steroids in hypertension should be explained to adolescents, and strongly discouraged.

Decision to start pharmacotherapy in children should be based on the severity and the underlying cause of hypertension in addition to target organ damage. The 2004 NHBPEP guidelines indicate that pharmacologic therapy should be initiated in the following categories of patients:

- Patients with symptomatic HTN (e.g. headache, seizures, chest pain, palpitations, or shortness of breath).
- End organ damage secondary to hypertension mostly left ventricle hypertrophy, or less frequently retinal changes.
- Stage 1 HTN should be treated only if failed 4–6 months trial of therapeutic life style modification or if associated with diabetes or other cardiovascular disease risk factor like smoking or dyslipidemia.
- Severe or Stage 2 HTN defined as BP levels that are 5 mmHg greater than the 99th percentile should be started on pharmacotherapy immediately.

Limited data is available regarding the choice of antihypertensive medications in children. Extrapolated data from adult studies suggest that first line medications in patients with essential hypertension should include thiazide diuretics or beta-blockers. ACE (angiotensin converting enzyme) inhibitors or angiotensin receptor blocker should be the first choice of medications in patients with hyperlipidemia, diabetes, chronic renal disease, or congestive heart failure due to their possible role in slowing the progression of diabetic and nondiabetic renal disease. On the other hand, ACE inhibitors should be avoided in patients with suspected secondary hypertension undergoing investigations or in patients with established diagnosis of renal artery stenosis either bilateral or in unilateral with single kidney, chronic renal failure with serum creatinine above 35% of the baseline, or hyperkalemia. ACE inhibitors are also known to be teratogenic and so they are not recommended in adolescent girls who might be pregnant. Please refer to drug doses and effects in the Pediatric Cardiology Pharmacopoeia chapter in this book.

The goal of therapy should be to correct blood pressure to be lower than the 95th percentile for age and height or the 90th percentile for age and height if hypertension is associated with other CVS risk factors. If the goal of therapy is not achieved with the initial dosage, then gradual increase in dose is recommended till maximum dose is reached. Failure to achieve target blood pressure with maximum dose should be followed by adding a second medication.

Case Scenarios

Case 1

History: A 14-year-old African American male was noted to have elevated blood pressure during physical examination prior to clearance for sports participation at school. Blood pressure taken from right arm was 130/85 mmHg. Family history is positive for myocardial infarction in a 55 y/o father.

Physical examination: This revealed normal physical examination. Blood pressure in upper and lower extremities were 133/92 and 136/92 mmHg, respectively. BMI was 29.

Diagnosis: This child has elevated blood pressure measurements; however, diagnosis of hypertension should not be made till repeat blood pressure measurements confirm diagnosis. Two months later blood pressure measurements were consistently elevated. Further work up should include urinalysis and basic metabolic panel, lipid profile, and fasting blood glucose to assess for secondary hypertension.

Treatment: Obesity in this child is a potential cause for hypertension; therefore healthy diet and increased physical activity are essential as first line therapy measures in this young man. Failure to control blood pressure with diet and physical activity may necessitate initiation of medical therapy with thiazide diuretics.

Case 2

History: A 4-year-old boy was found to have elevated blood pressure during a well child examination. The child was a product of full-term gestation with no complications. Past medical history is not significant.

Physical examination: Heart and respiratory rates were within normal limits. Oxygen saturation is 99% while breathing room air. Blood pressure in right upper extremity is 121/77 and in the right lower extremity 122/73 mmHg. The peripheral pulses were strong and the capillary refill was brisk. No hepatomegaly was detected. Heart sounds were normal with no murmurs detected.

Diagnosis: The blood pressure in this child is significantly elevated. Repeat measurements are warranted, however, this is unlikely due to anxiety.

Urinalysis and culture and a basic metabolic panel were obtained, these revealed elevated BUN and creatinine (30 and 1.3, respectively). Therefore renal hypertension is suspected.

Treatment: referral to a pediatric nephrologist is warranted for further work up of renal pathology. Renal ultrasound and Doppler was performed and revealed small kidneys, no signs of renal artery stenosis. Echocardiography was performed to assess for left ventricular hypertrophy secondary to hypertension. Treatment is directed to cause of renal disease as well as antihypertensive therapy using pharmacological agents.

Chapter 34
Syncope

Yolandee R. Bell-Cheddar and Ra-id Abdulla

Key Facts

- Neurocardiogenic syncope is the most common type of syncope; it is caused by reduced pre-load to the heart, such as with standing up and exaggerated by conditions of dehydration. The dominant heart rate feature in these patients at the time of syncope is bradycardia.
- Postural orthostatic tachycardia syndrome (POTS) is caused by excessive tachycardia when moving from supine to upright position causing reduction in blood pressure leading to dizziness or syncope. Unlike neurocardiogenic syncope, the dominant heart rate feature at time of syncope is tachycardia.
- Patients with prolonged QT syndrome are prone to ventricular arrhythmias which may present as syncope or sudden death.
- Brugada syndrome typically presents in adults but may present in children. Patients may present with syncope or sudden death. Diagnosis is made by typical ECG finding of ST elevation in the right precordial leads as well as right bundle branch block type picture.
- Left ventricular outflow obstructive lesions such as hypertrophic cardiomyopathy or severe aortic stenosis may present with syncope or sudden death due to acute drop in cardiac output.
- Abnormal origin of coronary arteries may cause these vital arteries to be compressed during periods of increase cardiac output, such as exercise, leading to syncope or sudden death.

Definition

Syncope is a transient, sudden, loss of consciousness. It is associated with a loss of postural tone, recovery tends to be spontaneous. The general etiology of syncope is cerebral ischemia, inadequate oxygen or glucose supply to the brain.

Y.R. Bell-Cheddar (✉)
Department of Pediatric Cardiology, Rush University Medical Center, 1122 N. Oakley Drive NW Apt. 107, Westmont, IL 60559, USA
e-mail: yollybeecee@yahoo.com

Ra-id Abdulla (ed.), *Heart Diseases in Children: A Pediatrician's Guide*,
DOI 10.1007/978-1-4419-7994-0_34, © Springer Science+Business Media, LLC 2011

Near Syncope (Presyncope) – includes the preceding symptomatology of syncope without the actual loss of consciousness. This includes dizziness, nausea, and sweating.

Incidence

Up to 20% of children would have experienced a syncopal episode by adolescence. In general females are more frequently afflicted than males.

Etiology

The etiology of syncope is wide and variable and often times poses a diagnostic dilemma to the clinician. In the pediatric population the etiological factors related to syncope are generally benign; however the most deleterious causes tend to be of cardiac origin; with an increased potential for sudden death.

Perhaps, the most useful approach would be to divide the causative factors into – cardiac vs. non-cardiac causes.

Cardiac causes: Dysrhythmias, obstructive lesions, coronary artery anomalies.
Non-cardiac causes: Vasovagal/neurocardiogenic; orthostatic hypotension; postural orthostatic tachycardia syndrome; neurological – seizures, migraine hyperventilation; electrolyte abnormalities.

Neurocardiogenic (Vasovagal Syncope)

This is the most common form of syncope in children – for this reason it is also called "Common Syncope." More than 60% of cases of childhood syncope is vasovagal in origin. It is characterized by a prodrome consisting of nausea, sweating, light-headedness. It may sometimes be recurrent and is precipitated by well-known triggers – sight of blood, heat, hunger, prolonged upright position. The duration is *typically* not long. Syncope occurs in the upright or sitting position and the recumbent/supine position often results in resolution of symptoms.

Pathophysiology

Neurocardiogenic syncope as the name suggests is neurally mediated. It is characterized by a reflex response which results ultimately in decreased cerebral perfusion and decreased systemic blood pressure. The final common pathway to diminished cerebral perfusion and decreased systemic blood pressure is through vasodilation and an associated tachycardia/bradycardia. Three types of neurally mediated responses exist; a cardioinhibitory response, vasodepressor response and a mixed response.

The cardio-inhibitory response involves increased parasympathetic tone which results in sinus bradycardia, and AV block. The vasodepressor response is due to decreased sympathetic activity – this leads to hypotension. The mechanism most frequently associated with neurocardiogenic syncope is the cardioinhibitory response.

Autonomic dysfunction can play a role in causing neurocardiogenic syncope. Some individuals may have an increased sympathetic response at rest with a decreased response with orthostatic stress. Carotid sinus and aortic arch receptors aid in controlling blood pressure and heart rate – as such a perceived increase in blood pressure would activate vagal pathways and result in decrease heart rate with decrease blood pressure. Activation of mechanoreceptors in the left ventricles and stretch receptors in the great vessels may stimulate C fibers which result in increased vagal tone. Normally the physiological response to an erect posture would result in less stretch on these receptors and hence a perception of hypotension which would in turn result in increased sympathetic drive and reflex increase heart rate and blood pressure. In individuals prone to syncope, a precipitous fall in venous return will result in sudden forceful ventricular contraction and this acts as a positive stimulus on the mechanoreceptors. The body's response to this will be to decrease sympathetic drive and increase vagal tone. This results in inadvertent decrease heart rate and blood pressure to a stimulus (erect posture) that should have otherwise increased heart rate and blood pressure – resulting in decreased cerebral blood flow and syncope.

Diagnosis

The diagnosis can often be made with a careful history (patients with classic triggers and sign), in which case no further work-up is necessary. Cardiac investigative studies – ECG, Echo, Holter are usually not helpful diagnostic tools in neurocardiogenic syncope. However patients in whom the diagnosis is uncertain may undergo the following work-up:

Tilt Table Test

This test is limited in its reproducibility. The angle of the tilt is 60–80°, and the duration of the tilt is variable. Early response to tilting is more indicative of neurocardiogenic syncope. Often times if there is no response with tilting alone then the test is done with isoproterenol. It is often times then even more difficult to determine a truly positive test.

Adenosine Administration

Administration of adenosine or its precursor has been used to simulate a cardioinhibitory response. The efficacy of the use of adenosine has been studied and the jury is still out on this. There remains conflicting results in various studies. This test is not routinely recommended and has been done in cases where there is diagnostic dilemma.

Management

General measures are usually the mainstay of treatment for infrequent neurocardiogenic syncope. It is important for the patient to comply with the body's attempt to maintain homeostasis – i.e., "assume the supine position at all cost." Attempts should never be made to keep the patient erect as this will only prolong the ordeal.

For patients with recurrent episodes of simple/common fainting medications may be used. These include:

- Beta-blockers which have negative inotropic effect.
- Disopyramide and scopolamine are two anti-cholinergic medications which work by decreasing vagal tone.
- Midodrine – is an alpha agonist and would work by preventing venous stasis and hypotension.

Pacemaker use in neurocardiogenic syncope is generally not recommended. It is conceivable that if the underlying mechanism of syncope is a cardioinhibitory one then a pacemaker may be beneficial, as opposed to syncope caused primarily by vasodepression. Often times it is difficult to distinguish between the two causes, and a lot of times one pt may have either or both of the pathophysiological mechanism occurring in them. There is therefore no recommendation at this time to use pacemaker as a form of therapy for neurocardiogenic syncope.

Postural Orthostatic Tachycardia Syndrome

Postural Orthostatic Tachycardia Syndrome (POTS) is defined classically as an increase in heart rate greater than 30 beats per minute when moving from supine to upright position. Concurrent with the increase in heart rate there must be associated symptoms – which may range from light headedness, fatigue, dizziness, pallor, to syncope and decreased daily functioning. Sometimes even acrocyanosis has been observed in affected individuals.

POTS affects mainly adolescent females and in general is not been seen in individuals <9 years of age. The normal response of the body to standing is an initial fall in thoracic blood volume with initial decrease in venous return to the heart. There is then a compensatory increase in heart rate and blood pressure through activation of several receptors – baroreceptors and stretch receptors in the heart, and carotid sinus. There is also neurohumoral activation which together with the stretch and baroreceptors also increase venous return, subsequently making heart rate and blood pressure normal. In patients with POTS this normal compensatory response is blunted. It has been hypothesized that the underlying etiology of POTS may be the existence of a relative hypovolemic state, or a relative hyperadrenergic state or possibly the presence of autoimmune antibodies to ganglionic acetylcholine receptors. It is quite possible that all three factors play a role.

The diagnosis of POTS remains a clinical diagnosis. Often times the history is one of a preceding debilitating illness – which somehow resulted in a decrease in the individual's usual activity level. Some viral illnesses have been associated with the development of POTS – Enteroviruses, Epstein–Barr virus and Parvovirus B19 are just a few of the commonly cited ones.

There is no single method to management of POTS especially in the pediatric population. The management of POTS is tailored toward reversing the proposed mechanisms of causation of symptoms. It is recommended that at least 2 l of water per day is consumed. Increasing salt intake will lead to intravascular expansion. An intake of at least 200 mEq of salt/5 g table salt per day is recommended. Supportive stockings will increase peripheral vascular resistance and increase venous return. In the same way regular exercise would also increase peripheral vascular resistance. The use of Beta blockers to blunt the increase in heart rate has been proposed – but with variable results. Alpha agonists, such as midodrine, will increase peripheral vascular resistance. As a method to mitigate the autoimmune pathway there has been the use of Intravenous immunoglobulins. Medications that would inhibit acetylcholinesterase, example pyridostigmine, would potentially increase the availability of acetylcholine hence increasing parasympathetic vagal tone and blunt the tachycardic response associated with POTS.

Orthostatic Hypotension

Orthostatic hypotension is defined as a fall in blood pressure of >10–15 mmHg when moving from supine to standing position. There is generally only slight increase in heart rate, if any at all. In orthostatic hypotension the normal response to standing is inappropriate and there is blunting of the adrenergic vasoconstrictive effect on the vasculature hence there is relative vasodilation upon assuming the upright position.

Patients with orthostatic hypotension may exhibit light headedness – but there is no associated prodrome prior to the episode as occurs in neurocardiogenic syncope. Occasionally these patients may faint.

Management of orthostatic hypotension includes counseling patients to assume the upright position very slowly – to give the body time to adapt to the postural change. Also the use of elastic stockings and adequate hydration has been tried;

each with variable results. If the condition is being exacerbated by the use of drugs (antihypertensives, calcium channel blockers, diuretics) then these drugs should be stopped, if at all possible.

Neurological Causes

Several neurological conditions may mimic syncope. These include seizures and pseudo-seizures. Migraine – especially of the basilar type is well known to cause syncopal type spells. It is conceivable that intracranial masses – vascular or otherwise could cause syncopal-type symptoms as they may affect cerebral perfusion and blood flow.

The management of each condition is tailored toward the specific diagnosis. However the importance of a good history and physical examination cannot be over-emphasized.

Cardiac Causes

Cardiac etiology remains the single most malignant form of syncope. These result either from structural heart lesions or arrhythmias. The latter group tends to be exclusively tachyarrhythmias – though in very rare circumstances a sudden bradyarrhythmia may result in syncope. Arrhythmias are less common in frequency than structural heart disease as a cardiac cause of syncope.

In general the common etiological pathway of cardiac origin of syncope is diminished cardiac output and subsequent decreased cerebral perfusion.

The classic features are syncope occurring on exertion or in the recumbent position. There are classically no premonitory signs – no pallor, nausea, sweating. The occurrence is abrupt. The history of underlying cardiac disease would be supportive. Family history may also be supportive (Table 34.1).

Table 34.1 Differentiating characteristics of cardiac and non-cardiac causes of syncope

Symptoms/signs	Neurogenic syncope	Cardiac syncope
Premonitory signs – nausea, light headedness	+	−
Occurs in the upright position	+	−
History of underlying cardiac disease	−	+
Significant family history of Long QT syndrome, sudden death, seizures, drowning	−	+
Association with exercise	−	+
Association with palpitations, chest pain	−	+

This table outlines the general differentiating features between cardiac and non-cardiac causes of syncope. This table is not meant to be all inclusive but instead offers a guide to the general practitioner

Arrhythmias

Long QT Syndrome

This is characterized by prolongation of QT interval on ECG. It is a disorder of repolarization of the myocardium. It may be congenital or acquired. Congenital Long QT syndrome has two classic forms: Romano–Ward syndrome and the Jervell and Lange Nielsen syndrome. The Romano–Ward syndrome – is inherited in an autosomal dominant fashion whereas Jervell and Lange Nielsen syndrome is inherited in an autosomal recessive fashion and is associated with sensorineural deafness.

Most cases are inherited by autosomal dominant transmission. Syncope occurs in approximately two-thirds of gene carriers, with sudden death in ~15% of untreated cases. Inherited Long QT cause syncope and sudden cardiac death due to ventricular tachyarrhythmias, causing torsades de pointes.

Clinical presentation includes syncope, seizures, palpitations, and unfortunately sudden death. A family history may be corroborative. Symptoms are precipitated by exercise.

Pathophysiology

Changes in the transmembrane potassium and sodium currents play a major role in the etiology of LQTS. In the congenital form the ion channel proteins are affected. The major problem is delayed recovery of the action potential. The delayed recovery predisposes to the development of early after-depolarizations and subsequent torsades de pointes arrhythmias. The torsade produces the syncope and sudden death. The torsade maintenance appears to be because of complex reentry or repetitive triggered beats, both of which can explain the unique and characteristic QRS morphology of torsade.

Diagnosis

An electrocardiogram with manual calculation of the QT interval should be performed on all patients with a suggestive history. The diagnosis of LQTS requires evaluation of all other family members. The signs of long QT syndrome are prolongation of the QT interval on the electrocardiogram and abnormalities of T wave morphology. The average QTc value is 0.49 s and vary somewhat by genotype. About 15% of long QT gene carriers have a normal QTc, < or =0.44 s. Therefore, a normal QTc interval does not exclude long QT syndrome. T wave morphology is important in making the diagnosis and is characteristic for each genotype (Fig. 34.1).

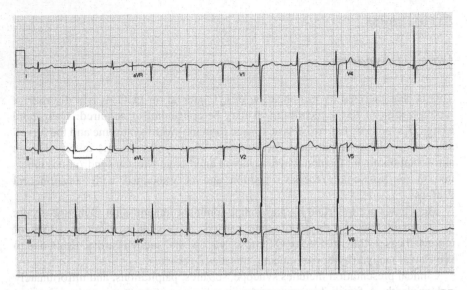

Fig. 34.1 Prolonged QTc. The QT interval in this ECG is 0.48 s (*12 small squares*), while the RR interval is 0.88 s (*22 small squares*). Therefore QTc + QT, RR = 0.48/0.9 = 0.53 s

Management

The mainstay of therapy is to prevent torsades de pointes or to prevent sudden death. Acute treatment include intravenous magnesium and potassium administration, and temporary cardiac pacing. Removal of any aggravating factors, correction of electrolyte imbalance, and intravenous isoproterenol administration are also additional forms of therapy. The long-term treatment is aimed at reducing the QT-interval duration includes use of oral beta-adrenergic blockers, implantation of permanent pacemaker/cardioverter-defibrillator, and left thoracic sympathectomy.

Brugada Syndrome

It is a syndrome of ST elevation in the right precordial leads, with associated risk for ventricular arrhythmias and sudden death. Most cases of arrhythmias occur between the 2nd and 4th decades of life. Some cases of sudden infant death are due to Brugada syndrome. In both children and adults the risk for sudden death is highest in sleep or at rest. There are some drugs which can induce a Brugada – type pattern on ECG – these include flecainide, procainamide, disopyramide, lithium, tricyclic antidepressants, and SSRIs.

Diagnosis

The diagnosis is made by typical ECG finding of ST elevation in the right precordial leads as well as right bundle branch block type picture. The typical ECG findings may not be present at all times in affected individuals.

Management

Implantable Cardioverter Defibrillator (ICD) device is the most effective therapy for Brugada syndrome.

Wolff–Parkinson–White Syndrome

It is the most common form of pre-excitation in children. It occurs as a result of an accessory pathway between the atrium and the ventricles – the bundle of Kent. The accessory pathway is a faster conduction path than the usual conduction in the AV node. Conduction via the accessory pathway, results in early depolarization of the ventricle and hence the classic "delta waves" on ECG. SVT – Supraventricular Tachycardia associated with Wolff–Parkinson–White syndrome is caused by retrograde conduction through the accessory pathway. The ECG then will show no evidence of pre-excitation but rather SVT only.

Diagnosis

The diagnosis is made by the ECG findings of short pr interval, initial slurring of QRS complex (delta wave) and subsequent widening of the QRS complex (Fig. 34.2).

Other Arrhythmias

There are other less common types of arrhythmias which may lead to syncope and sudden cardiac death. Congenital short QT syndrome – as the name suggests is characterized by a short QT interval on ECG, and absence of the ST segment on ECG. Patients are prone to atrial fibrillation and ventricular fibrillation. Management strategies include quinidine and flecainide. Catecholaminergic polymorphic ventricular tachycardia is an infrequent cause of syncope in children and adolescent. Arrhythmias are induced by exercise, emotional stress and catecholamine infusion.

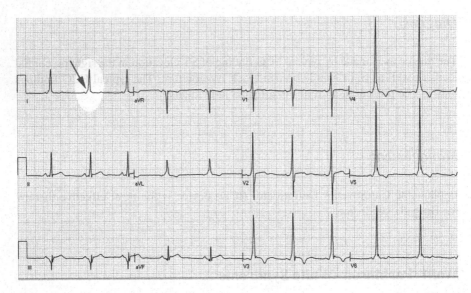

Fig. 34.2 *Arrow points* to delta wave. The QRS is prolonged secondary to early depolarization due to accessory pathway

Beta blockers and restriction from exercise are the mainstay of treatment. A defibrillator is sometimes needed. *Arrhythmogenic right ventricular dysplasia* is a genetic condition marked by ventricular arrhythmias and right ventricular abnormalities. There is a fibro-fatty infiltration of the right ventricular myocardium. The ECG findings – left bundle branch block is common during the tachycardia. T wave inversion over the right precordial leads is seen when patients are in sinus rhythm. Patients who have sustained Vtach or a history of aborted sudden cardiac arrest are candidates for ICD. The use of Beta-blockers have resulted in variable responses.

Hypertrophic Cardiomyopathy

Hypertrophic cardiomyopathy (HCM) is an inherited cardiac disease. It is inherited in an autosomal dominant pattern. It occurs in 1 in 500 individuals. It results in left ventricular hypertrophy, involving the interventricular septum. Hypertrophy may be present in infants, but typically develops during childhood and adolescence.

Patients may exhibit syncope on exertion. It is a very common cause of sudden death with exercise. The underlying pathophysiology is decreased cardiac output secondary to left ventricular outflow tract obstruction and arrhythmias. There is an association with WPW (Wolff–Parkinson–White) syndrome Family history of sudden death at a young age, LV hypertrophy >3 cm, unexplained syncope, nonsustained ventricular tachycardia in Holter monitoring, and abnormal blood pressure response during exercise are all clinical risk factors for sudden death.

Management of children with HCM aims to provide symptomatic relief and prevention of sudden death, which is the primary cause of death. Medical therapy with beta-adrenoceptor antagonists (beta-blockers), or verapamil is the first treatment option in all symptomatic patients. Surgical myectomy may be effective. It reduces symptoms in children with left ventricular (LV) obstruction who are unresponsive to medical treatment. Repeat surgical intervention may be needed in a moderate proportion of patients due to recurrence of LV obstruction. The absence of non sustained ventricular tachycardia during Holter monitoring has a high negative predictive value in adults but this has not been proven in children or adolescents. Amiodarone has been used as therapy in high risk patients by itself or in combination with ICD. HCM is one of the few pediatric indications for ICD implantation. Patients should be restricted from vigorous exercise since most cases of sudden death occurs shortly after exertion.

Aortic Stenosis

Aortic Valvar Stenosis is due to decreased valvar size resulting from thickening of the valve leaflets. If severe enough it will result in obstruction of left ventricular outflow and decreased cardiac output.

The pathophysiology of aortic stenosis results in obstruction of left ventricular outflow and compensatory increase ventricular wall size. The subendocardium and the papillary muscles are hence most susceptible to ischemia. At rest the compensatory coronary artery vasodilation is near maximal, hence with exertion there is very little coronary reserve. Exercise creates an inbalance in oxygen supply and demand which results in ischemia and infarction.

The clinical features of severe aortic valve stenosis are easy fatiguability, syncope with exertion and sometimes angina type symptoms. On examination there is a an ejection systolic murmur heard best at the aortic region (upper right sternal edge). An ejection click may be heard as well. ECG may show left ventricular hypertrophy. An echocardiogram confirms the diagnosis.

The management of severe aortic valve stenosis includes exercise restriction and subsequent balloon valvuloplasty. Aortic valve replacement is required in patients who develop recurrent stenosis after valvuloplasty or who have significant regurgitation after valvuloplasty.

Coronary Artery Anomalies

Congenital anomalies of the coronary artery may result in syncope and sudden cardiac death in the adolescents. The origin of the left coronary artery from the right main coronary artery is the most common coronary anomaly. When the anomalous branch passes between the aorta and the right ventricular infundibulum the association with sudden death is increased.

Patients present with recurrent syncopal attacks or chest pain with exercise or exertion. Unfortunately, for some, sudden death is their only mode of presentation. Death is due to myocardial ischemia. The diagnosis is made from an echocardiogram. However MRI and CT SCAN is more sensitive.

Management is surgical correction of the anomaly.

Summary

In summary; syncope may be an indicator or precursor of sudden death, and a good history, physical examination and evaluation are important for the patient. The history is by far the most important clue to identify the patient with syncope who is at risk for sudden death. Any patient presenting with syncope should have a careful cardiac and neurological examination. Judicious use of laboratory testing and cardiac monitoring may assist the physician in making the diagnosis. Most common cause of syncope is neurocardiogenic cause; however the most malignant life threatening causes of syncope are of cardiac origin. Patients are often times misdiagnosed with seizures as seen in our case 3 scenario. The circumstances of the events (onset, precipitating factors, aggravating factors, relieving factors) and knowledge of the ECG features are important in arriving at the correct diagnosis. Effective treatment modalities are available and with prompt diagnosis appropriate treatment has proven to be life-saving.

Case Scenarios

Case 1

18-year-old female presents to the clinic with a 3-year history of recurrent syncopal and pre-syncopal episodes. Syncope in her is often times triggered by anxiety, long standing and is more frequent around the times of her menses. She often times gets nauseated, with profuse sweating, blurred vision and light headedness prior to fainting. These she calls "warning signs." She has learnt over the last year to abort the syncopal episodes by squatting whenever she gets the "warning signs."

Physical examination: Adolescent female, well nourished, in no distress. Vitals were normal BP-110/76 SITTING, 96/70 – STANDING, HR-88/min SITTING, 86/min STANDING. Examination of her precordium revealed normal heart sounds and no cardiac murmur.

Diagnosis: Neurocardiogenic syncope. Possibility of Orthostatic intolerance was also entertained – based on blood pressure change with position at the time of her clinic visit

Treatment: Adequate daily oral hydration was recommended. Awareness of her triggers and prodrome was lauded in this patient and it was recommended that should these symptoms recur; that she assumes the recumbent position as much as is possible.

Case 2

12-year-old male was referred for school physical – at which time he was found by his primary care doctor to have an irregular heartbeat. He has no symptomatology, and has always been well. He was therefore referred to the cardiologist for further evaluation.

Physical examination: Heart rate was 92/min-irregular, Respiratory rate was 14/min. Blood pressure in the right upper limb was 104/68. Oxygen saturation was 100% on room air. There was no increased precordial activity and no murmur was heard. Rest of physical examination was within normal limits.

His baseline ECG revealed a QTc –0.458. An echocardiogram done was within normal limits.

He was referred for exercise stress test and was noted to have prolongation of his QTc during the recovery time. To date he remains totally asymptomatic and has no positive family history.

Treatment: He was subsequently evaluated by a pediatric electrophysiologist who has recommended genetic testing. Because he had remained asymptomatic no medication was started at the time of his last visit.

Case 3

16-year-old male athlete presents with a history of recurrent fainting episodes for the past 4 years. Fainting episodes are always preceded by palpitations. He gives no history of nausea, or light headedness prior to fainting but does attest to scotomas just prior to the episodes. He says the episodes are of sudden onset and often times are triggered by playing basketball. There is no chest pain with exertion. He says he tries to abort the episodes of palpitations by "holding his breath" for a long time. He has been seen several times in the past and was diagnosed with pseudo-seizures. He was taken to the ER once again after such an "attack."

Physical examination: Adolescent male – coherent with good recollection of the event. A bruise was noted to the forehead. Heart rate –76/min, BP-100/70, oxygen saturation –98% on room air. On examination of the precordium there was no increased activity. Normal heart sounds were heard without murmur. A detailed neurological examination revealed no neurological deficit.

Diagnosis: CT BRAIN – Normal. CXRAY – normal and ECG revealed "delta waves" suggestive of Wolff–Parkinson–White syndrome. He was transferred to a tertiary center where he subsequently had an echocardiogram done – which was within normal limits.

Treatment: He had EP study and evaluation and a lateral accessory pathway was found and ablated. He has been followed in clinic and has had no recurrence of his symptoms.

Chapter 35
Chest Pain

Ismael Gonzalez and Ra-id Abdulla

Definition

Chest pain is the second most frequent reason for referral of children and adolescents to a pediatric cardiologist despite the fact that chest pain is an unlikely manifestation of heart diseases in children as the majority of cases are benign in nature. However, the association of chest pain with fatal heart disease in adults creates undue anxiety leading many pediatricians to refer children with heart diseases to

I. Gonzalez (✉)
Department of Pediatric Cardiology, Rush University Medical Center,
1150 N. Lake Shore Dr., Apt 9J, Chicago, IL 60611, USA
e-mail: ismael_gonzalez@rush.edu

Ra-id Abdulla (ed.), *Heart Diseases in Children: A Pediatrician's Guide*,
DOI 10.1007/978-1-4419-7994-0_35, © Springer Science+Business Media, LLC 2011

pediatric cardiologists to rule out cardiac anomalies. Pediatricians should become familiar with causes of chest pain in children and how to assess this complaint to be able to provide reassurance to patients and families in the majority of such cases.

Incidence

Chest pain is a common complaint in pediatric patients. It accounts for 6 in 1,000 visits to pediatric emergency services. In addition, chest pain is the second most prevalent reason for referral to pediatric cardiologists. The male to female ratio appears to be equal and the average age of presentation is 13 years. Cardiac assessment is normal in the majority of patients and most cases are caused by noncardiac structures within the chest.

Etiology

The cause of chest pain in children and adolescence is noncardiac in most cases. The cause of chest pain in this age group is usually due to other structures within the thorax and respiratory system. Patients more than 12 years old are more likely to have a psychogenic cause. However, *psychological* causes of pain should be made carefully and only after excluding other causes of chest pain.

   Organ systems responsible for causing chest pain in children include musculoskeletal, pulmonary, psychiatric, gastrointestinal and cardiac. In most instances an etiology is difficult to identify, these are grouped as idiopathic and tend to be the most common category of chest pain.

Musculoskeletal Conditions

Costochondritis

Definition: Costochondritis is an inflammatory process of the costochondral or costosternal junction causing localized pain and tenderness. Any of the seven pairs of costochondral junctions may be affected. Typically more than one site is affected (90% of cases). The second to fifth costochondral junctions are most commonly involved.

Costochondritis Is More Common in Females

Presentation: Patients usually complain of insidious, sharp anterior chest pain, unilateral in the majority of cases. The pain is typically restricted to the affected costochondral junction (s), however, it may radiate to the back. The pain is exacerbated by movement of the trunk, deep breathing, exercise (basketball, baseball, and weight lifting) or unusual physical activity that involve upper extremities. The pain can be easily reproduced in the office by palpating the costochondral or costosternal junctions affected, although the majority of patients are typically not aware of the chest wall tenderness until physical examination.

Diagnosis: The sharp nature of the pain, its distinctive location and reproducibility through palpation makes diagnosis relatively easy. Further investigative studies are typically not warranted.

Treatment: This involves the use of nonsteroidal anti-inflammatory drugs to reduce pain and inflammation in the costochondral or costosternal joints. This should be used for 5–7 days to reduce inflammation. This could be repeated if pain is to reoccur. Patients should be advised to avoid repetitive motions that may exacerbate the pain. Reassurance that the pain is musculoskeletal in nature is important as most patients and families fear cardiac causes of pain.

Tietze's Syndrome

Definition: Unlike costochondritis, it is characterized by swelling of the costosternal junctions. It tends to affect only one joint, particularly the second and third junctions. This may become chronic in nature and last for years.

Presentation: Pain is typically localized to the affected junctions; however, at times it radiates rendering localization of pain difficult. Affected junctions are swollen and tender to touch

Diagnosis: The sharp nature of the pain, swelling of junctions and tenderness to palpation makes diagnosis relatively easy. Further investigative studies are typically not warranted.

Treatment: Nonsteroidal anti-inflammatory drugs help to reduce the pain; but physical therapy, steroid injections, ice packs and/or heat, TENS (transcutaneous electrical stimulation), acupuncture, have been reported to be effective as well.

Idiopathic Chest-Wall Pain

Definition: This is also known as nonspecific chest-wall pain; this disorder is one of the common causes of chest pain in children.

Presentation: The pain is sharp, lasts for a few seconds to minutes, localized to the middle of the sternum or the inframammary area, and is exacerbated by deep breathing or by manual pressure on the sternum or rib cage. Signs of inflammation are absent.

Diagnosis: This is a diagnosis of exclusion and most often resolves on its own over time.

Treatment: Reassurance and regular follow-up examinations.

Slipping-Rib Syndrome

Definition: This is characterized by intense pain in the lower chest or upper abdominal area caused by excess mobility of the eighth to tenth ribs. These ribs do not directly insert into the sternum.

Presentation: Patient presents with dull pain in between the scapulae or in the chest area. It may develop to intermittent sharp pains sometimes simulating a heart attack. It can also be associated with shortness of breath. Hence any young person who has a negative cardiac work up after having severe sharp chest pain with shortness of breath may be suffering from slipping rib syndrome.

Diagnosis: The pain can be reproduced by placing the fingers under the inferior rib margin and pulling the rib edge outward and upward. This is a rare finding in children.

Treatment: Many patients with slipping rib syndrome will have spontaneous resolution of their symptoms in about a week. Improvement may also be seen after short course of treatment and several options may be considered. Chiropractic manipulation often provides complete resolution after a few sessions. Massage also helps relieve muscle spasm and tightness. Topical analgesic balms sometimes help in pain palliation. Ice or cold packs likewise provide quick, soothing relief.

Trauma and Muscle Strain

Definition: This is seen more frequently in the adolescent population who are involved in sports, particularly weightlifting. The pain is due to damage to thoracic muscles and tendons.

Presentation: The pain is localized to the site of injury and usually is associated with swelling or erythema. In severe trauma to the chest, patients will present with shortness of breath, severe chest pain and arrhythmia and you should rule out myocardial injury and hemopericardium.

Diagnosis: Findings in the physical exam (erythema, bruises, hematomas), make the diagnosis straightforward. Chest X-ray is necessary if trauma is severe to rule out rib fractures, lung injury (hemothorax, pneumothorax) or cardiac injury (hemopericardium).

Treatment: According to the severity of the trauma and other organs affected. If mild trauma and no other lesions associated, nonsteroidal anti-inflammatory drugs help to reduce the pain.

Precordial Catch

Definition: This is also known as "Texidor twinge," is a frequent cause of chest pain in healthy adolescents and young adults. It is often associated with exercise, and is described as sharp, short duration, and located in the left substernal region. Pain occurs when the ligaments supporting the heart are stretched. Characteristics that distinguish it from angina are its sudden onset, localized nature, and short duration.

Presentation: This is characterized by sudden pain in the anterior left side of the chest and occurs at rest or during mild activity and can last for few seconds to several minutes. The *pain occurs* exclusively with inspiration, and resolves quickly and completely. It may recur several times in a day. The pain can sometimes disappear by forcing an inhalation. The cause of precordial catch syndrome remains unknown.

Diagnosis: Diagnosis is made through clinical presentation.

Treatment: No specific treatment is recommended, other than reassurance. There are no known significant complications of this condition. The frequency of events can be expected to decline through adolescence.

Respiratory Conditions

Reactive Airway Disease (Asthma)

Definition: Chest pain due to overuse of chest wall muscles secondary to reactive airway disease is a common cause of chest pain in the pediatric cage group.

Presentation: Vague muscular pain, typically bilateral occurring just after worsening of respiratory distress due to reactive airway disease exacerbation.

Diagnosis: History of reactive airway disease and occurrence of chest pain after exacerbation of reactive airway disease should alert the physician to this diagnosis.

Treatment: management of this condition should focus on management of reactive airway disease with inhalation bronchodilators to eliminate pain caused by overuse of accessory respiratory muscles.

Lung/Pleural Infections

Definition: Infections of the bronchial tree or lung, including bronchitis, pleurisy, pleural effusion, pneumonia, empyema, bronchiectasis and lung abscess, can cause acute chest pain.

Presentation: Patients present with history of an upper respiratory infection, fever, decrease activity, decrease appetite, and *vague* chest pain which is difficult to localize. Pain may radiate to the back and increase with deep inspiration.

Diagnosis: This is made through history, findings of rales, tachypnea, or decreased breath sounds.

Treatment: Antibiotics and drainage of the abscess or pleural fluid is the main treatment, some patients will benefit of additional O_2 and hospitalization.

Pleural Disease

Definition: Pleural space has the potential to collect large amount of fluid, air and consequent irritation of the phrenic nerve with posterior pleural irritation and chest pain.

Presentation: Spontaneous pneumothorax or pneumomediastinum can present with sudden respiratory distress and severe none localize chest pain. Children at high risk for these conditions are those who have asthma, cystic fibrosis, and Marfan syndrome, but previously healthy children may rupture an unrecognized subpleural bleb as well.

Diagnosis: Chest X-ray is helpful to make the diagnosis.

Treatment: Drainage of the fluid or air out of the pleural cavity will resolve this condition.

Skin Lesions

Definition: Skin lesions of the thorax may result in pain. Many skin lesions may cause pain in this region, such as Herpes zoster. Children may not be able to make the distinction of pain caused by a cutaneous lesion versus true chest pain.

Presentation: Pain is localized over cutaneous lesions. Herpes zoster is caused by the varicella zoster virus reactivation and posterior inflammation in the dorsal root ganglion accompanied by hemorrhagic necrosis of nerve cells. Patients complain of severe pain usually unilateral and restricted to a dermatomal distribution. It is important to note that initial chest pain is usually not associated with a vesicular rash; this will appear in the next 24–48 h of initial presentation.

Diagnosis: Careful inspection of skin over the thorax is essential when evaluating chest pain as it may reveal skin lesions causing the pain.

Treatment: This should focus on treatment of the skin lesion. In Herpes zoster pain can be reduced with NSAIDS, or opioids if very severe or antiviral therapy if given within 48–72 h of the appearance of the rash.

Pericardial Conditions

Definition: Pericarditis is characterized by swelling and irritation of the parietal and visceral pericardial surfaces, with an infiltration of polymorphonuclear leukocytes, lymphocytes, and pericardial vascularization, and may develop a serous, hemorrhage, or pyogenic effusion.

Presentation: Pericarditis presents with a sharp, stabbing pain that improves when the patient sits up and leans forward. The child is usually febrile, in respiratory distress, and has a friction rub heard through auscultation. Distant heart sounds, neck vein distention and pulsus paradoxus can occur when fluid accumulates rapidly. Large volume of fluid accumulation may cause cardiac tamponade. However, it should be noted that chest pain typically resolves when pericardial fluid accumulates as it serves to separate the two pericardial surfaces and prevent their friction which is the cause of pericardial pain.

Diagnosis: History and physical examination is helpful in making the presumptive diagnosis. Chest X-ray will show cardiomegaly with blunting of cardiac silhouette features. ECG may show nonspecific ST, T wave changes. Echocardiography is important to assess extent of fluid accumulation and need for intervention to prevent cardiac tamponade.

Treatment: This should focus on cause of inflammation. Antibiotics is used when bacterial infection is suspected, however, this is rare. Nonsteroidal anti-inflammatory agents are typically used to reduce inflammation and to assist with pain. Steroids may be indicated if fluid accumulation is significant and there is urgent need to reverse inflammatory process. Pericardiocentesis is indicated if pericardial fluid accumulation is excessive and interfering with cardiac output.

Cardiac Conditions

An essential goal for evaluating any child with chest pain is to rule out cardiac anomalies. Cardiac cause of chest pain is rare; however, it is primary concern of families of children with chest pain and if left undiagnosed may lead to significant complications. The role of any primary care physician confronted with a child with chest pain is to develop a list of differential diagnosis based upon history of illness, family history and physical findings on examination. In making the determination whether the cardiovascular system is the cause of chest pain it is helpful to identify on one hand red flags pointing towards cardiac disease and on the other hand signs which indicate etiologies of chest pain other than the cardiovascular system.

Features suggesting cardiac disease (red flags)

Abnormal findings in history

- Syncope
- Palpitations

- Dizziness
- Exertional chest pain
- Evidence of drug abuse

Abnormal findings in past or family history

- History of Kawasaki disease
- History of diabetes mellitus
- Prior heart surgery
- Family history of sudden death

Abnormal findings on cardiac examination

- Poor peripheral pulses and perfusion
- Hepatomegaly
- Abnormal RV and LV (apical) impulses
- Hyperactive precordium
- Abnormal heart sounds
- Abnormal heart murmurs

Features suggesting disease process other than cardiac in origin:

- Pain with motion/cough
- Bilateral distribution
- Recent change in exercise
- Non exertional chest pain

Cardiac Causes of Chest Pain

More details are available regarding the lesions discussed here in their respective chapters.

Severe pulmonary or aortic valve stenosis: This can lead to ischemia and results from increase myocardial oxygen demand from tachycardia and increase pressure work by the ventricle. These disorders almost always are diagnosed before the child presents with pain, and the associated murmurs are found on physical examination. Chest X-ray may show a prominent ascending aorta or pulmonary artery trunk, echocardiogram is the key in the diagnosis. The treatment is surgical or cardiac cath for ballooning of the valve.

Anomalous coronary arteries: Such as anomalous origin of the left or right coronary arteries, coronary artery fistula, coronary aneurysm/ stenosis secondary to Kawasaki disease. These can result in myocardial infarction without evidence of underlying pathology. However, chest pain is not typical in any of these conditions in the pediatric cage group. These conditions are associated with significant murmurs such as pansystolic, continuous or mitral regurgitation murmur or gallop rhythm that suggests myocardial dysfunction. Treatment of these conditions is surgical.

Arrhythmias: This can present with syncope and palpitations, and forceful heart beats that can be interpreted by a child as chest pain. Diagnosis can be done with an ECG, or a 24 h Holter monitor. Supraventricular tachycardia is the most common of these arrhythmias, but PVC's or ventricular tachycardia also can lead to brief, sharp chest pain and palpitations. These patients should be referred for evaluation by a pediatric cardiologist for assessment and treatment.

Mitral valve prolapse (MVP): This may cause chest pain due to papillary muscle or left ventricular endocardial ischemia; a midsystolic click and late systolic murmur are found in many cases. Majority of Marfan patients have MVP, however, if chest pain is experienced by these patients, prompt evaluation is crucial as this may represent aortic root dissection.

Hypertrophic obstructive cardiomyopathy: This hereditary lesion has an autosomal dominant pattern and patients have positive family history of the same disorder or a history of sudden death. Children with this disorder have a harsh systolic ejection murmur that is exaggerated with standing up or performing Valsalva maneuver. The patients are at risk for ischemic chest pain, especially when exercising. Echocardiogram is the study of choice to evaluate this condition, referral to a pediatric cardiologist should be done to evaluate patient and his/ her family.

Case Scenarios

Case 1

History: A 14-year-old girl previously healthy comes to your office complaining of chest pain that started 6 months ago. Pain is not constant and when it occurs it is localized to the precordial area. Pain lasts for few seconds, sometimes related with exercise but without difficulty in breathing. There appears to be no other associated symptoms. Past medical history *and family history are unremarkable*. The young lady denies the use of illicit drugs or cigarettes. Medical attention was sought due to chest pain and desire to join school's basketball team.

Physical exam: Vital signs are within normal limits, physical examination is normal except for tenderness when palpating the left 3, -4, -5 costochondral junctions.

Diagnosis: History and the physical examination are highly suggestive of costochondritis. The nature of pain, lack of any significant findings through history and physical examination and the ability to induce chest pain while pressing on affected costochondral junctions point to the diagnosis of costochondritis.

Treatment: Reassurance that the pain is benign and is not related to the heart is essential. Pain and inflammation of the affected costochondral junction can be eliminated through a 5–7 days course of nonsteroidal anti-inflammatory agent such as ibuprofen 400 mg PO three times a day. Patient can be advised to repeat the course if pain reoccurs in the future.

Case 2

History: A 6-year-old boy presents to the emergency room with a 1 day history of severe chest pain localize to the left side of the chest. Pain improves in the upright position, and worsens when taking a deep breath. The mother states that the child was noted to have fever and decrease in appetite of 1 day duration. In addition, he was noted to have shortness of breath over the past few hours.

Past medical history is significant for surgical repair of sinus venosus atrial septal defect 2 weeks ago. Surgical repair was uneventful and the child was discharged home 4 days after surgery in stable condition. He is currently on no medications.

Physical examination: the child exhibits mild respiratory distress. Vital signs demonstrate rapid respiratory and heart rates, normal oxygen saturation and normal blood pressure measurements. Peripheral pulses and perfusion were within normal limits. Heart sounds were normal with no murmurs detected. A friction rub was audible over the precordium.

Diagnosis: the past medical history and finding of friction rub is suggestive of pericarditis. Chest X-ray was unremarkable. ECG showed diffuse ST elevation and PR depression in aVF-V4-V6. Echocardiography revealed small pericardial effusion. The cause of pericarditis and chest pain in this child is post-pericardiotomy or Dressler's syndrome.

Treatment: In view of the small volume of pericardial effusion, compromise of cardiac output is not a present concern. Control of inflammation and fluid accumulation is essential. This could be achieved through the use of nonsteroidal anti-inflammatory agents. Steroids can be used if the first line of treatment is not effective. If pericardial effusion continues to enlarge despite medical therapy then pericardiocentesis can be used to remove pericardial fluid.

Chapter 36
Innocent Heart Murmurs

Ra-id Abdulla

Key Facts

- Innocent heart murmurs are encountered in 50% of all children.
- Innocent heart murmurs are not associated with any other cardiac symptoms of signs which may indicate cardiac pathology.
- Innocent heart murmurs are systolic and may be continuous in the case of venous hum, but never purely diastolic in nature.
- Typical innocent heart murmurs are 1–2/6 and never more than 3/6 in intensity.
- If the child is cooperative, it is essential to evaluate the change in intensity of heart murmurs through maneuvers that decrease cardiac preload such as moving the child from supine to sitting to standing positions and with Valsalva maneuver.
- Children with innocent heart murmurs should have normal findings on ECG and cheat X-ray.

Definition

Innocent heart murmurs are common in normal children. By definition, innocent heart murmurs do not reflect cardiac pathology. Instead, mild turbulence of blood flow, combined with the rapid heart rate and thin chest wall in children allow normal blood flow through normal cardiovascular structures to be audible. Innocent heart murmurs are also termed normal or physiological murmurs. Approximately 50% of all children have heart murmurs during childhood. Heart murmurs resolve spontaneously as child grows older with slower heart rate and thicker chest wall.

Ra-id Abdulla (✉)
Center for Congenital and Structural Heart Diseases, Rush University Medical Center,
1653 West Congress Parkway, Room 763 Jones, Chicago, IL 60612, USA
e-mail: rabdulla@rush.edu

Ra-id Abdulla (ed.), *Heart Diseases in Children: A Pediatrician's Guide*,
DOI 10.1007/978-1-4419-7994-0_36, © Springer Science+Business Media, LLC 2011

Origins of Murmurs

Blood flow through the heart and blood vessels is laminar in nature. Laminar flow of fluid is silent. Narrowing of passageways of blood results in turbulence which is characterized by eddies or recirculation. Eddies produces vibrations which can be heard through auscultation and in severe cases palpable as a thrill. On the other hand, laminar flow of blood is relatively silent and not audible through auscultation.

Narrowing of blood vessels or cardiac valves results in rapid change (drop) in pressure, also referred to as pressure gradient, this causes fluid to accelerate which in turn results in eddies or recirculation phenomenon. Eddies produce the vibrations which result in murmurs or when significant a thrill which can be felt by hand through palpation.

Types of Innocent Heart Murmurs

Innocent heart murmurs are defined by the cardiac structure producing the murmur. Different types of innocent heart murmurs are caused by different physiological processes (Table 36.1). When examining a child with a heart murmur features of pathological murmurs should be carefully examined to rule out presence of congenital heart disease (Table 36.2). Heart murmurs conforming to any type of innocent heart murmurs do not necessarily require referral to a pediatric cardiologist. On the other hand, lack of clarity of the nature of the murmur examined or in the presence of any feature that may indicate that the murmur is pathological in nature, referral to a pediatric cardiologist for further evaluation is necessary (Table 36.3).

Table 36.1 Features of innocence of a heart murmur

No evidence of cardiac disease form history and physical examination

Normal heart sounds

Murmur is systolic

Murmur is soft, vibratory or musical in quality

Murmur is suppressed by Valsalva maneuver or changing position from supine to sitting to standing positions

Table 36.2 Features of pathology of a heart murmur

Findings in history or physical examination which are consistent with heart disease

Presence of a thrill over the precordium or suprasternal notch

Second heart sound may be single or fixed in its splitting throughout respiration

Heart murmur is diastolic

Murmur is harsh, or loud

No significant change in quality of murmur with Valsalva maneuver or changing in position

Table 36.3 When to refer a child with a heart murmur for further evaluation?

History or physical examination consistent with pathological murmur
History of frequent respiratory infections or history of atypical reactive airway disease
Patients with syndromes which may be associated with heart diseases such as trisomy 21, Turner
    syndrome, Noonan syndrome, William's syndrome
Family history of congenital heart disease
Change in nature of murmur, such as becoming louder, or becoming systolic and diastolic
Evidence of cardiac disease by chest X-ray or electrocardiography

Peripheral Pulmonary Stenosis

This is the most common type of innocent heart murmurs in newborn children and infants younger than 2 months of age. Turbulent blood flow in relatively small peripheral pulmonary arteries cause this type of innocent heart murmur.

The pulmonary arteries while in-utero carry small volume of blood to the collapsed lungs. Approximately 5–10% of blood ejected from the right ventricle travels through the pulmonary circulation; while the majority of blood ejected from the right ventricle crosses the patent ductus arteriosus to supply blood to the descending aorta. Immediately after birth the entire right ventricular output is ejected to the right and left pulmonary arteries, thus increasing blood flow through each pulmonary artery by approximately sevenfold. This will result in relative stenosis of these normal pulmonary arteries which require approximately 6–8 weeks to reach a size suitable for this increase in blood flow thus resulting in elimination of this innocent heart murmur by 6–8 weeks of age.

The murmur is systolic ejection in type, typically 1–2/6 in intensity, although it may be as loud as 3/6. As all innocent heart murmurs, it is vibratory in nature. The murmur is best heard over the left upper sternal border with radiation into one or both axillae.

Peripheral pulmonary stenosis (PPS) due to normal developmental changes in the first few weeks of life should not be confused with pathological PPS as seen in congenital rubella, Williams syndrome, Alagille syndrome, and Noonan syndrome. Pathological PPS tends to be more significant than innocent PPS with louder murmur and worsening stenosis with time.

Physiologic Pulmonary Flow Murmur

Blood flow through the pulmonary valve may be audible in children due to relative hyperdynamic status of blood circulation secondary to faster heart rate as well as thin chest wall allowing easier detection of normal blood flow through the pulmonary valve.

This type of murmur is typically 1–2/6 in intensity and occasionally as loud as 3/6. The murmur is soft and vibratory (or musical) in quality. The murmur is heard best over the left upper sternal border in supine position and is significantly reduced in intensity or completely resolves when the child sits or stands up as well as with

Valsalva maneuver due to reduction in blood volume returning to the chest (decrease in pre-load).

Stills Murmur

Stills murmur is similar to physiologic pulmonary flow murmur, but in this case the murmur is due to blood flow across the aortic valve. The murmur is due to relative hyperdynamic status of blood circulation secondary to faster heart rate as well as thin chest wall allowing easier detection of normal blood flow through a normal aortic valve.

This type of murmur is typically 1–2/6 in intensity and occasionally as loud as 3/6. The murmur is soft and vibratory (or musical) in quality. The murmur is heard best over the right upper sternal border in supine position and is significantly reduced in intensity or completely resolves when the child sits or stands up as well as with Valsalva maneuver due to reduction in blood volume returning to the chest (decrease in pre-load).

Venous Hum

This is a soft continuous murmur heard over the lateral aspect of the neck generated by blood flow in the internal jugular vein. The close proximity of the internal jugular vein to the skin allows normal blood flow to be heard through auscultation even though there is no significant turbulence. Venous hum is soft, typically 1–2/6 in intensity and heard throughout systole and most diastole. An important distinction between venous hum and murmur produced by a patent ductus arteriosus or collateral vessels include the following:

- Intensity: Venous hum murmur is soft, while that of patent ductus arteriosus is harsh.
- Location: Venous hum murmur is supraclavicular and on either sides of the neck, while murmurs caused by patent ductus arteriosus is infraclavicular and on the left side.
- Change in quality: Venous hum murmurs can be diminished or eliminated by applying pressure to the jugular veins higher in the neck, while that of ductus arteriosus are not affected by this maneuver.

Mammary Soufflé

This murmur is caused by engorged arteries in the breasts due to rapid growth such as seen during pregnancy or adolescence. The murmur is systolic or continuous and heard over a wide area over the anterior chest. These murmurs tend to be 1–2/6 in intensity and do not change with Valsalva maneuver or patient's position.

Case Scenarios

Case 1

History: A 2-year-old boy presents to a pediatrician's office for a well child care visit. The child is thriving well with no significant medical problems except for reactive airway disease with occasional need for albuterol inhalation. He is currently on no medications.

Physical examination: Heart rate was 100 bpm, regular, respiratory rate was 30/min and blood pressure in the right upper extremity was 90/55 mmHg. Child appeared in no respiratory distress, mucosa was pink with good peripheral pulses and perfusion. The femoral and brachial arterial pulses were equal and full. No hepatomegaly was detected. Palpation of the precordium reveals normal location and intensity of the left ventricle and right ventricle impulses. Auscultation demonstrates a normal first heart sound, second heart sound split and varied with respiration. A 2/6 systolic ejection murmur was heard over the right upper sternal border with no radiation. Murmur was soft and vibratory in quality with significant reduction in intensity while standing, while becoming well heard in supine position.

Assessment: The child appears to be healthy; the physical examination is within normal limits. The heart murmur is consistent with Still's murmur, an innocent heart murmur. The quality of murmur and its diminished intensity in upright position suggests innocence of the heart murmur. This pediatrician's records indicate that previous examination revealed similar murmur.

Plan: It is reasonable for the pediatrician at this point to choose to continue observing this heart murmur without referral to a pediatric cardiologist. Some pediatricians will choose to obtain a chest X-ray and ECG, relatively inexpensive test modalities to ensure no evidence of heart disease to support the diagnosis of innocent heart murmur.

Case 2

History: A 2-week-old child is seen by a pediatrician for the first time for a well child care visit. The child is a product of 37 week gestation with no complication other than premature onset of labor. Delivery was by spontaneous vaginal deliver with no complications. Apgar scores were 9 and 9 at 1 and 5 min. The child remained at the hospital for 3 days and discharged in good condition. Mom reports that the child nurses well with no significant medical problems.

Physical examination: Heart rate was 140 bpm, regular, respiratory rate was 35/min and blood pressure in the right upper extremity was 80/45 mmHg. Child had normal feature and appeared in no respiratory distress, mucosa was pink with good peripheral pulses and perfusion. The femoral and brachial arterial pulses were equal and full. No hepatomegaly was detected. Palpation of the precordium reveals normal location and intensity of the left ventricle and right ventricle impulses. Auscultation demonstrates a normal first heart sound, second heart sound most probably split, however was difficult to evaluate due to rapid heart rate. A 2/6 systolic ejection murmur was heard over the left upper sternal border with radiation into left axilla.

Assessment: The heart murmur in this child is consistent with PPS, a frequently encountered innocent heart murmur encountered in the first few weeks of life. This type of murmur radiates, or even heard exclusively in one or both axillae. It is difficult to subject these types of murmurs to assessment while in different position or with Valsalva maneuver due to child's age. It is important to make sure that the child does not have history or physical features supporting pathological PPS such as with William, Noonan, Alagille syndromes or due to congenital rubella.

Plan: The pediatrician may choose to see the child again in 2 weeks for re-evaluation of heart murmur. An innocent heart murmur due to PPS should disappear by 6–8 weeks of life. On the other hand, if the murmur becomes louder, or if the child shows any features of heart disease, then referral to a pediatric cardiologist is essential to rule out pathological causes for this murmur.

Chapter 37
Obesity and Dyslipidemia

Kathryn W. Holmes and Jacquelyn Busse

Key Facts

- The prevalence of obesity among school age children is increasing exponentially over the past 3 decades.
- Dyslipidemia is defined as:

  - Total cholesterol (TC) >200 mg/dL
  - HDL-C <45 mg/dL
  - LDL-C >130 mg/dL
  - Triglycerides >150 mg/dL in adolescents and >130 mg/dL in children

- Early screening (between 2 and 8 years of age) should be done in all of the following high-risk groups:

  - Family history of early coronary artery disease or stroke
  - Familial dyslipidemia
  - BMI >85‰
  - History of Kawasaki disease
  - Active kidney disease or who have received a kidney transplant
  - After heart transplant
  - Type I or II diabetes
  - Congenital heart disease
  - Cancer treatment survivors

(continued)

K.W. Holmes (✉)
Department of Pediatric Cardiology, John Hopkins Medical Institutes, 600 N. Wolfe St.,
Brady 5, Baltimore, MD 21287, USA
e-mail: kwholmes@jhmi.edu

Ra-id Abdulla (ed.), *Heart Diseases in Children: A Pediatrician's Guide*,
DOI 10.1007/978-1-4419-7994-0_37, © Springer Science+Business Media, LLC 2011

Key Facts (continued)

- Pharmacotherapy should be used in patients greater than 8 years of age with total cholesterol persistently higher than 190 mg/dL despite changes in lifestyle and diet.
- Pharmacotherapy includes agents such as:

  - Bile acid sequestrants
  - Niacin
  - Fish oil or omega-3 fatty acids
  - HMG Co-A reductase inhibitors: such as Statins
  - Cholesterol absorption inhibitors

Definition

Obesity is a term that refers to an excess of body fat. However, since accurate measurements of body fat are difficult to obtain, indirect anthropomorphic measurements have been substituted for measurement of body fat. Obesity in children is determined by the weight in relation to height or by body mass index (BMI) adjusted for age and sex (BMI charts are available through the CDC). Obesity is defined as a BMI >95‰ for age and overweight is defined as a BMI >85‰. While there is additional evidence suggesting that abdominal obesity in particular is a marker for increased cardiovascular risk (as an indirect measure of visceral fat), a practical definition for clinical practice in the pediatric setting has not been formulated.

Incidence

The prevalence of obesity among school age children is increasing exponentially. Over the past 3 decades, one-third of children are either overweight or obese by the time they are adolescents. These trends continue into adulthood and numerous adult studies have suggested increased risk of cardiovascular disease in obese patients.

Obesity is associated with many comorbidities, affecting nearly every body system. Some examples include:

1. Endocrine – impaired glucose tolerance, diabetes mellitus, hyperandrogenism, and abnormalities of growth and puberty.
2. Cardiovascular – hypertension, hyperlipidemia, and early coronary artery disease.
3. Gastrointestinal – nonalcoholic fatty liver disease, and cholelithiasis.
4. Pulmonary – obstructive sleep apnea.

5. Musculoskeletal – slipped capital femoral epiphysis and tibia vara (Blount's disease).
6. Neurologic – idiopathic intracranial hypertension.
7. Dermatologic – furunculosis and acanthosis nigricans.
8. Psychosocial – low self-esteem, poor or distorted body image.

Dyslipidemia is defined as an abnormal fasting lipid profile. For clinical purposes, dyslipidemia in a child is defined by the American heart association as one or more of the following fasting laboratory values:

1. Total cholesterol (TC) >200 mg/dL
2. High-density lipoprotein cholesterol (HDL-C) <45 mg/dL
3. Low-density lipoprotein cholesterol (LDL-C) >130 mg/dL
4. Triglycerides >150 mg/dL in adolescents and >130 mg/dL in children

Originally, dyslipidemias were classified by phenotype. The Fredrickson's criteria were most often used, but are now largely outdated as the specific genetic defects related to these disorders are better understood. Traditionally, familial dyslipidemias were considered the most significant childhood disorders conferring increased risk of cardiovascular disease in children and so needed to be screened for early in suspected patients. We now appreciate that there are many other diseases that predispose children to early development of cardiovascular disease and so must also be recognized and screened for. Such diseases include Kawasaki disease with coronary involvement, diabetes, solid organ transplants, kidney disease and, of course, obesity.

Pathophysiology of Energy Balance and Cholesterol Metabolism

Energy balance is a complex interaction of neuroendocrine signals that integrate appetite, food intake, satiety, and energy stores. Lipids are needed in a number of important metabolic pathways including the use and storage of energy, the formation of steroids, and the building of cell walls. Lipids are hydrophobic and therefore insoluble in plasma and so must be transported to their destinations via lipoproteins. There are five major categories of lipoproteins: chylomicrons, very low density lipoproteins (VLDL), intermediate density lipoproteins (IDL), low-density lipoproteins (LDL) and high-density lipoprotein (HDL). Lipoproteins consist of cholesterol, triglycerides, phospholipids, and apolipoproteins. Therefore, abnormalities in lipoprotein or apolipoprotein metabolism can lead to derangements in cholesterol storage and metabolism.

Lipoprotein metabolism consists of two pathways – exogenous and endogenous. The exogenous pathway starts with absorption of dietary cholesterol and fatty acids from the intestinal lumen. Pancreatic enzymes and bile acid salts hydrolyze and emulsify these fats into micelles that are transported into the intestinal cell. Within the intestinal cell, fatty acids combine with glycerol to form triglycerides and cholesterol is esterified to form cholesterol esters. Triglycerides and cholesterol are then repackaged into chylomicrons and enter the portal circulation. Once in the circulation, chylomicrons travel until they reach their destination at which point the fatty acids are cleaved from the glycerol by lipoprotein lipase, an enzyme present on the luminal surface of epithelial cells. The free fatty acids are readily taken up by muscle cells while adipose cells take up and store fatty acids in the form of triglycerides. Fatty acids can also bind to fatty acid-binding proteins which are then taken up by the liver and repackaged into VLDL.

The endogenous pathway of lipid metabolism begins with the synthesis of VLDL in the liver. VLDL molecules contain a core of triglycerides and cholesterol esters and, once synthesized, follow a similar metabolic pathway to the chylomicrons, providing muscle cells with free fatty acids. The metabolism of VLDL generates particles that can either be cleared from the circulation, transferred to HDL, or remodeled to form LDL. Hepatic LDL can be converted to bile acids and secreted into the intestinal lumen for excretion.

LDL is internalized by hepatic and nonhepatic tissues. Nonhepatic LDL can be used for hormone production and cell membrane synthesis or it can be stored. A defective cellular LDL receptor is the genetic basis for familial hypercholesterolemia. In these patients, LDL is ineffectively taken into cells, resulting in increased plasma levels of LDL and total cholesterol.

As a small molecule, LDL can penetrate the endothelial layer of blood vessels and contribute significantly to the progression of atherosclerosis including disruption of the endothelial surface, impairment of endothelial function, and increased platelet aggregation. In addition, circulating LDL can be taken up by macrophages to become foam cells that contribute to athermanous plaque formation.

In contrast to the other lipoproteins, HDL has antiatherogenic properties that include the reversal of cholesterol transport, antioxidation, preservation of endothelial function, and maintenance of low blood viscosity. The main function of HDL appears to be reverse cholesterol transport from intracellular cholesterol back to the liver. As there is a suspected inverse relationship between the development of an atherosclerotic plaque and the ratio of LDL to HDL, increasing the levels of HDL will be a future management strategy.

IDL, VLDL, and a number of other smaller apolipoproteins such as apo E and apo B also play a role in the development of atherosclerosis. However, more research is needed before specific statements about their role in plaque formation can be made.

Elevated triglycerides also increase atherosclerotic risk by a number of pathways including increased blood viscosity and inflammation.

Clinical Manifestations

Patients presenting with one of the familial hypercholesterolemias may have no external signs. Some may demonstrate xanthomas on extensor surfaces. Family history is key to identifying patients for screening.

Patients presenting with obesity are self-evident and may have associated comorbidities described above.

Diagnosis

Early screening (between 2 and 8 years of age) with a fasting lipid profile should be done in all of the following high-risk groups:

1. Patients with a family history of early coronary artery disease or stroke.
2. Patients with familial dyslipidemia.
3. Patients with a BMI >85‰.
4. Patients with a history of Kawasaki disease.
5. Patients with active kidney disease or who have received a kidney transplant.
6. Patients who have had a heart transplant.
7. Patients with type I or II diabetes.
8. Patients with congenital heart disease.
9. Patients who are cancer treatment survivors.

Additional screening is recommended every 3–5 years through adulthood for these high-risk groups. The American Academy of Pediatrics currently does not recommend universal cholesterol screening. In addition, thresholds for elevated cholesterol differ by age with slightly higher total cholesterol levels tolerated in early adolescence.

Treatment

Management of obesity: Management of obesity is difficult as behavioral and dietary modification can be challenging for many patients. In general, the goal weight for a patient should be a BMI less than or equal to the 85th percentile for age and gender. For patients with BMI between 85 and 95‰, a goal of maintaining current weight will gradually reduce the BMI. For patients with BMI >95‰, a slow weight reduction plan with a goal loss of 1–2 pounds per week is reasonable. Weight reduction programs need to emphasize lifestyle and behavioral changes including reduced caloric intake and increased physical activity. All plans that involve weight reduction should be made in consultation with a dietitian and exercise specialist. Children will be more successful if their parents are involved in this process. This is especially important in cases where one or both parents are also obese or overweight.

Management of hyperlipidemia: Management focuses on reduction of cholesterol as well as total risk factor reduction. There is some controversy regarding what level of cholesterol pharmacotherapy should be initiated. However, it is generally accepted that patients greater than 8 years of age with total cholesterol persistently higher than 190 mg/dL despite changes in lifestyle and diet, should be started on pharmacotherapy. Controversy remains whether first line treatment should be HMG Co A reductase inhibitors (Statins) or one of the other more traditional therapies such as Bile acid sequestrants. Less controversial are high-risk groups such as patients with diabetes, history of kidney disease, or solid organ transplants. In these groups, pharmacotherapy is initiated when LDL is >130 g/dL and Statin therapy is the first line treatment. Note that pharmacological recommendations will likely continue to change in the future as the safety and efficacy of long-term Statin use is evaluated in the general population.

Pharmacotherapy

Bile acid sequestrants: Bile acid sequestrants work in the intestinal lumen by binding the cholesterol within the bile acids thereby preventing absorption. They can lower cholesterol by an average of 10–20% and while they do not have systemic side effects (as they are not absorbed), abdominal boating and increased stool frequency are common. These medications are difficult to take as they are either in the form of large tablets or a dissolvable powder. They are generally not well tolerated by children and compliance is often poor.

Niacin: Niacin works by decreasing the production of VLDL and thus increasing production of HDL while lowering LDL and triglyceride concentrations. While it is quite effective, the substantial side effect profile of Niacin limits its use. Side effects include hepatic failure, myopathy, glucose intolerance, and hyperuricemia.

Fish oil or omega-3 fatty acids: Fish oils are fatty acids that lower plasma triglycerides levels and have antithrombotic properties.

HMG co A reductase inhibitors: HMG Co-A reductase inhibitors (Statins) interfere with the rate-limiting step in endogenous hepatic cholesterol synthesis. Intracellular cholesterol levels decline and LDL receptors are unregulated. More LDL is taken into the cells so plasma levels decline. Statins are better tolerated than other pharmacologic options and can lower total cholesterol by 20–50%. Adverse effects include elevated hepatic transaminases. There are rare reports of rhabdomyolysis and there is some risk of teratogenicity. Stains should be used with caution in females of reproductive age and these patients should be specifically counseled about the risks of the medication in pregnancy.

Cholesterol absorption inhibitors: This is a relatively new class of drug, introduced in the 1990s, that inhibits cholesterol absorption from the intestinal lumen. They are most often used in combination therapy. Though these medications may be better tolerated than bile acid sequestrants, there is only limited data for their use in pediatrics.

Case Scenarios

Case 1: Familial Hypercholesterolemia

An 8-year-old male presents with his mother for routine health care maintenance. His mother reports that her husband died suddenly of a myocardial infarction at age 37 and was known to have elevated cholesterol. The boy is quite active and participates in soccer and basketball without cardio respiratory complaints. He appears healthy with height and weight in the 50th percentile for age. Physical examination is unremarkable except for a few Achilles tendon xanthomas. You obtain a fasting lipid panel, which shows total cholesterol of 323, HDL of 44, LDL of 262, and triglycerides of 86.

This patient has a familial hypercholesterolemia with an LDL receptor defect. He is likely a heterozygous, as total cholesterol for patients with homozygous mutations can be as high as 700–800. Because this diagnosis confers a high risk of early cardiovascular disease, intervention is necessary at this time. The patient should be started on a low cholesterol diet and pharmacotherapy should be initiated. Dietary modification alone is not effective in lower total cholesterol in this disorder. A statin would be the first line agent. The patient will then need hepatic enzymes checked in 1 month, then every 6 months after that. As rhabdomyolysis is a rare complication of statin therapy, any new muscle soreness, especially soreness not related to exercise, needs to be taken seriously.

Case 2: Obesity

A 14-year-old female comes in for her annual well child check. She voices no complaints this year. Family history is notable for mild obesity and hypertension in both parents. Her father also has non-insulin-dependent diabetes mellitus. A maternal grandmother suffered a stroke at age 60 and a paternal grandfather has diabetes, hypertension, and is status post coronary artery stent placements at age 50. The patient is not taking gym this year in school and has been overweight since age 8. Mom complains that her daughter is tired all the time and snores loudly at night. Physical examination demonstrates an obese adolescent female with weight 87 kg (>97‰), height 163 cm (50‰), BMI 47 (>98‰), and BP 140/75 (one time measurement). HEENT exam is remarkable for an obese patient with prominent acanthosis nigricans on her neck. Chest is clear, Cardiac examination is normal. Abdomen is soft without masses. She is tanner stage IV for breast and pubic hair. She has stria in her arms, neck, back, and hips. Neurological examination is grossly normal; however, you notice that she has some difficulty maneuvering on and off the examination table. You obtain a fasting lipid panel, which shows total cholesterol of 190, HDL of 40, LDL of 150, and triglycerides of 120. Hemoglobin A1C is at the upper limits of normal. Other laboratory values (thyroid function tests, renal and hepatic function panels) are normal.

At age 14, this girl represents an all too common presentation of childhood obesity with associated risk factors for early coronary artery disease including positive family history, obesity, possible hypertension, and elevated cholesterol and triglycerides. She is at high risk for development of diabetes and given her history of snoring, may already have obstructive sleep apnea.

The first step in management of this patient is a comprehensive weight reduction program that includes dietary modification and increased physical activity for at least 3 months. This patient would benefit greatly from a family approach to care given her parents are also obese. Hypertension cannot be diagnosed with a single blood pressure measurement. At least three ambulatory measurements are required before considering pharmacotherapy. In addition, given her size, it may be appropriate to use either a large adult cuff or potentially a thigh blood pressure cuff. Her possible sleep apnea should be addressed with further questions regarding her sleep and diagnostic sleep study. Pharmacotherapy targeted at her hypertension and hyperlipidemia could be considered after 3 months if there is no improvement.

Drugs in Pediatric Cardiology

Paul Severin, Beth Shields, Joan Hoffman, Sawsan Awad, William Bonney,
Edmundo Cortez, Rani Ganesan, Aloka Patel, Steve Barnes, Sean Barnes,
Shada Al-Anani, Umang Gupta, Yolandee Bell-Cheddar, Ra-id Abdulla

Key Facts

- Whenever possible, medications given to children with heart diseases are best started at low doses, then titrated to effect.
- In infants and children with severe diarrhea and or vomiting it may be advisable to hold diuretic therapy during this time.
- Use of intravenous calcium infusion should be done through central venous lines since extravasation is likely to lead to tissue necrosis.
- Patients on any combination of spironolactone, potassium supplements, and angiotensin converting enzyme inhibitors (captopril, enalapril) should have their serum potassium levels monitored at regular intervals.
- If digoxin is prescribed correctly, serum levels are not necessary. Serum levels should be obtained if there is lack of compliance, acute changes in renal function, or signs of digoxin toxicity.
- Epinephrine infusion should be limited to very ill children, due to broad spectrum effect.
- Milrinone improves myocardial contractility and reduces vascular resistance, thus reducing afterload effect.
- Neo-synephrine (Phenylephrine hydrochloride) is used in severe hypercyanotic spells due to tetralogy of Fallot. It is typically used after all other pharmacological measures have failed.
- Development of a dry cough after use of ACE inhibitor (captopril or enalapril) may be due to these agents. Replacement medication may be considered.
- Amiodarone is an anti-arrhythmic agent with broad spectrum effect. The half life of the medication is very long and therefore, its effect lasts days or even weeks after discontinuation.
- Esmolol is a rapid acting intravenous beta blocker with prompt effect when started and quick cessation of effect when discontinued.

Ra-id Abdulla (ed.), *Heart Diseases in Children: A Pediatrician's Guide*,
DOI 10.1007/978-1-4419-7994-0, © Springer Science+Business Media, LLC 2011

Inotropes and vasopressors

Drug	Pharmacology	Route	Dose	Frequency	Comments
Calcium Chloride	Onset: immediate Mode of action: enhances contractility through regulation of action potential Half-life: short	IV	Hypocalcemia: 10–20 mg/kg (maximum dose=1 g)	Q4–6 h for hypocalcemia Infuse slowly over 10 min Q10 min for cardiac arrest	Side effects: bradycardia, hypotension, peripheral vasodilation, hypercalcemia, hypermagnesemia, hyperchloremic acidosis; ventricular fibrillation Caution: central venous access preferred due to high risk of extravasation injury; use with caution in patients who are being digitalized Contraindication: hypercalcemia, ventricular fibrillation
Calcium Gluconate	Onset: rapid Mode of action: enhances contractility through regulation of action potential	PO, IV	Hypocalcemia: 50–100 mg/kg (maximum dose=3 g)	QID	Side effects: bradycardia, hypotension, peripheral vasodilation, hypercalcemia, hypermagnesemia Caution: central venous line administration recommended. Maximum concentration for infusion is 50 mg/ml. Extravasation may lead to tissue necrosis, use local hyaluronidase if occurs, may precipitate arrhythmia in digitalized patient Contraindication: hypercalcemia, ventricular fibrillation

| Digoxin (Lanoxin, Lanoxicaps) | Onset: PO 30 min–2 h; IV 5–30 min

Mode of action:
Inhibition of Na$^+$–K pump resulting in increase Ca^{2+} intracellular influx

Decreases conduction through AV and sinus nodes by inhibiting ATPase

Increase parasympathetic cardiac and arterial baroreceptor activity leading to decreased sympathetic outflow

Half-life: preterm 60–170 h; full term 35–45 h; toddler 18–25 h; children 35 h | PO

IV | Loading: note: 1st half initially administered followed by one-fourth of calculated dose q8 × 2 doses
Infants: preterm: 20 μg/kg total; term: 30 μg/kg total
Maintenance: preterm: 5–8 μg/kg/day; term: 6–10 μg/kg/day

Loading: Follow same schedule as above (for oral loading) with following doses: preterm: 15 μg/kg; term: 20 μg/kg
Maintenance: preterm: 3–4 μg/kg/day; term: 5–8 μg/kg/day (maximum (adult) dose: 250 μg/day) | BID | Side effects: dysrhythmia, AV block, fatigue, headache, nausea, anorexia, feeding intolerance, neuralgias, blurred vision, photophobia, somnolence, fatigue
Caution: cardioversion or calcium infusion may cause VF in patients receiving digoxin (pretreatment with Lidocaine may be helpful)
Therapeutic level: 0.8–2 ng/ml, not reliable in neonates, since they may have falsely elevated levels (due to maternal digoxin like substances in serum)
Contraindication: subaortic obstruction; hypertrophic cardiomyopathy; severe electrolyte abnormalities more specifically hypokalemia and alkalemia; hypothyroidism; renal failure (cannot be removed with dialysis)
Toxicity: usually associated with digoxin level 2 ng/ml; symptoms include AV block, arrhythmias; hyperkalemia |

(continued)

Drug	Pharmacology	Route	Dose	Frequency	Comments
Dobutamine Dobutrex	Onset: 1–10 min Peak: 10–20 min Mode of action: stimulates beta 1 adrenergic receptors (minimal beta 2 and alpha), resulting in increase myocardial contractility and heart rate Half-life: 2 min	Infusion	2–20 μg/kg/min		Side effects: atrial/ventricular arrhythmias, hypertrophic cardiomyopathy, tachycardia, hypertension, angina, palpitation, headache Contraindication: IHSS, tachycardia, arrhythmias, hypertension Caution: central venous infusion preferred due to high risk of extravasation injury
Dopamine Intropin	Onset: 5 min Peak: Mode of action: precursor of norepinephrine; dose dependent stimulation of DA1, DA2, B1, and alpha Half-life: 2 min	Infusion	Low dose (DA1 and DA2 resulting in splanchnic, renal, and coronary vasodilation): 1–5 μg/kg/min Intermediate dose (dopaminergic + b adrenergic resulting in increased renal blood flow, inotropic and chronotropic): 5–15 μg/kg/min High dose (predominant alpha with vasoconstriction): 15–20 μg/kg/min		Side effects (dose dependent): tachyarrhythmias, ectopic atrial/ventricular beats, hypertension, headache, nausea, increases pulmonary vascular resistance, mydriasis Contraindication: pheochromocytoma, ventricular fibrillation Caution: central venous infusion preferred due to high risk of extravasation injury

Drug	Pharmacology	Route	Dose	Interval	Side effects/Contraindications
Epinephrine HCl Adrenaline	Onset: IV: 1–5 min (<1 min) SQ: 5–10 min Mode of action: dose dependent stimulates alpha 1, beta 1, beta 2 receptors Half-life: 2–3 min	IV/IO (Arrest)	Bradycardia/hypotension: 1:10,000 0.01 mg/kg (max = 1 mg)	Q3–5 min	Side effects: tachyarrhythmias, hypertension, headache, nervousness, nausea, vomiting, sudden death, decrease renal blood flow, leukocytosis Contraindication: Acute coronary artery disease, angle closure glaucoma Caution: central venous infusion preferred due to high risk of extravasation injury; use with caution in cases of myocardial ischemia
		Endotracheal	Bradycardia/hypotension: 1:1,000 0.1 mg/kg	Q3–5 min	
		SQ/IM	Asthma/Anaphylaxis 1:1,000 (0.01 mg/kg) (max = 0.3 mg)	Q5–10 min	
		Infusion	0.05–1 µg/kg/min		
Milrinone Primacor	Onset: IV 5–15 min Mode of action: inodilator with lusitropy properties; myocardial cAMP phosphodiesterase inhibitor resulting in increased intracellular cAMP; lowers both systemic and pulmonary vascular resistance Half-life: 3 h	Infusion	Load: 50 µg/kg, over 10–15 min Maintenance: 0.25–1 µg/kg/min		Side effects: arrhythmia, headache, hypotension, thrombocytopenia; angina; hypokalemia; bronchospasm; transaminitis Contraindication: severe right and left ventricular outflow obstruction Caution: adjust dose in patients with renal dysfunction; use with caution in patients with history of atrial fibrillation or flutter

(continued)

Drug	Pharmacology	Route	Dose	Frequency	Comments
Phenylephrine HCl Neo-synephrine	Onset: IV immediate; IM/SQ 10–15 min Mode of action: Alpha adrenergic receptors agonist resulting in potent vasoconstriction Half-life: IV 2.5 h; IM/SQ 2.5 h	IV SQ/IM Infusion	5–20 µg/kg, (maximum dose = 0.5 mg) 0.1 mg/kg (maximum dose = 5 mg) 0.1–0.5 µg/kg/min, (maximum = 4 µg/kg/min)	Q10–20 min Q1–2 h	Side effects: tremor, insomnia, palpitation, hypertension, angina, excitability, headache, tremors, sinus bradycardia, reflux, photophobia Caution: central venous access preferred with high risk of extravasation injury Contraindication: pheochromocytoma, severe hypertension, ventricular tachyarrhythmias, myocardial disease, narrow angle glaucoma
Norepinephrine Levophed	Onset: very rapid Mode of action: alpha and beta adrenergic receptor agonist (predominantly alpha effect) resulting in significant vasoconstriction Half-life: 1–2 min	Infusion	0.05–2 µg/kg/min (maximum = 2 µg/kg/min)		Side effects: arrhythmias, palpitation, hypertension, angina, headache, anxiety, vomiting, uterine contractions, respiratory distress, diaphoresis Caution: central venous access preferred with high risk of extravasation injury Contraindication: pheochromocytoma, severe hypertension, ventricular tachyarrhythmias, severe coronary artery disease
Vasopressin (DI, gastrointestinal bleeding, refractory hypotension)	Onset: 1 h Mode of action: binds to AVPR1 receptors resulting in increased intracellular Ca levels; vasoconstriction Half-life: 10–20 min	IV Infusion	0.0003–0.002 U/kg/min (vasoplegic shock)		Side effects: hypertension, bradycardia, arrhythmia, venous thrombosis, vasoconstriction, angina, cardiac arrest, heart block; seizures; hyponatremia Contraindications: Caution: use with caution in patients with kidney, hepatic, and cardiac dysfunction; also use with caution in the presence of seizures

Vasodilators and antihypertensives

Drug	Pharmacology	Route	Dose	Frequency	Comments
Captopril Capoten	Onset: 15–60 min Peak effect: 60–90 min Mode of action: angiotensin converting enzyme inhibitor Duration: dose related Half-life: 1–12 h	PO	Premature: 0.01 mg/kg/dose PO/NG q8–12 h Neonates: Initial dose: 0.05–0.1 mg/kg/dose (titrate dose to maximum = 0.5 mg/kg/dose) q8–24 h Infants and children: Initial dose: 0.15–0.5 mg/kg/dose (titrate dose to max = 6 mg/kg/day) q8–24 h Adolescents: 6.25–12.5 mg PO q12–24 h Adults: 12.5–25 mg q8–24 h (usual dose range 25–100 mg/day divided BID)	TID, BID, QD TID, BID, QD BID	Side effects: hypotension, rash, proteinuria, neutropenia, tachycardia, cough, diminution of taste, reduce aldosterone production causing increased potassium renal absorption causing hyperkalemia Caution: Adjust with renal dysfunction Creatinine clearance 10–50 ml/min/1.73 m^2 administer 75% of recommended dose Creatinine clearance <10 ml/min/1.73 m^2 administer 50% of recommended dose Drug interactions: NSAIDs, e.g., indomethacin, may decrease the antihypertensive effect of captopril. Potassium sparing agents potentiate hyperkalemic effect Note: doses for all patients should be titrated to desired effect. Lowest possible dose should be used. Lower doses are indicated for patients treated with diuretics

(continued)

Drug	Pharmacology	Route	Dose	Frequency	Comments
Carvedilol	Onset: alpha blockade 30 min; beta blockade 60 min Peak effect: Mode of action: alpha and beta antagonist	PO	Infants and children: Initial dose: 0.03–0.8 mg/ kg/dose BID (maximum initial dose=3.125 mg) Maintenance dose: to be increased every 2 weeks for average dose 0.3–0.9 mg/kg/dose BID (maximum dose=25 mg PO BID) Adults: Initial dose: 3.125 mg PO BID (x2 weeks) Maintenance dose: double dose q2 weeks to maximum 25 mg PO BID (<85 kg) and 50 mg PO BID (>85 kg)	BID	Side effects: hypotension, cardiac arrest, AV block, bradycardia, syncope, peripheral edema, withdrawal and postural hypotension, dizziness, hyperglycemia, hypertriglyceridemia, weight gain, hyperkalemia, bone marrow suppression, liver dysfunction, myalgia, fatigue, headache, insomnia, somnolence, microalbuminuria, erectile dysfunction, bronchospasm, rhinitis, pharyngitis, dyspnea Caution: concomitant use with amiodarone, dihydropyridine calcium channel blockers, withdrawal of clonidine. Digoxin, diltiazem, insulin, phenoxybenzamine, verapamil Contraindication: severe liver failure Note: dose adjust in hepatic insufficiency

| Enalapril (Vasotec) | Onset: PO 30–60 min; IV: 10–15 min
Peak effect: PO 1 h; IV 15 min
Mode of action: angiotensin converting enzyme inhibitor
Half-life: PO depends on age or presence of CHF (2–10 h)
IV depends on age (10–38 h) | PO (enalapril) | Infants/children: 0.05–0.1 mg/kg/dose initial PO QD (titrate as required every 3–5 days to maximum of 0.5 mg/kg/day)
Adults: 2.5 mg PO initial PO QD-BID (titrate by 2.5 mg/dose to maximum of 40 mg/day) | QD, BID | Side effects: neutropenia, hyperkalemia, hypoglycemia, chronic cough, hypotension, tachycardia, dyspnea, eosinophilic pneumonitis, fatigue, vertigo, dizziness, headache, insomnia, cholestatic jaundice, fulminant hepatic necrosis, renal insufficiency, erectile dysfunction, muscle cramps, hyperkalemia, bone marrow suppression, rash, angioedema
Caution: reduce dose in renal failure
Creatinine clearance 10–50 ml/min/1.73 m^2 administer 75% of recommended dose
Creatinine clearance <10 ml/min/1.73 m^2 administer 50% of recommended dose
Contraindications: idiopathic/hereditary angioedema
Drug interactions: NSAIDs, e.g., indomethacin, may decrease the antihypertensive effect. Potassium sparing agents potentiate hyperkalemic effect. May also increase serum lithium levels |
| | | IV, slow over 5 min (enalaprilat) | Infants/children: 5–10 µg/kg (titrate to response maximum = 1.25 mg/dose)
Adults: 0.625 mg/dose initial IV q6 (maximum dose = 20 mg/day) | QD–Q8H | Note: doses for all patients should be titrated to desired effect. Lowest possible dose should be used. Lower doses are indicated for patients treated with diuretics
With the presence of benzyl alcohol in enalaprilat, it may cause an allergic reaction and potentially fatal toxicity in neonates called "gasping syndrome."
Gasping syndrome presents with metabolic acidosis, respiratory distress, CV collapse, and intracranial hemorrhage |

(continued)

Drug	Pharmacology	Route	Dose	Frequency	Comments
Hydralazine (Apresoline)	Onset: PO: 10–30 min; IV: 5–20 min Mode of action: direct acting peripheral vasodilator with precise mechanism unknown Half Life: 2–8 h Duration: PO 2–4 h; IV 2–6 h	PO	Infants/children: Initial: 0.75–1 mg/kg/day NG (maximum 25 mg/dose). Increase every 3–4 weeks by 5 mg/kg/day to maximum final daily dose=200 mg/day Adults: Initial: 10 mg PO QID increase 10–25 mg/dose every 2–5 days (max 300 mg/day)	BID, QID	Side effects: SLE like syndrome (reversible), palpitation, flushing, rash hematological changes. Hypotension, tachycardia, headache, anorexia, nausea, dizziness, nausea, vomiting, diarrhea, arthralgias Caution: severe renal failure and cardiac disease, CVA Dose adjustment in renal impairment recommended
		IV, IM	Infants/children: Initial: 0.1–0.2 mg/kg/dose (maximum=20 mg/dose) Adults: Initial: 10–20 mg/dose (maximum dose=40 mg/dose)	Q4–Q6 h	Contraindication: coronary artery disease, dissecting aortic aneurysm, mitral valve rheumatic heart disease Drug interactions: concomitant use with MAO inhibitors may cause profound hypotension. May increase the levels of metoprolol and propranolol

| Labetolol (Normodyne) | Onset: IV 5–10 min; PO 20–120 min
Peak effect: IV 5–30 min; PO 1–4 h
Mode of action: combined beta (B1/B2) and alpha adrenergic receptor antagonist
Duration: IV 2–6 h; PO 8–12 h (dose dependent) | PO (100, 200, 300 mg)

IV | Children: 1.5 mg–10 mg/kg/dose (maximum dose = 40 mg/kg/day and a maximum dose of 2.4 g/day)
Adult: 100 mg PO BID to increase by 100 mg/dose every 2–3 days (maximum dose = 2.4 g/day)
Children: 0.2 mg–1 mg/kg/dose bolus; 0.4–1 mg/kg/h continuous infusion
Adult: 20 mg IV bolus over 2 min; may repeat 20–80 mg IV every 10 min (total dose = 300 mg)
Continuous infusion: 2 mg/min (max = 300 mg/h) | BID

q10 min PRN | Side effects: orthostatic hypotension, hypotension, bradycardia, dyspnea, syncope, dizziness, weight gain, diaphoresis, tremor, vomiting, altered mental status, jaundice, abdominal pain, arrhythmia
Drug Interactions: Concomitant use with insulin and oral antidiabetic medications potentiates hypoglycemia
Contraindications: hypersensitivity
Caution: Avoid in patients with asthma, COPD, CHF, bradycardia, or greater than first-degree heart block |

(continued)

Drug	Pharmacology	Route	Dose	Frequency	Comments
Lisinopril	Onset: 1 h Peak effect: 6–8 h Mode of action: ACE inhibitor Half life: 11–13 h	PO	Children (6 years old): initial dose: 0.07 mg/kg/dose PO QD (maximum initial dose 5 mg PO QD); titrate dose every 1–2 weeks to desired effect (maximum dose = 40 mg/day) Adults: initial: 5–10 mg PO QD; titrate dose every 1–2 weeks by 5–10 mg to desired effect (maximum dose = 40 mg/day)	QD	Side effects: hypotension, angina, orthostatic hypotension, tachycardia, cough, dyspnea, syncope, eosinophilic pneumonitis, headache, dizziness, fatigue, diarrhea, nausea, vomiting, loss of taste, angioedema, cholestatic jaundice, hepatitis, fulminant hepatic necrosis, renal insufficiency, hyperkalemia, bone marrow suppression, rash, anaphylactoid reactions Drug interactions: consider the cessation of any potassium supplements or potassium sparing drugs as concomitant use may increase serum potassium levels Contraindications: patients with idiopathic or hereditary angioedema Caution: doses for all patients should be titrated to desired effect. Lowest possible dose should be used. Lower doses indicated for patients are being treated with diuretics

| Losartan | Onset: 6 h
Peak effect: 1 h
Mode of action: angiotensin II receptor antagonist
Half life: 1–2 h | PO | Infants: no data
Children (6–16 years old): 0.7 mg/kg PO QD (maximum dose 50 mg/day)
Adults: initial: 25–50 mg PO QD (maximum dose 100 mg PO QD) | QD | Side effects: angina, hypotension, orthostatic hypotension, tachycardia, cough, bronchitis, rhinitis, sinusitis, fatigue, dizziness, hypoesthesia, insomnia, diarrhea, dyspepsia, nausea, UTI, weakness, arthralgias, myalgias, hypoglycemia, hyperkalemia, anemia, cellulitis, fever, infections, flu-like syndrome
Drug interactions: consider the cessation of any potassium supplements or potassium sparing drugs as concomitant use may increase serum potassium levels
Contraindications: bilateral renal artery stenosis; pregnancy
Caution: fetal death, avoid use in nursing mothers |
| Metoprolol (Lopressor) | Onset: 15–30 min
Mode of action: β adrenergic receptor blockade | PO | 0.5–1 mg/kg, (maximum = 200 mg) | BID | Side effects: hypoglycemia, hypotension, nausea, vomiting, abdominal pain, CNS symptoms (depression, weakness, dizziness) bronchospasm, heart block, bradycardia, negative inotropic effect
Caution: in lung disease, heart, hepatic or renal failure
Drug interactions: barbiturates, rifampin increase clearance of metoprolol. Metoprolol metabolism decreases with cimetidine, amiodarone, diltiazem, propafenone, quinidine, hydralazine, chlorpromazine, or verapamil
Contraindication: asthma, heart block with concurrent use of verapamil |

(continued)

Drug	Pharmacology	Route	Dose	Frequency	Comments
Nesiritide (Natrecor)	Onset: rapid; Peak effect: Mode of action: a recombinant human B-type natriuretic peptide that regulates cardiovascular homeostasis and fluid volume during states of volume and pressure overload; Half-life:	Infusion	Load (optional): 1 µg/kg, over 1 min; Maintenance (increase by 0.005 µg/kg/min increments): 0.005–0.02 µg/kg/min		Side effects: hypotension, headache, hypotension, nausea, arrhythmia; Caution: greater risk of hypotension when coadministered with ACE inhibitors; Contraindication: significant valvular stenosis; restrictive or obstructive cardiomyopathy; constrictive pericarditis; pericardial tamponade; suspected low cardiac filling pressures; atrial, ventricular arrhythmias/conduction defects (has not been evaluated in these patients); hypotension
Nicardipine (Cardene)	Onset: IV rapid; PO 30–120 min; Peak effect: IV rapid; PO 1–7 h; Mode of action: a calcium channel blocker structurally related to nifedipine; Half-life: PO 2–4 h; IV	Infusion	Load: none; Maintenance: 0.5–5 µg/kg/min		Side effects: reflex tachycardia, hypotension; Caution: continuous blood pressure monitoring required; Contraindications: neonates with asphyxia
Nitroglycerin (Tridil, Nitro-Bid)	Onset: rapid; Mode of action: vasodilation, venous more than arterial	Infusion; Ointment	Initial: 0.25–0.5 µg/kg/min; Then: 0.5–10 µg/kg/min; Usual dose 1–3 µg/kg/min; 1–2 in.	Q8 h	Side effects: flushing, headache, hypotension, tachycardia, nausea, perspiration, tolerance; Caution: increase ICP, hypovolemia; Contraindication: glaucoma, severe anemia

	Route	Dose	Interval	Onset/Mode of action	Side effects
Nitroprusside (Niprid, Nitropress)	Infusion	0.5–10 μg/kg/min Usual dose is 3 μg/kg/min Neonates maximum = 6 μg/kg/min		Onset: rapid Mode of action: peripheral vasodilator	Side effects: profound hypotension, metabolic acidosis, weakness, psychosis, headache, increased ICP, thyroid suppression, nausea, sweating, cyanide and thiocyanate toxicity Caution: monitor thiocyanate level, if used >48 h. Keep level <35 mg/l Contraindication: reduced cerebral perfusion, coarctation of the aorta, AV shunts
Phenoxy-benzamine	PO/IV	PO: Infants/children: initial dose: 0.2 mg/kg/dose PO QD-BID. May increase dose gradually to 10 mg/dose	Q6–8 h	Onset: rapid Peak effect: rapid Mode of action: nonspecific, long-acting, irreversible alpha adrenergic antagonist – potent peripheral vasodilator Half-life: PO not well-known; IV 24 h	Side effects: tachycardia, arrhythmia, hypotension, shock, vomiting, sodium and water retention, dizziness, miosis, nasal congestion, fatigue, lethargy Contraindications: concomitant use with beta adrenergic receptors may cause profound hypotension with reflex tachycardia Toxicity: treatment of overdose – drug elevation, IV fluid resuscitation, recumbent position with leg elevation, infusion with norepinephrine or vasopressin (epinephrine contraindicated) for severe hypotension
		PO: Adults: 5–10 mg PO; titrate every 48 h to maximum dose = 40 mg/day	Q8 h		

(continued)

Drug	Pharmacology	Route	Dose	Frequency	Comments
Phentolamine	Onset: immediate Peak effect: 2 min Mode of action: reversible, competitive, nonselective alpha adrenergic antagonist – systemic vasodilator Half-life: 19 min	IV	Infants/children: initial dose: 0.05–0.1 mg/kg (maximum dose = 5 mg) infused over 10–30 min Adults: initial dose: 2.5–5 mg IV	Infusion	Side effects: hypotension, tachycardia, arrhythmia, shock, ischemia, vomiting, nausea, abdominal pain, diarrhea, peptic ulcer, fatigue, flushing, dizziness, nasal congestion Contraindications: ischemic cerebral and myocardial disease; concomitant use with beta adrenergic receptors may cause profound hypotension with reflex tachycardia Toxicity: treatment of overdose – drug withdrawal, recumbent position with leg elevation, IV fluid resuscitation, infusion with norepinephrine or vasopressin (epinephrine contraindicated) for severe hypotension

Antiarrhythmics medications

Drug	Pharmacology	Route	Dose	Frequency	Comments
Adenosine (Adenocard)	Onset: very rapid Half-life: seconds Slows AV node conduction	IV, rapid push followed by saline flush	0.1 mg/kg/dose. Increase to 0.15 and 0.2 mg/kg/dose with successive doses. Maximum dose is 0.3 mg/kg (maximum dose = 12 mg)	Rapid IV push Q2 min PRN	Side effects: palpitations, flushing, headache, dyspnea, nausea, chest pain, lightheadedness, bradycardia Caution: bronchospasm in asthmatics. Atrial fibrillation (usually nonsustained) results in about 10% of patients Drug interactions: dipyridamole potentiates effects, carbamazepine may increase heart block, theophylline antagonizes effect of adenosine
Amiodarone (Cordarone)	Onset: 3 days–3 weeks with oral loading. May see effect within 30 min with IV Mode of action: class III, inhibits alpha and beta adrenergic receptors, prolongs action potential and refractoriness	PO Infusion	Loading: 10–15 mg/kg/day (maximum dose = 1,600 mg) Maintenance: 2.5–5 mg/kg/day (maximum dose = 800 mg) Load: 5 mg/kg over 20–60 min. May repeat X4 (maximum 20 mg of all 4 loading doses) Maintenance: 5–15 μg/kg/min	QD X 7–14 days	Side effects: long half life. Worsening AV block and bradycardias especially in infants. Pulmonary fibrosis alters thyroid (hypothyroidism) and liver dysfunction. Anorexia, nausea, vomiting, dizziness, paresthesia, ataxia and tremor, corneal deposits, blue discoloration of skin, photosensitivity Caution: increases digoxin (reduce digoxin dose by 1/2), warfarin, flecainide, procainamide, quinidine and phenytoin serum levels, thyroid disease Therapeutic level: 0.5–2.5 mg/L Contraindications: AV block, sinus node dysfunction, sinus bradycardia

(continued)

Drug	Pharmacology	Route	Dose	Frequency	Comments
Atenolol (Tenormin)	Onset: 60–120 min Mode of action: class II antiarrhythmic agent, long acting selective β Blocker	PO	0.5–1 mg/kg/dose (maximum dose = 100 mg/day)	QD or BID	Side effects: hypoglycemia, hypotension, nausea, vomiting, depression, weakness, less bronchospasm than propranolol, heart block, bradycardia, negative inotropic effect Caution: CHF, adjust dose in renal failure Contraindication: cardiogenic shock, pulmonary edema
Esmolol (Brevibloc)	Onset: rapid Route: IV only Mode of action: class II. Selective β₁ blocker	Infusion	Loading: 500 µg/kg rapid IV bolus Maintenance: 50 µg/ kg/min, increase by 50 µg/kg increments to a maximum of 200 µg/ kg/min. Reload with each increase. Titrate to effect	Over 1 min Continuous infusion	Side effects: hypoglycemia, hypotension, nausea, vomiting, depression, phlebitis, bronchospasm at higher doses, heart block, bradycardia, negative inotropic effect Caution: skin necrosis may occur with extravasation, maximum concentration is 10 mg/ml due to hyperosmolarity. May increase digoxin or theophylline serum levels Contraindication: cardiogenic shock, heart block, severe asthma
Flecainide (Tambocor)	Onset: rapid Mode of action: class Ic antiarrhythmic agent, sodium channel blocker, cell membrane depression	PO (IV not available in USA)	0.5–1 mg/kg/dose Maximum 8 mg/kg/day Maximum adult 400 mg/day	TID	Side effects: proarrhythmia (VT or incessant SVT). Negative inotropic effect, arrhythmias, rash Caution: monitor for proarrhythmia in hospital during drug initiation. Heart failure, heart block, hepatic impairment, reduce dose by 25–50% in renal failure. Milk may inhibit absorption in infants if given concurrently Contraindication: 2nd or 3rd degree AV block Therapeutic level: 0.2–1 µg/mL

Drug	Onset/Mode of action	Route	Dose	Frequency	Notes
Lidocaine (Xylocaine)	Onset: rapid. Mode of action: class Ib antiarrhythmic agent, sodium channel blocker, local anesthetic depressing myocardial irritability	IV	1 mg/kg loading dose	Repeat after 5 min, PRN	Side effects: hypotension, shock, nausea, seizures, respiratory depression, anxiety, euphoria, drowsiness, agitation. Caution: hepatic disease, heart failure. Levels must be monitored carefully to prevent neurotoxicity. Contraindication: AV block. Therapeutic level: 2–5 μg/mL
		Infusion	20–50 μg/kg/min	Continuous infusion	
Phenytoin (Dilantin)	Onset: minutes. Mode of action: not well defined	IV (arrhythmia dose)	Load: 1.25 mg/kg (may repeat to total dose of 15 mg/kg)	Q 5 min	Side effects: phlebitis if given through a peripheral IV. Gingival hyperplasia, hirsutism, exfoliative dermatitis, osteomalacia, ataxia, drowsiness, blood dyscrasias, SLE-like syndrome, Stevens–Johnson syndrome, peripheral neuropathy, lymphadenopathy, hepatitis, nystagmus, hypotension, bradycardia, folic acid deficiency. Note: useful for treating arrhythmias caused by digitalis toxicity. Caution: oral absorption reduced in neonates, serum levels are increased by cimetidine, chloramphenicol, INH, sulfonamide, trimethoprim. Rapid injection may cause hypotension and bradycardia. Contraindication: heart block or sinus bradycardia
		PO	5–10 mg/kg/day	Divided BID or TID	

(continued)

Drug	Pharmacology	Route	Dose	Frequency	Comments
Procainamide	Onset: IV rapid; PO 2–4 h; IM 10–30 min Mode of action: class Ia antiarrhythmic agent, Sodium channel blocker depressing myocardial excitability and conduction	Oral form discontinued by manufacturer IV Infusion	4–12 mg/kg (maximum = 1 g/dose or 4 g/day) Load: 3–6 mg/kg/dose, may repeat up to 15 mg/kg (maximum dose = 100 mg/dose) Maintenance: 20–80 µg/kg/min, maximum dose = 6 mg/min, maximum = 2 g/day	Q3–6 h Over 5 min Continuous infusion	Side effects: hypotension, prolongs QRS and QT durations, SLE-like symptoms, fever, positive coombs' test, thrombocytopenia, rash, myalgia, arrhythmias, GI symptoms, confusion Caution: monitor closely for hypotension during loading and stop infusion if hypotension occurs or QRS complex widens by >50%. Toxicity when QRS >200 ms, do not routinely administer procainamide and amiodarone together Therapeutic level: 4–10 mg/L of procainamide, or 10–30 mg/L of procainamide and NAPA levels combined Drug interactions: PA and NAPA levels are increased with cimetidine, ranitidine, amiodarone, beta blockers, trimethoprim. Anticholinergic agents enhance effect Contraindication: Myasthenia gravis, complete heart block
Propafenone Rhythmol, Rhythmol SR	Onset: rapid Mode of action: Class Ic antiarrhythmic agent, also blocks sodium channels and β Blocker effect	PO	150–200 mg/m²/day, maximum dose 400–500 mg/m²/day	TID	Side effects: AV block, palpitations, bradycardia, CHF, conduction disturbances, dizziness, drowsiness, dry mouth, altered taste, dyspnea, flatulence, blurred vision, dyspepsia Caution: recent MI, CHF, hepatic or renal dysfunction, rarely proarrhythmia and/or VT Contraindication: cardiogenic shock, bronchospastic disorder, conduction disorder

Drug	Mode of action / Onset	Route	Dose	Frequency	Side effects / Caution / Contraindication
Propranolol (Inderal)	Onset: PO 40–120 min; IV rapid. Mode of action: β blocker, class II antidysrhythmic agent	PO IV (over 10 min)	1–4 mg/kg/day 0.01–0.15 mg/kg dose over 15–30 min (maximum = 1 mg/dose for infants and 3 mg/dose for children)	QID Q6 h	Side effects: hypo- or hyperglycemia, hypotension, nausea, vomiting, depression, weakness, bronchospasm, heart block, bradycardia, negative inotropic effect. Caution: in lung disease, heart, hepatic or renal failure. Barbiturates, rifampin, or indomethacin increases clearance, cimetidine, hydralazine, chlorpromazine, or verapamil causes decrease in clearance and enhanced effect. IV dose must be given slowly. Contraindication: asthma, cardiogenic shock, and heart block
Verapamil (rapid release)	Onset: PO 60–120 min; IV rapid. Mode of action: Class IV Calcium channel blocker	PO IV over 2–3 min	2–8 mg/kg/day (maximum dose = 80 mg) Children 1–16 years: 0.1–0.3 mg/kg/dose given over 2 min. May repeat in 30 min (maximum dose = 5 mg)	TID Q30 min PRN If stable: TID, BID (for rapid release only)	Side effects: negative inotropic effect, constipation, hypotension, dizziness, fatigue. Caution: avoid use in neonates and young infants and in WPW due to severe apnea, bradycardia, hypotensive reactions, and cardiac arrest. Do not use with other negative inotropes (e.g., beta-blockers). To reverse hypotension use calcium, and IV volume. Reduce digoxin by 1/3 to 1/2. Contraindication: CHF, hypotension, shock, AV block, right to left shunt lesions, atrial fibrillation, sinus bradycardia. Drug interactions: may increase serum level of digoxin, quinidine, carbamazepine, cyclosporin. Phenobarbital and rifampin may increase metabolism of verapamil

Emergency medications

Drug	Pharmacology	Route	Dose	Frequency	Comments
Atropine	Onset: Rapid Mode of action: blocks acetylcholine activity	IV, ET	0.01–0.02 mg/kg (minimum single dose = 0.1 mg and maximum single dose = 1 mg)	PRN	Side effects: dry mouth, blurred vision, tachycardia, dry hot skin, restlessness, fatigue, difficult micturition, impaired GI motility, CNS symptoms, hyperthermia, palpitation, delirium, headache, tremor Contraindication: glaucoma, tachycardia, thyrotoxicosis, GI obstruction, uropathy
Diphenhydramine (Benadryl)	Onset: PO 20–40 min; IV 10–20 min Mode of action: histamine 1 receptor antagonist	PO, IV, IM	1–2 mg/kg (maximum = 50 mg)	QID	Side effects: sedation, drowsiness, insomnia, vomiting, anorexia, constipation, diarrhea, anticholinergic effect, hypotension, palpitation, tachycardia, paradoxical excitement, fatigue, photosensitivity, rash, dry mouth, urinary retention, blurred vision, thickened bronchial secretions Caution: peptic ulcers, hyperthyroidism Contraindication: angle closure glaucoma, GI or urinary tract obstruction
Calcium Chloride	Onset: rapid Mode of action: enhances contractility through regulation of action potential	IV	Cardiac arrest: 20 mg/kg (maximum dose = 500 mg (5 ml))	Q10 min PRN	Side effects: bradycardia, hypotension, peripheral vasodilation, hypercalcemia, hypomagnesemia, hyperchloremic acidosis, hypercalcemia Caution: central venous line recommended. Maximum concentration is 20 mg/ml infusion. Extravasation may lead to tissue necrosis, use local hyaluronidase if occurs, may precipitate arrhythmia in digitalized patient Contraindication: hypercalcemia, ventricular fibrillation

Epinephrine Hydrochloride (Adrenaline)	Onset: rapid Mode of action: stimulates alpha, beta 1 and 2 adrenergic receptors	IV (1:10,000) ET	(1:10,000) 0.01 mg/kg (maximum dose=1 mg) (1:10,000) neonates: 0.01 mg/kg (maximum dose=1 mg) (1:1,000) infants/children: 0.1 mg/kg (maximum dose=1 mg)	PRN	Side effects: anxiety, tremor, headache, tachycardia, hypertension, arrhythmias
Lidocaine (Xylocaine)	Onset: rapid Mode of action: class Ib antiarrhythmic agent, sodium channel blocker, local anesthetic depressing myocardial irritability	IV, ET Infusion	0.5–1.0 mg/kg 20–50 μg/kg/min	Q5 min, PRN PRN	Side effects: hypotension, shock, nausea, seizures, respiratory depression, anxiety, euphoria, drowsiness, agitation Caution: hepatic disease, heart failure Contraindication: AV block Therapeutic level: 2–5 μg/ml
Magnesium sulfate	Onset: rapid Mode of action: exerts antiarrhythmic action	IV	Torsades de pointes: 25–50 mg/kg (maximum dose 2 g)		Side effects: confusion, sedation, depressed reflexes, flaccid paralysis, weakness, respiratory depression, hypotension, bradycardia, heart block, cardiac arrest, nausea, vomiting, cramps, flushing, sweating, hypermagnesemia Caution: rapid bolus may cause severe hypotension and bradycardia Contraindication: renal failure

(continued)

Drug	Pharmacology	Route	Dose	Frequency	Comments
Sodium Bicarbonate	Onset: IV rapid Mode of action: alkalization	IV, ET	Cardiac arrest: 0.5–1 mEq/kg	PRN	Side effects: increased oxygen affinity to Hgb, alkalosis, edema, hyperosmolality, hypernatremia, cerebral hemorrhage, hypokalemia, hypocalcemia Caution: in infants under 3 months, use concentration of 0.5 mEq/ml. Do not mix with calcium salts or catecholamines. Extravasation may cause tissue necrosis, infiltrate with hyaluronidase to minimize tissue necrosis Contraindication: inadequate alveolar ventilation
Vasopressin	Onset: rapid Mode of action: stimulates vasopressin receptors	IV	0.5 U/Kg/dose Adult dose: 40U/dose	Once	Use following two doses of epinephrine (limited data) Side effects: excessive vasoconstriction, regional ischemia, hyponatremia, fluid retention Caution: potent peripheral vasoconstrictor which may provoke cardiac ischemia and angina Contraindication: not recommended for responsive patients with coronary artery disease

Anticoagulation

Drug	Pharmacology	Route	Dose	Frequency	Comments
Acetylsalicylic acid (Aspirin)	Inhibits prostaglandin synthesis and formation of platelet aggregating thromboxane A2	PO, PR	Antiplatelet: 3–10 mg/kg/dose daily (maximum single dose: 325 mg) Anti-inflammatory/Kawasaki Disease: 20–25 mg/kg/dose. In Kawasaki, while febrile use anti-inflammatory dose, then 3–5 mg/kg/day once daily (duration based on coronary artery abnormalities). Round doses based on tablet sizes of 81 mg and 325 mg and dosing recommendations above Adult maximum dose: 4 g/day	Daily to q6 h per indication	Caution: GI bleeding, bronchospasm, GI distress, tinnitus, inhibit platelet aggregation Do not use in infants and children less than 16 years of age with viral illness due to the association with Reye's syndrome Monitor serum salicylate concentrations when using high doses
Clopidogrel (Plavix)	Irreversibly modifies ADP platelet receptor thereby inhibiting ADP-dependent platelet aggregation	Oral	0.2–1 mg/kg/dose Adult dose: 75 mg QD	Daily	Monitor for signs of bleeding More recent data demonstrates that infants and young children (less than 24 months of age) require lower mg/kg doses then older children and adults, begin with lower end of dosing range. Discontinue concomitant treatment with protonics

(continued)

Drug	Pharmacology	Route	Dose	Frequency	Comments
Dalteparin (Fragmin)	Potentiates the effect of antithrombin III and inactivates coagulation factor 10a and IIa (but to a lesser degree)	Subcutaneous	Prophylaxis: Infants/children: 92 U/kg/ dose q24 h Adults: 5,000 U q24 h Treatment: Infants/children: 129 U/kg/ dose q24 h; Adults: 100–120 U/kg/dose q12 h (maximum 10,000 U/dose)	Daily or q12 h (see specific dosing)	Peak anti-10a levels 2–6 h following sq dose. Monitor levels in infants and children Antidote: protamine sulfate
Enoxaparin (Lovenox)	Potentiate the effect of antithrombin III and inactivates coagulation factor 10a and IIa (but to a lesser degree)	Subcutaneous	Prophylaxis: <2 months: 0.75 mg/kg/ dose q12 h >2 months: 0.5 mg/kg/ dose q12 h Adults: 40 mg daily or 30 mg q12 h Treatment: <2 months: 1.5 mg/kg/dose (neonates may have higher dose requirements) >2 months: 1 mg/kg/dose Adults: 1 mg/kg/dose (maximum single dose: 150 mg) or 1.5 mg/kg/dose	Daily or q12 h (see specific dosing) Q12 or QD	Peak anti-10a levels 2–6 h following sq dose. Monitor levels in infants and children Antidote: protamine sulfate

Drug	Mechanism	Route	Dose	Frequency	Comments
Heparin (unfractionated heparin, UFH)	Potentiates antithrombin III which inactivates several activated clotting factors including XIIa, Xia, IXa, Xa, and IIa (thrombin) and prevents the conversion of fibrinogen to fibrin	IV infusion	Loading dose: 75 U/kg/dose over 10 min. Continuous infusion: <1 year (infants up to 2 months corrected for gestational age): 28 U/kg/h continuous infusion (adjust dose to maintain desired APTT) >1 year: 20 U/kg/h continuous infusion (adjust dose to maintain desired APTT) Older children/adults: 18 U/kg/h	Once; Continuous infusion	Monitor for: bleeding, allergy, heparin-induced thrombocytopenia, osteopenia. Ideal monitoring assay for UFH in infants and children remains unknown. Monitor therapy with APTT, anti-10a levels or ACT based on particular patient. A subcutaneous injection of UFH may be used when poor venous access – total daily IV requirements administered two to three times daily. Antidote: protamine sulfate
Warfarin (Coumadin, Sofatin)	Inhibits hepatic synthesis of vitamin K-dependent factors (II, VII, IX, X)	PO	0.2 mg/kg/dose (maximum initial dose: 5 mg)	Daily	Round dose to nearest quarter, half, or whole tablet. Adjust to desired INR. Target INR 2–3 (see specific indications for exact target goal). Close monitoring for drug–drug and drug–dietary interactions. Antidote: vitamin K

Diuretics

Drug	Pharmacology	Route	Dose	Frequency	Comments
Acetazolamide (Diamox)	Mode of action: carbonic anhydrase inhibitor, diuretic	PO, IV	Diuretic: 5 mg/kg/dose (maximum single dose = 375 mg)	Daily	Side effects: paresthesias, hypokalemia, acidosis, reduced urate secretion, polyuria, and development of renal calculi Contraindicated: hepatic failure, severe renal failure, and sulfa hypersensitivity
Bumetanide (Bumex)	Onset: IV 5–10 min; PO 30–60 min Mode of action: loop diuretic, prevent reabsorption of Cl as ascending loop of Henle	IV, IM, PO	Neonates: 0.01–0.05 mg/kg/dose Infants/children: 0.015–0.1 mg/kg/dose Maximum single dose = 2 mg Maximum daily dose = 10 mg	Daily (neonate) Every 6–24 h (older infants and children)	Side effects: Hypotension, hypoglycemia, increase serum creatinine, hyperurecemia, hypokalemia, hypocalcemia, hyponatremia, hypochloremia, hypercalciuria, metabolic alkalosis Caution: Sulfonamide hypersensitivity
		Continuous Infusion	Continuous infusion: 0.05 mg/kg/h Adults: 0.5–1 mg/h	continuous	
Chlorothiazide Diuril	Onset: IV: 5–10 min PO: 1–2 h Mode of Action: Inhibits renal tubular reabsorption of Na⁺ in distal tubule	PO	10–20 mg/kg/dose maximum daily dose = infants less 6 months = 375 mg Infants greater 6 months and children = 1,000 mg	BID	Side effects: Hypokalemia, hypochloremia, alkalosis, hypotension, hyperlipidemia, cholestasis, muscle weakness, paresthesia, pre-renal azotemia, hyperuricemia, hyperglycemia Caution: Sulfonamide hypersensitivity. Avoid use if Creatinine clearance less than 10 ml/min
		IV	1–4 mg/kg/dose (Adults: 100–500 mg/day)	BID	

Ethacrynic Acid Edecrin	Onset: IV: 5 min PO: 10–30 min Mode of Action: Potent loop diuretic, prevent reabsorption of Cl at ascending loop of Henle	PO	1–3 mg/kg/dose (start low and titrate) (Adult maximum dose = 200 mg)	Daily
		IV	0.5–1 mg/kg/dose repeat IV doses not routinely recommended (Adult maximum dose = 100 mg)	Daily to q12 h if indicated
			Side effects: Hypovolemia, hypokalemia, hypochloremic alkalosis, pre-renal azotemia, hyperuricemia, abnormal LFT's, agranulocytosis or thrombocytopenia, anorexia, dysphagia, GI bleeding, GI irritation, rash, hypotension, vertigo, hyponatremia, hyperglycemia, hepatotoxicity, ototoxic, tinnitus, hematuria, hypomagnesemia Caution: Renal dysfunction		
Furosemide Lasix	Onset: IV: 5 min PO: 30–60 min Mode of action: Loop diuretic, prevent reabsorption of Cl at ascending loop of Henle. Oral bioavailability is poor, consequently oral doses much larger than IV.	PO	2–4 mg/kg/dose – start at lower end of dosing range and titrate. (maximum initial dose: 20 mg)	Every 6–24 h scheduled or prn as clinically indicated
		IV	1–2 mg/kg/dose (maximum initial dose = 20 mg)	
		Continuous Infusion	0.1–1 mg/kg/h, titrate to desired effect	
			Side effects: Hypovolemia, hypokalemia, hypochloremia, hypocalcemia, hypochloremic metabolic alkalosis. Hyperuricemia, dermatitis, hyperglycemia, azotemia, anemia, ototoxicity especially when used with aminoglycosides, hypotension, pancreatitis, interstitial nephritis, hypercalciuria Caution: Prolonged use in neonates may cause nephrocalcinosis. Renal or hepatic failure		

(continued)

Drug	Pharmacology	Route	Dose	Frequency	Comments
Hydrochlorothiazide Hydrodiuril	Onset: PO: 60–120 min Mode of action: inhibits sodium reabsorption in the distal renal tubule	PO	1–2 mg/kg/dose maximum daily dose= infants less 6 months = 37.5 mg infants greater 6 months, children, and adults = 200 mg	BID	Side effects: hypokalemia, hyperlipidemia, hypochloremic metabolic alkalosis, nausea, muscle cramps, pancreatitis, agranulocytosis, hemolytic anemia, hepatitis, paresthesia, pre-renal azotemia, hyperuricemia, hyperglycemia, allergic reaction Caution: Sulfonamide cross sensitivity. Avoid use if ClCr less than 10 ml/min
Metolazone Zaroxolyn	Onset: PO: 60 min Mode of Action: Blocks sodium reabsorption at distal renal tubules	PO	0.1–0.2 mg/kg/dose Maximum single dose = 5 mg	Every 12–24 h	Side effects: hepatic dysfunction, calcium retention, GI upset, orthostatic hypotension, hypokalemia, hypochloremic metabolic alkalosis, hyperglycemia, hypomagnesemia, hyperuricemia, tinnitus Caution: Hepatic disease, oral absorption varies between products, sulfonamide cross sensitivity

| Spironolactone Aldactone | Onset: Hours to days Mode of action: Aldosterone blocker, therefore decrease potassium loss | PO | 0.5–1.5 mg/kg/dose Maximum single dose = 50 mg in children and 100 mg in adults | Every 12–24 h | Side effects: Potassium retention, GI irritation, rash, gynecomastia, hyperchloremic metabolic acidosis, amenorrhea, anorexia, agranulocytosis, hyponatremia Contraindications: Renal failure Caution: Avoid use if ClCr less than 10 ml/min Drug interactions: Hyperkalemia when used with other potassium sparing drugs or potassium supplements |

Ductal Management

Drug	Pharmacology	Route	Dose	Frequency	Comments
Ibuprofen Lysine NeoProfen	Mode of action: Nonsteroidal anti-inflammatory agent Prostaglandin synthesis inhibitor	IV	Closure of ductus arteriosus: Initial 10 mg/kg, then 5 mg/kg	Q24 h X 3 doses total (including higher initial dose), then reevaluate	Side effects: Drowsiness, fatigue, headache, GI irritation, inhibition of platelet aggregation, hepatitis, acute renal dysfunction, blood dyscrasias. Caution: Monitor renal and hepatic function. Keep urine output >1 ml/kg/h. Pulmonary hypertension, CHF, renal disease, hepatic disease, may displace bilirubin from albumin, increased risk of gastrointestinal perforation when given in combination with corticosteroids. Contraindication: Neonates with BUN >40 mg/dl, Cr ≥1.6 mg/dl, thrombocytopenia, recent IVH, NEC, or active bleeding, coagulopathy, congenital heart disease requiring patency of ductus arteriosus
Indomethacin Indocin	Mode of action: Prostaglandin synthesis inhibitor	IV	Closure of ductus arteriosus: 0.1–0.2 mg/kg	Q12–24 h X 3 doses, then reevaluate	Side effects: Decrease platelet aggregation, GI disease: ulcers, diarrhea, blood dyscrasias, GI bleeding, hypertension, oliguria, renal failure, dilutional hyponatremia, hyperkalemia, hypoglycemia, hepatitis. Caution: Monitor renal and hepatic function. Keep urine output >1 ml/kg/h. Increased risk of gastrointestinal perforation when given in combination with corticosteroids. Contraindication: Neonates with BUN >40 mg/dl, Cr ≥1.6 mg/dl, thrombocytopenia, recent IVH, NEC, or active bleeding

| Prostaglandin E₁ (Alprostadil) Prostin | Onset: minutes Mode of action: Direct effect on vascular smooth muscles causing pulmonary, systemic, and ductus arteriosus vasodilatation | Infusion | Initial: 0.05–0.1 µg/kg/min Maintenance: 0.01–0.4 µg/kg/min | Side effects: Apnea, Hypotension, flushing, Bradycardia, tachycardia, fever, seizure-like activity, hypocalcemia, diarrhea, hypoglycemia, inhibition of platelet aggregation, cortical hyperostosis (chronic therapy) |

Sedatives/Analgesics/Muscle Relaxants

Drug	Pharmacology	Route	Dose	Frequency	Comments
Chloral Hydrate (Noctec)	Onset: 10–20 min Mode of action: CNS depressant	PO, PR	20–100 mg/kg max dose = 2,000 mg	Q6–8 h PRN	Side effects: Irritates mucosa causing upset GI, laryngospasm if aspirated. Myocardial and respiratory depressant. CNS depression Contraindications: Hepatic or renal impairment Caution: Heart disease
Cisatracurium (21) (Nimbex)	Onset: 2–3 min Mode of action: A nondepolarizing skeletal muscle relaxant of intermediate onset and duration of action; metabolized by organ-*independent* Hofmann elimination and ester hydrolysis (i.e., metabolism and excretion are not dependent upon renal or hepatic function); no major effects on mean arterial pressure or heart rate when used in children with heart disease	Infusion	Load: 0.1 mg/kg Maintenance: 0.1–0.5 mg/kg/h		Monitoring: Nerve stimulator recommended to monitor neuromotor end-plate function Side effects: Myopathy (rare; associated with coadministration of corticosteroids) Caution: Concomitant administration of drugs that may potentiate effect include aminoglycosides, corticosteroids, calcium-channel blockers, procainamide, and vancomycin; not recommended for rapid-sequence intubation (intermediate acting) Contraindications: Hypersensitivity to cisatracurium or other bis-benzylisoquinolinium agents

Drug	Onset/Mode of action	Route	Dose	Frequency	Side effects/Contraindications/Caution
Clonidine (Catapres)	Onset: Slow. Mode of action: central alpha$_2$-adrenergic agonist	PO	1–2 µg/kg	Q6 h	Side effects: Dry mouth, dizziness, drowsiness, fatigue, constipation, anorexia, arrhythmia, hypotension. Caution: Do not abruptly discontinue; signs of sympathetic overactivity may occur. May need dosage adjustment in renal impairment
Dexmedetomidine (Precedex)	Onset: Rapid. Mode of action: Selective alpha$_2$-adrenoceptor agonist	Infusion	Load: 0.5–1 µg/kg Maintenance: 0.2–0.7 µg/kg/h	Infusion <24 h	Side effects: Hypotension, bradycardia, nausea. Contraindications: Hypersensitivity to dexmedetomidine. Caution: Load dose over 10 min, hepatic insufficiency, cardiac and respiratory disease
Diazepam (Valium)	Onset: Rapid. Mode of action: CNS depression through enhanced GABA at the limbic system	IM, IV PO	0.05–0.25 mg/kg 0.05–0.25 mg/kg Q8	PRN Q 8 h, PRN	Side effects: Hypotension, CNS and respiratory depression, physical dependence. Contraindications: Narrow angle glaucoma. Caution: Glaucoma, shock, depression, hypoalbuminemia, hepatic dysfunction. No faster than 1–2 mg/min(IV)
Etomidate (Amidate)	Onset: Rapid. Modes of action: Nonbarbiturate hypnotic	IV	0.2–0.6 mg/kg	Once	Side effects: Pain at injection site, myoclonus, hiccups, blocks normal stress-induced increase in adrenal cortisol production for 4–8 h. Contraindications: Hypersensitivity to etomidate or any component of the formulation. Caution: Hepatic and renal insufficiency

(continued)

Drug	Pharmacology	Route	Dose	Frequency	Comments
Fentanyl (Sublimaze)	Onset: Rapid Mode of action: Semisynthetic opiate analgesic	IV, IM Infusion	1–3 µg/kg 1–5 µg/kg/h	Q2 h, PRN	Side effects: Respiratory depression (beyond period of analgesia). Chest wall rigidity with large bolus doses. Bradycardia, functional ileus, physical dependence Contraindications: Increase ICP and IOP Caution: IV dose over 3–5 min, hepatic and renal insufficiency, respiratory disease
Ketamine (Ketalar)	Onset: Rapid Mode of action: Dissociative anesthesia by direct action on the cortex and limbic system	IV PO IM Infusion	0.5–2 mg/kg 6–10 mg/kg 3–7 mg/kg 0.5–2 mg/kg/h	Q 2 h PRN Q 2 h PRN Q 2 h PRN	Side effects: Hypertension, tachycardia, respiratory depression, laryngospasm, hypersalivation, delirium. CNS symptoms (dream-like state, confusion, agitation) Contraindications: Elevated ICP, thyrotoxicosis, CHF, angina and psychosis disorder Caution: Must be used in conjunction with antisialagogue due to increased secretions
Ketorolac (Toradol)	Mode of Action: NSAID, inhibits cyclooxygenase thereby preventing the production of peripheral analgesic mediators (i.e., prostaglandins). May also induce analgesia centrally by triggering the release of endogenous opiods	IM, IV	IM, IV: 0.5 mg/kg/dose max single dose: 30 mg Do not use for more than 5 days	Q 6–8 h	Side Effects: Edema, somnolence, dizziness, headache, dyspepsia, nausea, diarrhea, GI pain, GI bleeding, peptic ulcer, impaired platelet aggregation, oliguria, acute renal failure, dyspnea, wheezing, pain at injection site Contraindications: hepatic or renal failure

Drug	Onset / Mode of action	Route	Dose	Frequency	Side effects / Contraindications / Caution
Lorazepam (Ativan)	Onset: Rapid. Mode of action: CNS depression through enhanced GABA at limbic system	IV, IM, PO	0.05–0.1 mg/kg (max = 4 mg/dose)	Q4–8 h PRN	Side Effects: respiratory depression, hypotension, bradycardia, physical dependence. Contraindications: narrow angle glaucoma, shock. Caution: Lower dose should be used with narcotics. Care should be observed in the postoperative cardiac surgical patient, and with hemodynamic instability. Benzyl alcohol may be toxic to newborns in high doses
Meperidine (Demerol)	Onset: Rapid. Mode of action: Semisynthetic opiate analgesic	IM, IV, SC, PO	1–2 mg/kg; max = 100 mg	Q 3–4 h PRN	Side effects: Nausea, vomiting, respiratory depression, smooth muscle spasm, physical dependence, seizures, constipation, lethargy, tachycardia. Contraindications: Cardiac arrhythmia, asthma, increased ICP, renal failure. Caution: potentiated by MAO inhibitors, phenothiazines, and other CNS depressants, biliary colic
Midazolam (Versed)	Onset: IV: Rapid, IM: 5–15 min, PO/PR: 15–30 min. Mode of action: CNS depression by inducing GABA at limbic system	IV; IN; PO; IM; PR; Infusion	0.05–0.1 mg/kg max-2.5 mg; 0.2 mg/kg; 0.3–0.75 mg/kg; 0.1–0.2 mg/kg; 0.5–1 mg/kg; 0.05–0.5 mg/kg/h	PRN; PRN; PRN; PRN; PRN; PRN	Side effects: Respiratory depression, hypotension, bradycardia, myoclonic jerking in neonates. Contraindications: Narrow angle glaucoma, shock, physical dependence. Caution: Lower dose by 25% when used with narcotics, cimetidine, or anesthetic agents. Care should be observed in the postoperative open-heart patient, and with hemodynamic instability

(continued)

Drug	Pharmacology	Route	Dose	Frequency	Comments
Morphine sulfate (Duramorph, Centin, Astramorph)	Onset: IV: Rapid, PO: 15–30 min Mode of action: Strongest narcotic analgesic. Unspecified aid with CHF, pulmonary edema, and anoxic spells	IV, IM, SC Infusion	0.05–0.2 mg/kg max = 10 mg/dose 0.01–0.1 mg/kg/h	Q2–4 h, PRN	Side effects: Physical dependence, CNS and respiratory depression, bronchospasm, nausea, vomiting, constipation, hypotension, bradycardia, increases ICP, miosis, biliary or urinary spasm Contraindications: Increase ICP and IOP (unless ventilated), shock Caution: Hepatic failure, renal failure
Pancuronium (Pavulon)	Onset: Rapid Mode of action: Postsynaptic acetylcholine receptor blocker	IV	0.1 mg/kg	PRN	Side effects: Tachycardia Caution: Secure airway prior to administration. Effect increased by hypothermia, acidosis, decreased renal function, volatile anesthetics, succinycholine, hypokalemia, and aminoglycoside
Propofol (Diprivan)	Onset: Rapid Mode of action: Hindered phenolic compound with intravenous general anesthetic	IV Infusion	1–2 mg/kg 50–200 μg/kg/min		Side effects: Hypotension, hypertlipidemia, metabolic acidosis, pain at injection site Contraindications: Hypersensitivity to propofol or any component of the formulation; hypersensitivity to eggs, egg products, soybeans, or soy products Caution: Hypotension, hemodynamic instability, or severe cardiac or respiratory disease

Drug	Onset / Mode of action	Route	Dose	Frequency	Caution / Side effects / Contraindications
Rocuronium (Zemuron)	Onset: Rapid Mode of action: postsynaptic Acetylcholine receptor blocker	IV Infusion	0.6–1.2 mg/kg (1–1.2 mg/kg for rapid sequence induction) 0.5–1 mg/kg/h	PRN	Caution: Hepatic impairment, neuromuscular disease. Effect increased by hypothermia, acidosis, volatile anesthetics, succinylcholine, aminoglycosides, clindamycin, tetracycline, magnesium sulfate, quinine, and quinidine
Thiopental (Pentothal)	Onset: Rapid Mode of action: CNS depression by inducing GABA activity, depresses reticular activating system	IV	3–5 mg/kg		Side effects: Decrease in cardiac output, cough/laryngospasm/bronchospasm, necrosis with IV extravasation Contraindications: Hypersensitivity to thiopental, pentobarbital, any component, or other barbiturates; porphyria Caution: Asthma/pharyngeal infection, hypotension or severe cardiac disease, hepatic or renal dysfunction
Vecuronium bromide (Norcuron)	Onset: Rapid Mode of action: Postsynaptic acetylcholine receptor blocker	IV Infusion	0.1 mg/kg 0.1 mg/kg/h	PRN	Caution: Hepatic impairment, neuromuscular disease. Longer recovery period in infant less than 1 year. Potency and duration of effect may be prolonged by volatile anesthetics, aminoglycoside, metronidazole, tetracycline, bacitracin, and clindamycin Antidotes: Neostigmine, pyridostigmine, or edrophonium

Index

Printed in the United States
By Bookmasters

Printed in the United States
By Bookmasters